Mosby's

Pediatric Assessment

Joyce K. Engel, RN, MEd, PhD

Dean of Students
Medicine Hat College
Medicine Hat, Alberta, Canada

Fifth Edition

with 100 illustrations

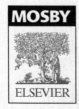

MOSBY

ELSEVIER

MOSBY
ELSEVIER

11830 Westline Industrial Drive
St. Louis, Missouri 63146

MOSBY'S POCKET GUIDE TO PEDIATRIC   ISBN-13: 978-0-323-04412-7
ASSESSMENT, FIFTH EDITION   ISBN-10: 0-323-04412-3

Notice

Knowledge and best practice in this field are constantly changing. As new research and experience broaden our knowledge, changes in practice, treatment and drug therapy may become necessary or appropriate. Readers are advised to check the most current information provided (i) on procedures featured or (ii) by the manufacturer of each product to be administered, to verify the recommended dose or formula, the method and duration of administration, and contraindications. It is the responsibility of the practitioner, relying on their own experience and knowledge of the patient, to make diagnoses, to determine dosages and the best treatment for each individual patient, and to take all appropriate safety precautions. To the fullest extent of the law, neither the Publisher nor the Author assumes any liability for any injury and/or damage to persons or property arising out or related to any use of the material contained in this book.

The Publisher

Previous editions copyrighted 2002, 1997, 1993, 1989

ISBN-13: 978-0-323-04412-7
ISBN-10: 0-323-04412-3

Acquisitions Editor: Catherine Jackson
Managing Editor: Michele D. Hayden
Publishing Services Manager: John Rogers
Senior Project Manager: Cheryl A. Abbott
Senior Design Manager: Bill Drone

Printed in the United States of America

Last digit is the print number: 9   8   7

Reviewers

Sherry D. Ferki, RN, MSN
Adjunct Faculty
Old Dominion University School of Nursing;
Adjunct Faculty
College of the Albemarle
Portsmouth, Virginia

Mary Ann McClellan, ARNP, CPNP, MN, CFLE
Assistant Professor
University of Oklahoma College of Nursing
Oklahoma City, Oklahoma

The author would also like to acknowledge consultants and reviewers who participated in previous editions of this book:

Barbara W. Berg, RN, PNP, MN
Head Nurse
Rose Children's Center at Rose Medical Center
Denver, Colorado

Dena K. Cuyjet, RN, MS, CPNP
Pediatric Nurse Practitioner
Newborn Discharge Coordinator
Kaiser Permanente San Francisco
San Francisco, California

Terry Fugate, RN, BSN
Formerly Adjunct and Associate Faculty
Texas Tech University, Health Sciences Center
Lubbock, Texas

Sarah G. Fuller, RN, CPNP, PhD

Associate Professor
College of Nursing, University of South Carolina
Columbia, South Carolina

Sandra L. Gardner, RN, MS, PNP

Director
Professional Outreach Consultation
Aurora, Colorado

Marilyn B. Hartsell, RN, MSN

Coordinator
Tri-Regional Education and Networking Development
    System
University of Delaware
Newark, Delaware

Karen Halvorson, RN, MN

Chief Patient Care Officer
Highline Medical Center
Seattle, Washington

Christina Bergh Jackson, RN, CPNP, MSN

Pediatric Nurse Practitioner
Pennsylvania School of the Deaf
Philadelphia, Pennsylvania;
Instructor
Eastern College
St. Davids, Pennsylvania

Carol A. Kilmon, RN, MSN, PhD, CPNP

Assistant Professor
The University of Texas Medical Branch
Galveston, Texas

Catherine F. Noonan, RN, MS, CPNP
Nurse Practitioner
Children's Hospital;
Assistant Professor
Nurse Education Department, Bunker Hill Community
    College
Boston, Massachusetts

Mary Ann Norton, RNC, PhD, CPNP
Associate Professor
North Michigan University
Marquette, Michigan

Margaret C. Slota, RN, MN
Pediatrics Consultant
Pittsburgh, Pennsylvania

Janet F. Sullivan, RN,C, PhD
Clinical Associate Professor
Parent Child Health Nursing
State of New York Health Sciences Center
Stony Brook, New York

Preface

As in previous editions, the goal of *Mosby's Pocket Guide to Pediatric Assessment* is to present the complexities of assessing the health of children within a portable, usable, accessible, and practical format. The emphasis of the pocket guide on children 1 month to late adolescence assumes the influences of families, culture, genetics, and of the prenatal and neonatal periods.

Organization and Approach

This edition continues to set about the physical assessment of children through a systematic, body systems approach. This approach is replicated in the family assessment model, which strongly reflects its foundations in systems. The presentation of approaches to the home environment, culture, communication, development, abuse, and psychosocial and mental health places assessment of the child within a broader and holistic framework related to the health of children and families. Sections on assessment methodologies and findings are usually preceded by discussion of developmental variations that assist in rooting the process of assessment within the context of the child. Clinical alerts draw the attention of beginning and advanced nurses to significant findings and/or deviations from normal that might commonly be found in pediatric clients. Nursing diagnoses complete the assessment.

The New Edition

Since the fourth edition was written, we have been confronted with global concern about diseases such as SARS and avian flu. These infectious diseases, along with West Nile virus, while perhaps less devastating among children than adults, reflect the global challenges that infections present for the young. Infections, suicide, and unintentional injuries represent leading causes of death among children and adolescents. In recognition of this, the fifth edition provides up-to-date information and assessments associated with the new viral infections and with athletic and head injuries. It also offers a new chapter on assessment of mental health in children and adolescents, as well as incorporation of mental health findings throughout the text, including those associated with eating disorders.

Nearly every chapter includes revised or new content. Expanded assessment material on the common childhood symptoms of fever, vomiting, and diarrhea has been incorporated into charts, similar to those included in earlier editions on cough, headaches, and abdominal pain, with the goal of providing nurses with information that is quickly available in these areas that often crop up in everyday practice with children.

Continued Journeys

The expansion of knowledge and the causes of illness are reminders that health is dynamic and complex, just as are families and children. It is my hope that *Mosby's Pocket Guide to Pediatric Assessment* will provide a concise, practical guide to assist in making sound decisions that will in turn help families and children toward making sense of their experience and toward positive coping.

Joyce Engel

Contents

UNIT I HEALTH HISTORY

1 **Beginning the Assessment, 3**
   Guidelines for Communicating with Children, 3
   Communicating with Infants, 4
   Communicating with Toddlers, 5
   Communicating with Preschool-Age Children, 6
   Communicating with School-Age Children, 6
   Communicating with Adolescents, 7
   Communicating with Parents, 7
   Communicating with Parents and Children from Diverse
      Cultures, 8
   Establishing a Setting for the Health History, 9

2 **Dimensions of a History, 32**
   Guidelines for Interviewing Parents and Children, 32
   Information for Comprehensive History, 34

3 **Family Assessment, 44**
   Rationale, 44
   General Concepts Related to Assessment, 44
   Stages in Family Development, 46
   Tasks and Characteristics of Stepfamilies, 47
   Guidelines for Communicating with Families, 47
   Assessment of the Family, 48
   Related Nursing Diagnoses, 56

4 **Home Visits and Assessments, 58**
   Making Home Visits, 58
   Making the Initial Visit, 59
   Assessment of the Home Environment, 59
   Related Nursing Diagnoses, 61

5   Physical Assessment, 63
Guidelines for Inspection, 63
Guidelines for Palpation, 63
Guidelines for Percussion, 65
Guidelines for Auscultation, 65

6   Preparation for Examination, 68
Preparation of Environment, 68
Preparation of Equipment, 68
Equipment for Physical Assessment, 68
Guidelines for Physical Assessment of Infant or Child, 69
Age-Related Approaches to Physical Assessment, 70

7   Dimensions of Nutritional Assessment, 73
Establishing Weight, 73
Establishing Height, 77
Assessment of Eating Practices, 78
Assessment of Physical Signs of Nutrition
    or Malnutrition, 80
Related Nursing Diagnoses, 80

UNIT II   MEASUREMENT OF VITAL SIGNS

8   Body Temperature, Pulse, and Respirations, 95
Measurement of Body Temperature, 95
Measurement of Pulse, 104
Measurement of Respirations, 106
Related Nursing Diagnoses, 110

9   Blood Pressure, 111
Rationale, 111
Anatomy and Physiology, 111
Equipment for Measuring Blood Pressure, 113
Preparation, 113
Guidelines for Measurement of Blood Pressure, 114
Auscultation Method of Blood Pressure Measurement, 116
Palpation Method of Blood Pressure Measurement, 118
Flush Method of Blood Pressure Measurement, 119
Related Nursing Diagnoses, 119

UNIT III   ASSESSMENT OF BODY SYSTEMS

10   Integument, 123
Rationale, 123
Anatomy and Physiology, 123
Preparation, 124
Assessment of Skin, 125
Assessment of Nails, 141
Assessment of Hair, 142
Related Nursing Diagnoses, 143

11   Head and Neck, 144
Rationale, 144
Anatomy and Physiology, 144
Equipment for Measurement of Head Circumference, 146
Preparation, 147
Assessment of Head, 147
Assessment of Neck, 149
Related Nursing Diagnoses, 151

12   Ears, 153
Rationale, 153
Anatomy and Physiology, 153
Equipment for Ear Assessment, 154
Preparation, 154
Assessment of External Ear, 156
Assessment of Hearing Acuity, 159
Preparation, 160
Equipment for Assessment of Hearing Acuity, 160
Otoscopic Examination, 164
Related Nursing Diagnoses, 167

13   Eyes, 168
Rationale, 168
Anatomy and Physiology, 168
Equipment for Eye Assessment, 170
Preparation, 171
Assessment of External Eye, 171
Assessment of Extraocular Movement, 177
Assessment of Color Vision, 179

Assessment of Visual Acuity, 180
Ophthalmoscopic Examination, 183
Related Nursing Diagnoses, 184

14   **Face, Nose, and Oral Cavity, 185**
Rationale, 185
Anatomy and Physiology, 185
Equipment for Face, Nose, and Oral Cavity
    Assessment, 190
Preparation, 190
Assessment of Face and Nose, 190
Assessment of Oral Cavity, 194
Related Nursing Diagnoses, 199

15   **Thorax and Lungs, 200**
Rationale, 200
Anatomy and Physiology, 200
Equipment for Assessment of Thorax and Lungs, 201
Preparation, 202
Assessment of Thorax and Lungs, 202
Related Nursing Diagnoses, 220

16   **Cardiovascular System, 221**
Rationale, 221
Anatomy and Physiology, 221
Equipment for Assessment of Cardiovascular System, 222
Preparation, 222
Assessment of Heart, 224
Assessment of Vascular System, 232
Related Nursing Diagnoses, 236

17   **Abdomen, 238**
Rationale, 238
Anatomy and Physiology, 238
Equipment for Assessment of Abdomen, 240
Preparation, 240
Assessment of Abdomen, 264
Assessment of Anal Area, 272
Related Nursing Diagnoses, 273

18 **Lymphatic System, 274**
    Rationale, 274
    Anatomy and Physiology, 274
    Equipment for Assessment of Lymphatic System, 275
    Preparation, 275
    Assessment of Lymph Nodes, 275
    Assessment of Spleen, 277
    Related Nursing Diagnoses, 277

19 **Reproductive System, 278**
    Rationale, 278
    Anatomy and Physiology, 278
    Equipment for Assessment of Reproductive System, 282
    Preparation, 282
    Assessment of Female Breasts, 283
    Assessment of Female Genitalia, 288
    Assessment of Male Genitalia, 290
    Related Nursing Diagnoses, 295

20 **Musculoskeletal System, 296**
    Rationale, 296
    Anatomy and Physiology, 296
    Preparation, 297
    Assessment of Musculoskeletal System, 297
    Related Nursing Diagnoses, 307

21 **Nervous System, 309**
    Rationale, 309
    Anatomy and Physiology, 309
    Equipment for Assessment of Nervous System, 310
    Preparation, 310
    Assessment of Mental Status, 311
    Assessment of Motor Function, 316
    Assessment of Sensory Function, 318
    Assessment of Cranial Nerve Function, 318
    Assessment of Deep Tendon Reflexes, 318
    Assessment of Infant Reflexes, 324
    Assessment of Pain, 324
    Related Nursing Diagnoses, 339

UNIT IV   GENERAL ASSESSMENT

22   Development, 343
Rationale, 343
Preparation, 343
Assessment of Development Using the Denver II, 344
Assessment of Growth and Development, 345
Assessment of Speech and Language, 365
Related Nursing Diagnoses, 368

23   Assessment of Child Abuse, 369
Rationale, 369
Development of Abuse, 369
Assessment of Abuse and Neglect in Children, 369
Related Nursing Diagnoses, 374

24   Assessment of Mental Health, 376
Rationale, 376
Preparation, 377
Assessment of Mental Health, 378
Related Nursing Diagnoses, 390

UNIT V   CONCLUDING THE ASSESSMENT

25   Completing the Examination, 395

APPENDIXES

A   Developmental Assessment, 399
B   Growth Charts, 405
C   Normal Laboratory Values, 422
D   Immunization Schedules for Infants and
Children, 443
E   Sample Documentation of a Child Health
History, 448

BIBLIOGRAPHY, 456

HEALTH HISTORY

I

Beginning the Assessment

1

This text focuses on health assessment of the child, beginning with the 1-month-old infant and ending with the teenager in late adolescence. Although the physical assessment process is broken down into evaluations of the various body systems, the nurse need not adopt a fragmented approach to physical assessment. In fact, physical assessment is continuous and occurs during the health interview, when the nurse is also able to observe the infant, child, or adolescent.

Assessment is facilitated for the child, parent (if present), and examiner if a rapport is established early. It might not be possible to erase all of a child's apprehension or discomfort, but creating an atmosphere of trust and communication can help make the assessment a more positive experience.

Guidelines for Communicating with Children

- Take time to become acquainted with the child and parents.
- Set up a physical environment that is appropriately warm, cheerful, and private. If possible, select an environment that is decorated in an age-appropriate manner; for example, adolescents might not appreciate Snow White pictures.
- Ask the parents how the child usually copes with new or stressful situations or what previous experiences the child has had with health care or caregivers. Knowing how the child might react enables the nurse to plan specific interventions to facilitate communication.
- Ask the parents what they have told the child about the health care encounter. The preparation children receive, especially males, is often inadequate or inappropriate. In such a case, more time might be necessary to prepare the child before beginning any aspect of the health assessment requiring active participation.
- Observe the child's behavior for clues to readiness. A child who is ready to participate in assessment will ask questions, make eye contact, describe past experiences, touch equipment, or detach willingly from the parent.

- Consider the child's developmental level and attention span, and use an imaginative approach when planning the examination.
- If a child is having difficulty accepting the assessment:

  Talk to the parent, ignoring the child.

  Compliment the child.

  Play a game (such as peek-a-boo) or tell a story.

  Use the third-person linguistic form: "Sometimes a guy can get really scared when his blood pressure is taken."

  Sequence the assessment from that causing least discomfort to that causing most discomfort.

  Start from toe to head.

  Undress the child gradually or allow the child to undress gradually.

  Briefly perform the technique on the parent first.
- Encourage the child to ask questions during the assessment, but do not pressure to do so. This allows the child some control over the situation.
- Explain the assessment process in terms consistent with the child's developmental level.
- Use concrete terms rather than technical information, particularly with young children: "I can hear you breathing in and out," not "I am auscultating your chest." "Do your ears ever hurt?" not "Have you had otitis media?"
- Present small amounts of information at a time. A rule of thumb is that no more than three items should be presented at once.
- Do not make rushed movements.
- Make expectations known clearly and simply: "I want you to be very still."
- *Do not offer choice where there is none.*
- Offer honest praise: "I know that hurt. You held your tummy very still." A positive experience helps build coping skills and self-esteem.
- If using an interpreter, it is critical to explain the purpose of the assessment and to introduce the interpreter to the family. Avoid medical jargon as much as possible, and ask one question at a time.
- When examining more than one child, usually begin with the oldest or most cooperative child.

Communicating with Infants

Infants (1 to 12 months) primarily communicate through nonverbal vocalization and crying and respond to nonverbal communication behaviors of adults such as holding, rocking, and patting. It is useful to observe the parent's or caregiver's interpretation of the infant's nonverbal cues and the nonverbal communications of the parents. These established communication patterns can aid the nurse in establishing rapport with the infant.

Young infants respond well to gentle physical contact with any adult, but older infants can demonstrate strong separation and stranger anxieties. If it is necessary to handle the older infant, do so firmly. Avoid preparatory gestures such as holding out hands or coaxing the child to come and abrupt movements. Although infants younger than 6 months usually tolerate lying on the examining table, older infants and toddlers are more comfortable when held or sitting in the parent's or caregiver's lap. As much as possible, carry out the assessment in a way that allows the infant to either keep the parent in view or to be held by the parent. Infants should be allowed security objects such as blankets and pacifiers, if they have them. The use of a high-pitched, soft voice and smile will also assist in gaining the infant's cooperation.

Communicating with Toddlers

Toddlers (12 months to 3 years) have not yet acquired the ability to effectively communicate verbally. Their communication is rich with expressive nonverbal gestures and simple verbal communications. Pushing the examiner's hand away and crying can be an eloquent expression of fear, anxiety, or lack of knowledge. Toddlers accept the verbal communications of others literally, so that saying, "I can see all the way to your tummy button when you open your mouth" will mean just that to toddlers. Toddlers have the beginnings of memory and imagination, but they are unable to understand abstractions and become frustrated and frightened by phrases that seem ordinary to adults. Perceptions of threat are amplified by inaccurate understandings of the situation and limited knowledge of the resources that are available.

Communication with toddlers requires that the nurse use short, concrete terms. Explanations and descriptions need to be repeated several times. Visual aids such as puppets and dolls assist explanations. Children of this age attribute magical qualities to inanimate objects, so it is useful to allow them to handle instruments and to tell them exactly, in concrete terms, what the instrument does and how it feels. The use of comfort objects and access to the parent should be encouraged throughout the assessment, as they are for the infant.

Communicating with Preschool-Age Children

Although preschoolers (3 to 6 years) generally use more sophisticated verbal communications, their reasoning is intuitive. Therefore many of the guidelines for communicating with toddlers apply to preschoolers as well. Because of the preschooler's increased verbal communication abilities, the nurse can successfully indicate to the child how and when cooperation is desired. The older preschooler, in particular, likes to conform, knows most external body parts, and might be interested in the purpose of various parts of the assessment. Allowing the preschooler to handle the equipment eases fears and helps answer questions about how the equipment is used.

Preschool-age children are often very modest. They should be exposed minimally during examination and requested to undress themselves. They need to know exactly what is being examined and benefit from opportunities for questions. Parental proximity is still important for this age group.

Communicating with School-Age Children

School-age children (6 to 12 years) think in concrete terms but at a more sophisticated level. Generally they have had enough contact with health care personnel that they can rely on past experiences to guide them. Depending on the quality of their past experiences, they might appear shy or reticent during health assessment. Children might fear injury or embarrassment. Allowing time for composure and privacy (perhaps even from parents) aids in communication. Reassurance and third-person speech are helpful in eliciting worries and anxieties and in allowing the child to express fear or pain.

The purpose of the health assessment should be related to the child's condition. It is useful to determine what the child already knows about the health contact and to proceed from there. Simple medical diagrams and teaching dolls are useful in explaining the assessment process. Specific information should be given about body parts affected by the assessment.

Children of this age are often curious about the function of equipment and its usefulness. An appropriate response to "How can you tell what my temperature is from the thermometer?" might be "Your body heat is picked up by a special sensor. The sensor reads your temperature as a number. I can then tell from the number how warm you are."

Communicating with Adolescents

Adolescents (12 years and older) use sophisticated verbal communication, although their behavior might not necessarily indicate an advanced level of communication, cognition, or maturity. Adolescents sometimes respond to verbal approaches with monosyllables, reticence, anger, or other behaviors, and the nurse might have to do more talking than is usual at the beginning of the interaction. The nurse must avoid the tendency to respond to less than desirable social behaviors with prying, confrontation, continuous questioning, or judgmental attitudes. Easing into the initial contact with discussion of friends, hobbies, school, and family can give the apprehensive adolescent time for self-composure. Disclosure might occur more easily when the adolescent and nurse are engaged in joint activity.

It is helpful to ask the adolescent what he or she knows about the health contact and to explain the rationale for the health assessment. Adolescents might be concerned about privacy and confidentiality, and opportunity should be provided for completing some or all of the assessment without the presence of the parent. The female nurse needs to be sensitive to the potential of embarrassment for male adolescents at being examined by a female and provide draping and minimal touching. The parameters of confidentiality should be explained; specifically, it should be explained that disclosure is confidential unless intervention is necessary. Adolescents tend to be preoccupied with body image and function, and when appropriate they should be given feedback from the assessment. Diagrams and models can enhance feedback. Although adolescents have a high level of comprehension and vocabulary, they might not consistently function at higher levels of cognition, and the nurse must avoid the tendency to become too abstract, too detailed, and too technical. The self-conscious adolescent might be reluctant to ask for clarification of an explanation that has not been understood.

Communicating with Parents

Parents are often an integral part of the health assessment of an infant or child. Parents are the primary source of information about the young child. The information that parents give can be considered reliable in most instances because of close contact with their children.

Broad questions are useful, especially in eliciting responses in sensitive areas, because the parent can assume control over the direction of the response: "Tell me what Jason did at 2 years" is less threatening than "Did Jason talk when he was 2?" or "Did you have trouble disciplining Jason when he was 2?" More focused and closed questions should be saved for later in the assessment process when specific information is desired.

Silence and listening are essential to reassure parents that what they are about to say is worthwhile. In a supportive, attentive atmosphere, parents often communicate information and feelings that might have little to do with the current problem but are significant in the overall care of the child.

The parents are members of the health team. If they believe the child has a problem, their concern must be treated seriously. The parents and the nurse must agree that the problem exists. Once agreement exists, the nurse can ask how the parents have tried to solve the problem. This approach reinforces the worth of the parents' solutions. Having accomplished this, the nurse can help the parents to find alternative solutions for the problem. Occasionally parents will select alternatives that are not preferred. If the alternative will not harm the child, it is best to allow the parents to carry out their plan.

The nurse must avoid the temptation to inundate the parents with anticipatory guidance. Parents need recognition, praise, and reassurance for their strengths. Too much information and advice can intimidate parents and effectively shut down communication.

Communicating with Parents and Children from Diverse Cultures

In communicating with parents and children from diverse cultures, it is critical to recognize that communication patterns, childrearing practices, and health practices might differ from those of the nurse (Table 1-1). Knowledge of these differences will assist in developing hypotheses about the family and in acquiring sensitivity to differences; however, the nurse must observe the family carefully for cues to family practices and relationships with children and each other. Further, the nurse must avoid the trap of assuming that because the family belongs to a specific ethnic or cultural group, they will behave and hold beliefs similar to those of the group as a whole.

When communicating with families from diverse cultures, watch their interactions with others (e.g., note whether eye contact is established and with whom) and observe what distance is generally assumed in communication. This will assist in determining what body gestures are appropriate; however, if unsure, ask. When addressing the family, it is important to learn and to use culturally appropriate forms of address. If the family has limited language comprehension, speak slowly and carefully, avoiding the tendency to speak loudly. If unsure as to what has been said, ask for clarification; if unsure whether information has been understood, repeat important points. If possible, use wording written in the family's own language and if necessary, use an interpreter. As with all families, convey caring and use active listening.

Establishing a Setting for the Health History

The health interview provides an ideal opportunity to establish communication and rapport and usually is the first step in an assessment. The interview should be conducted in a room that is private, bright, and nonthreatening. Toys and drawing materials are useful for distracting the young child, so that the parent can give the interviewer full attention.

Before beginning the health interview, nurses must introduce themselves and ask the names of family members. Family members are then addressed by name. Unless an infant, the child is usually included in the interview; the extent of involvement varies with age and culture.

Nurses must clarify their roles in the assessment process because in some health settings many health practitioners see the child. The purposes of the health interview and physical assessment are clarified because parents might wonder about the relevance of the information they are about to give. Parents, and the child, as appropriate, are also told who has access to the information and are assured about the limits of access. After the parameters of the interview and physical assessment have been set, the parents are better able to decide how and what they want to communicate.

Table 1-1   Cultural Variations in Family and Health Practices

Ethnic Group	Family Structure	Child Rearing	Traditional Health Care Beliefs/Practices	Relationship with Professionals	Prevalent Health Concerns
Asian Indians	Family most important social unit. Extended family tend to live in one household. Lifestyle collectivistic rather than individualistic. Earnings shared in the extended family. Head of household	Children relatively more controlled and protected than North American children. Compliance achieved through threats, treats, and occasional spanking. Independence not	Illnesses result from imbalance in body humors (bile, wind, phlegm). Dietary imbalance most common cause of sickness. Hot/cold classification used for foods, depending on how they affect the body. Food is to be eaten in a quiet room and with warm water. Bathing, massage,	Physician expected to have all the answers, make all decisions, and go beyond questions. Medication is expected. Formal dress expected of caregivers. Females tend to be uncomfortable with male caregivers. Health decisions	Tuberculosis Parasites Hepatitis Malaria Cardiac disease

is the most established and financially secure male; head of household makes most decisions but consults close relatives on matters of importance.

encouraged. No fixed schedule for young children. Male children are preferred and have special roles. Education highly valued. Careers and marriage partners selected for children although this is changing.

ritual oils, herbs, and foods are used to treat ailments.

about children made by senior family members. Care of ill family members is responsibility of wife, grandparents. Leisurely style of communication preferred. Small talk significant; rushing considered rude; a direct "no" is impolite.

Continued

Table 1-1 Cultural Variations in Family and Health Practices—cont'd

Ethnic Group	Family Structure	Child Rearing	Traditional Health Care Beliefs/Practices	Relationship with Professionals	Prevalent Health Concerns
Blacks	Strong kinship ties and interactions with extended family. Kinship network not necessarily limited to blood lines; unrelated persons found in same household.	High emphasis on peoplehood or collective consciousness. Strong emphasis on ambition and work.	Self-care, folk medicine important. Tend to seek help from "old lady," priest, root doctor, spiritualist, or minister when ill. Prayer important to healing and treatment. Illness seen as "will of God." Might believe in voodoo and religious healing.	Sensitive to any evidence of discrimination. Might disguise health concern initially to "test" health care professional's ability to see real problem. Nonverbal behavior important in interactions. Might deny need for help to avoid appearing	Sickle cell disease Hemoglobin C disease Diabetes Pneumonia Asthma Cardiovascular disease Lactose intolerance (preschoolers and older) Obesity Drug/alcohol use

Continued

Rigid sex roles deemphasized. Men and women share in household and family responsibilities. Turn to neighbors, or minister in time of crisis. Discussion of family concerns outside of family is major breach of family ethics.

Might wear copper and silver bracelets to prevent illness. Prevention important through cleanliness, laxatives, rest, and diet.

helpless or dependent.

Table 1-1   Cultural Variations in Family and Health Practices—cont'd

Ethnic Group	Family Structure	Child Rearing	Traditional Health Care Beliefs/Practices	Relationship with Professionals	Prevalent Health Concerns
Cambodians/ Laotians	Family key social and economic unit. Extended family source of support and assistance. Husband is head of household, decision maker. Family problems	Physical discipline rare; discipline occurs through verbal reprimand. Respect for older siblings, adults predominant. Children learn through observation	Coin rubbing, using a coin or metal spoon, is used to treat a variety of common ailments. Pinching involves pinching area between eyebrows until it turns red. Pinching and coin rubbing might leave bruising. Ginseng, Tiger Balm are common self-treatments.	Tend to seek professionals only if very ill. Passive role in therapeutic relationship. Expect treatments and medications. Might see blood tests as life threatening.	Tuberculosis Intestinal parasites Anemia Hepatitis B Dental caries Lactose intolerance

		are considered private.	and imitation. Infants carried a great deal; not allowed to cry, walk later than Western children.	
Chinese	Large extended families in a single household; unmarried children live at home until marriage.	Discipline might seem harsh to Westerners. Open affection rarely displayed. Toilet training	Practices based on combination of folk, traditional, and modern medicine. Word of mouth, family practices, magic, and religion important. Health professionals highly respected; Chinese patient might not question out of respect. Might find team approach confusing as	Hepatitis Tuberculosis Intestinal parasites Lactose intolerance Dental caries

Continued

Table 1-1 Cultural Variations in Family and Health Practices—cont'd

Ethnic Group	Family Structure	Child Rearing	Traditional Health Care Beliefs/Practices	Relationship with Professionals	Prevalent Health Concerns
Chinese—cont'd	Husband is breadwinner, takes care of finances, and disciplines children. Wife takes care of household and usually makes health decisions.	initiated early. High value placed on success in school and at work.	Illness results from disequilibrium of opposing forces. Cures are sought from substances associated with perceived deficiencies (e.g., eating brains to get wiser). Food is essential to harmony with nature and is used	Chinese are more familiar with having a close relationship with one or two professionals. Prefer older professionals and Chinese physicians, if available. Strong respect for intactness	

Divorce
considered a
disgrace.
Serious
decisions can
involve all
family
members.
Young
obliged to
take care
of elderly.

to explain causes of
illness and to treat
disease.

of body so might
refuse surgery.
Might become
intensely
distressed by
drawing of blood
as blood is consid-
ered source of
all life and is
not believed to
regenerate.
High expectations
of treatment; might
not understand
limitations.
Prevention difficult
because many
Chinese seek
help only if ill.

Continued

Table 1-1   Cultural Variations in Family and Health Practices—cont'd

Ethnic Group	Family Structure	Child Rearing	Traditional Health Care Beliefs/Practices	Relationship with Professionals	Prevalent Health Concerns
Filipino	Family highly structured. Extended family is central and contains maternal and paternal relatives. Kinship extended to neighbors and friends and is initiated through sharing of Roman	Children adored. Children indulged until age of 6 years when they begin to be socialized through negative feedback. Children expected to be obedient, respectful, to contain emotions,	God's will and supernatural forces govern universe. Misfortunes such as ill health are result of violating God's will. Head considered sacred. Feet lowest part of body so considered rude to show bottom of shoes. Some illnesses considered imbalance of hot and cold. Need to treat hot illnesses with cold	Communication polite and formal. Loud talking considered rude. Elders never addressed by first name. Sensitive topics such as income and personal health avoided. Direct eye contact avoided as can be considered sexually aggressive, but if eye contact made, it is appropriate	Dental caries Lactose intolerance

Continued

Catholic rituals. Community obligations shared through extensions of kinship and include shared labor, food, and financial resources. Conflict is avoided in relationships through use of euphemisms. Go-between selected in sensitive situations.	and to be polite. Children might appear shy and quiet.	foods and cold illnesses with hot foods. Diarrhea and fevers considered hot illnesses; chills and colds considered cold illnesses. Some health practices based on imitative qualities (e.g., nursing mothers avoid dark foods so that babies will have light skin). Fish heads and onions considered brain foods. Honey and certain herbs used to treat diabetes.	to return it.

Table 1-1   Cultural Variations in Family and Health Practices—cont'd

Ethnic Group	Family Structure	Child Rearing	Traditional Health Care Beliefs/Practices	Relationship with Professionals	Prevalent Health Concerns
Hispanics	Couple expected to set up independent household but has close ties with extended family. Extended family includes blood relatives and godparents. Husband responsible	More physical aggression present in urban than in rural families. Children tend to play in groups and to roam neighborhood. Children highly desired and valued.	Might associate hospitalization with death. Might resist bathing a fevered child. Health is achieved through equilibrium of temperature. Some medications, such as antibiotics, are seen as "hot" and therefore undesirable for a fever. Disabled might be restricted to	Physicians are held in high esteem; nurses might not hold much status. Health professional needs to avoid going directly into health concerns; talk first about unrelated matters. Prescriptions are expected. Careful explanations about alternative measures,	Malnutrition Dental caries Scabies Fevers Bronchitis Asthma Eczema Worms Parasites Diabetes Lead poisoning

for work outside the home and the wife for household duties. Physical force is acceptable in arguments. Men give orders to women and older give orders to younger. Grandparents often involved in major decisions. Family honor is important.

Children might react strongly to separation from mother.

privacy of home.

diagnostic assessments, and preventive measures are beneficial. Might be late for appointments because of present time orientation. Females will bring female relative when visiting male professionals. Discussion of sexuality is taboo for a female in the presence of a male.

Continued

Table 1-1   Cultural Variations in Family and Health Practices—cont'd

Ethnic Group	Family Structure	Child Rearing	Traditional Health Care Beliefs/Practices	Relationship with Professionals	Prevalent Health Concerns
Iranians	Extended family considered important for advice, support, and for employment, security, and influence. Paternal influence strong. Sex roles very strong. Children are least respected in family.	Verbal abuse can be common; spanking is less common. Children have many limits. Children have little say in family matters.	Highly fatalistic; what occurs is will of God. Hot and cold used to treat minor illnesses. Thin children believed to be unhealthy; children tend to be overfed.	Older, male health professionals (especially physicians) generally preferred. Health visits need to allow time for undivided attention and to listen to long accounts of health and personal matters. Personal relationship sought with	

Japanese	Extended families more common in traditional family units. Husband is breadwinner; role of wife is to respect and honor the husband and care	Babies encouraged to be passive and not to cry. Toilet training initiated before a year. Infant sleeps with adults.	Humans inherently good; illnesses caused by polluting agents. Evil removed through purification. Believe in removing diseased part. Use acupuncture, herbs,	caregiver. Diagnostic tests and medications expected. Several family members might contact health professional about patient. Physicians held in high esteem; other health care professionals less so. Tend to prefer physicians from own culture. Expect thorough examination at health visit, medication, and	Cleft lip/cleft palate Cardio-vascular diseases Oguchi's disease Acatalasemia

Continued

Table 1-1   Cultural Variations in Family and Health Practices—cont'd

Ethnic Group	Family Structure	Child Rearing	Traditional Health Care Beliefs/Practices	Relationship with Professionals	Prevalent Health Concerns
Japanese—cont'd	for the children. Wife might consult with older family members regarding decisions related to the children. Mother-in-law might assume responsibility for ensuring daughter-in-law meets	Discipline is permissive until child reaches school age. Discipline involves consideration for child and use of example. Light spanking is acceptable. Tidiness and good manners are	moxibustion, and Western and Chinese medicine. Fear of stomach ailments is stronger than any other fear.	explanation of illness. Only exception is when diagnosis is cancer, when family and not patient is told. Family and friends expect to visit in hospital and to take active part in care.	

Continued

all her
obligations.
Woman
responsible to
care for all
members,
young and
old, in
family.
Woman is not
encouraged
to work
outside home.
Etiquette and
conduct
of family
members very
important.
Problems are
not shared
outside
family.

encouraged.
Children
taught to
respect
elders and to
distinguish
between
family and
non-family.

Table 1-1   Cultural Variations in Family and Health Practices—cont'd

Ethnic Group	Family Structure	Child Rearing	Traditional Health Care Beliefs/Practices	Relationship with Professionals	Prevalent Health Concerns
Koreans	Loyalty to family more important than individual needs. Generational ties more important than marriage ties, although this is changing. Male is always head of family; if father unable to fulfill role, then eldest	Parents very close to child. Birth order determines privileges; oldest males receive more privileges than younger children. Opinions of elders must be respected.	Might adhere to shamanism. Good appetite means good health. Foods such as ginseng and ginger tea given to promote good health. Food taboos during pregnancy related to imitative beliefs (e.g., eating bruised fruit can cause baby to have poor skin).	Communication quiet. Excessive laughter might indicate embarrassment. Direct disagreement is uncommon. Disagreement indicated by tipping head back and hissing through teeth. Direct eye contact expected. Touching uncommon.	Dental caries Lactose intolerance

son assumes head, even if still a child. Women assume full responsibility for child care and housekeeping Elders held in high esteem and are expected to relax and enjoy life once they reach 60 years. Rising expected when elders enter room.

Continued

Table 1-1   Cultural Variations in Family and Health Practices—cont'd

Ethnic Group	Family Structure	Child Rearing	Traditional Health Care Beliefs/Practices	Relationship with Professionals	Prevalent Health Concerns
Native Americans	Many variations in family structure and values. Tribe and extended family tend to come before self. Elders are source of wisdom. Extended family structures.	Children learn through observation, imitation, legends. Male child held in higher esteem than female child.	Health is a state of harmony with nature. Spirituality interwoven with medicine. All disorders believed to have element of supernatural. Native healers used in some tribes. Do not believe in germ theory. Illness prevented through religious	Going to hospital associated with illness. Native American healers ask few questions. Present, not future oriented, therefore preventive practices difficult to understand. Time is on a continuum, therefore set intervals (e.g., with medication	Tuberculosis Suicide Lactose intolerance Drug/alcohol abuse Accidents Ear infections Obesity

Continued

					Asthma
Puerto Ricans	Families usually large; home important. Father is head of household; wife and children subordinate. Father makes decisions for family.	Children valued, seen as gift from God. Children expected to obey. Corporal punishment considered acceptable.	rituals and charms. Believe in hot-cold theory of causation of illnesses. Use hot and cold treatments to treat illnesses. Evil spirits can cause illness. Use folk healers, herbs, rituals.	dosing) may need careful explanation. Take time to form opinions of health professionals. Silence, avoiding direct eye contact show respect. Suspicious of hospitals and use health care systems infrequently. Relaxed sense of time and might not be on time for appointments.	

Table 1-1   Cultural Variations in Family and Health Practices—cont'd

Ethnic Group	Family Structure	Child Rearing	Traditional Health Care Beliefs/Practices	Relationship with Professionals	Prevalent Health Concerns
Vietnamese	Family main source of identity. While traditional households often include grandparents, unmarried children, an adult couple, and children, traumatic circumstances might have separated many from	Children are highly valued. Most training is through example. Discipline might include quiet verbal admonitions, shouting, or slapping. Beatings, although rare, are	Herbal remedies, isolation of sick, and visits to shrines practiced. Ideas of health center around hereditary causes of illness, supernatural causes of illness, hot and cold equilibrium, and good and bad wind and water. Being "hot" might refer to having a symptom believed caused by heat	Regard physicians very highly; public health nurses more highly regarded than any other nurses because they are government employees. Visits are expected to be formal, unhurried,	Hepatitis B Pulmonary tuberculosis Intestinal parasites Incomplete immunization Constipation Malnutrition Anemia Dental caries Lactose intolerance

family in Vietnam. Might limit ability to become established in new surroundings. Women have fewer rights than men. Males are main decision makers.

considered to be private family matters. Quiet compliance is expected of children; open anger rare although children might express anger through stubbornness or passive non-cooperation.

imbalance in body— not necessarily fever. Might use rituals to prevent illness. Coin rubbing or placing a hot cup on the body might leave bruises.

without detailed questions about health or social background. Touching or removal of clothing produces discomfort. Stoical with illness and pain; some illnesses are to be ignored. More accepting of prescriptions than changes in behavior.

Dimensions of a History

2

Obtaining a health history is an important component of the health assessment process. The health interview assists in establishing rapport with the parent and child, provides data from which tentative nursing diagnoses can be made, offers an opportunity for the nurse and family to establish goals, and affords the opportunity for the nurse to provide education and support to the family.

The purposes and extent of the health interview vary with the nature of the health care contact. For example, in an emergency situation it is necessary to focus on the chief complaint and the details of past health care contacts. The prenatal and postnatal histories and the psychosocial dimensions can be left for later, unless they are the focus for the concern. When a child has repeated contacts with a health care facility, it is necessary only to update a health history if it has been completed on initial contact. The course of an interview must be modified to fit the situation and the setting. A home setting, for example, can include many distractions and will require adaptation to the family's environment.

Generally, a direct interview is preferred for a health history, as it facilitates the building of a relationship between the family and the nurse and enables the nurse to make rich observations related to behavior, interactions, and environment. However, if an indirect method, such as a questionnaire, is used, then it is important to review the written responses and follow up any unusual responses with the family.

Guidelines for Interviewing Parents and Children

- Follow principles of communication during the interview (see Chapter 1).
- Before beginning the interview the nurse must thoroughly understand the purposes of the health history and of the questions that are asked.

- If a specific illness or health concern is the reason for the interview, knowledge of the diagnosis helps focus questions related to the chief complaint. The nurse must also be alert to concerns raised by the parent or child that are not related to the diagnosis.
- Explain the purpose of the interview, before starting, to the parents and to the child. Cooperation and sharing are more likely to occur if the parents understand that the questions facilitate better care for their child. For the adolescent, understanding the parameters of confidentiality can be crucial to what is shared.
- Write brief notations about specific details. *Do not try to write finished sentences* and *keep writing to a minimum.* The flow of contact is lost if the nurse spends an extended amount of time writing or staring at a form. Further, the nurse might miss important opportunities to observe behaviors and family interactions if overly committed to recording during the interview.
- Know what information is necessary so that the parents and child are not asked for the same type of information repeatedly. *Repeat questions only if further clarification is desired.*
- Give broad openings at the beginning of the interview, such as, "Tell me why you came to see me today." Use direct questions, such as, "Are the stools watery?" to assist the parent to focus on specific details.
- Do not interrupt the parent, child, or parent and interpreter.
- Accept what is being said. Nodding, reestablishing eye contact, or saying "uh-huh" provides encouragement to continue. If parents have difficulty recalling specific details (e.g., when specific developmental milestones were achieved), move on to other areas in the history. When this happens, it is important *not* to make the parents feel that they are "bad parents" because they are unable to remember.
- If an interpreter is being used, avoid commenting about the family in the presence of the family.
- Listen, and attend to nonverbal cues. The presenting complaint might have little to do with the real concern.
- Convey empathy and an unhurried attitude. Sit at eye level, if possible. If the family is from another culture, observe to determine what behaviors are acceptable and therefore empathic to them. Eye contact, for example, is considered disrespectful in some cultures (e.g., Native Americans) rather than indicative of active listening and empathy.

- Ensure mutual understanding. *Clarify* if unsure, and summarize for the parent and child what has been understood.
- Integrate the child when possible and when culturally appropriate. Even the very young can answer the question "What do you like to eat?"
- Be sensitive to the need to separately interview parents and child, particularly if the child is an adolescent.
- Be sensitive to the need to consider who is responsible for health decisions in the family and for child care (see Chapter 1).

Information for Comprehensive History

Information	Comment
Date of History	Identifying Data
Include name of child and nickname (if any), names of parents and guardians, home telephone number, work numbers and hours when parents or guardians work, child's date of birth, age (months, years), sex, race, language spoken, language understood.	Much of this information might already be on a child's nameplate or chart.
Source of Referral, if Any	
Source of Information	
Include relationship of inform-ant to child (child, parent, other) and judgment about reliability of information. If an interpreter has been used, note this as well.	Hesitations and vague or contradictory answers might raise concerns about reliability.
Chief Complaint	
Use broad opening statements, such as, "What concerns bring you here today?" Record parents' or child's	Note who identified the chief complaint. In some instances a schoolteacher or physician might have

Information	Comment

Chief Complaint—cont'd

own words: "Running to the bathroom since Saturday."

expressed the concern. Agreement between parents and another referral source is important to note. Adolescents and parents might differ regarding perception of complaint.

Present Illness

Include a chronologic narrative of the chief complaint. The narrative answers questions related to *where* (location), *what* (quality, factors that aggravate or relieve symptoms), *when* (onset, duration, frequency), and *how much* (intensity, severity). The parent or child should also be asked about associated manifestations. Include significant negatives: "The parent denies that the child has experienced undue fatigue, bruising, or joint tenderness." Ask what home and formal health care interventions have been tried to manage the concern and the effectiveness of these interventions. Inquire specifically about natural or homeopathic remedies as well. Use direct questions to focus on specific details, as necessary.

Reasons for seeking care can provide valuable information about changes in the status of the child's health concern. This information can aid in diagnosis and care planning Parents might need assistance in sorting out details. Prior knowledge of diagnosis aids in planning specific questions; however, care must be taken to avoid premature closure or diminished openness to possibilities not presented by the diagnosis. In a primary care setting, the nurse often begins by addressing health maintenance or health-promoting issues. Information about previously tried home and health care interventions provides important data about parent/child knowledge of interventions, self-care abilities, motivation, and

Information	Comment

Present Illness—cont'd

cultural practices. Some folk remedies can be harmful. For example, two folk remedies from Mexico that are used to treat colic contain lead (azarcon and greta).

Clinical Alert

Persistent denial in the face of unexplained or vaguely defined injuries can signal child abuse. Denial might also indicate nonacceptance of a concern such as a developmental delay or behavior problem.

Insistent presentation of symptoms (especially by mother) in the absence of objective data might be suggestive of Munchausen syndrome by proxy.

Medical History

General State of Health

Inquire about appetite, recent weight losses or gains, fatigue, stresses.

Do not include information that might have been elicited for chief complaint or present illness.

Birth History

Include prenatal history (maternal health; infections; drugs taken, including prescription and illegal; tobacco and alcohol use; abnormal bleeding; weight gain; duration of pregnancy; attitudes toward pregnancy; birth; duration of labor; type of delivery; complications; birth weight; condition of

Birth history is especially important if the child is younger than 2 years or is experiencing developmental or neurologic problems.

Information	Comment
Birth History—cont'd	

infant at birth), and neonatal history (respiratory distress, cyanosis, jaundice, seizures, poor feeding, patterns of sleeping).

Dietary History

For infants, include type of feeding (bottle, breast, solid foods), frequency of feedings, quantity of feeds, responses to feeding, types of foods, specific problems with feeding (colic, regurgitation, lethargy). For children, include self-feeding abilities, likes and dislikes, appetite, and amounts of food taken. For adolescents, include usual eating patterns and daily caloric intake.

Guidelines for a more complete nutritional history are supplied in Chapter 7.
Clinical Alert
Patterns and responses to feeding as an infant or as a child can be indicators of underlying concerns. For example, difficulty breastfeeding and/or slow eating as a preschooler and overwhelming preference for certain foods can be an indication of autism spectrum disorder. Skipping meals can be the strongest predictor of inadequate calcium intake in adolescents.

Previous Illnesses, Operations, or Injuries

Ask parents about other illnesses the child has had. Parents are likely to recall significant illnesses but might need guidance to talk about common childhood illnesses and details of these illnesses, such as tonsillitis and earaches. Include dates of hospitalizations, reasons for hospitalizations, and responses to illnesses.

Knowing how a child reacted during past hospitalizations can help in planning interventions for a current hospitalization.
Negative or frightening experiences with illnesses or care need to be considered when approaching assessment and planning care.

Information	Comment

*Previous Illnesses, Operations,
or Injuries—cont'd*

Clinical Alert
If the child has experienced
frequent accidents such as
injuries or poisoning, this
might indicate a need
for teaching and guidance.

Childhood Illnesses
Include the common communicable diseases, such as
measles, mumps, and
chickenpox. Inquire about
recent contact with persons
with communicable diseases.

Immunizations
Include specific details
about immunizations (dates,
types) and untoward reactions.
If a child has not been
immunized, note the reason.
Note desensitization
procedures.

Fainting, stable neurologic
conditions, and mild
illnesses are not contra-
indications for adminis-
tration of immunizations.
Clinical Alert
Anaphylactic reactions such
as hives, wheezing,
difficulty breathing, or
circulatory collapse (not
fainting) after an
immunization are
contraindications to
further doses.
An anaphylactic reaction to
eating eggs is a
contraindication for
administration of influenza
vaccine; an anaphylactic
reaction to eating gelatin is
a contraindication for
administration of MMR.
Encephalopathy within 7 days
of receiving DTP/DTaP
is a contraindication for
administering DTP/DTaP.

Information	Comment
Current Medications	
Include prescription and nonprescription drugs (ask specifically about use of vitamins, cold medications, herbs), dose, frequency, duration of use, time of last dose, and understanding of parents and/or child about the prescribed drugs.	Although herbs and vitamins are sometimes seen as natural substances, not as medications, parents and other caregivers need to consider these substances when asked about medications. Some herbs have powerful interactions with prescription medications (e.g., garlic can increase bleeding tendencies and therefore needs to be considered if medications are given that affect clotting times).
Allergies	
Include agent *and* reaction.	Knowing the reaction is useful because reactions might not be indicative of allergic manifestations.
Growth and Development	
Physical	
Include approximate height and weight at 1, 2, 5, and 10 years, and tooth eruption/loss.	A thorough history of growth and development is important in planning nursing interventions appropriate to the child's level and in screening for developmental and neurologic problems. A social history can identify the need for anticipatory guidance.
Developmental History	
Include ages at which child rolled over, sat alone, crawled, walked, spoke first words, spoke first sentences, and dressed without help.	

Information	Comment
Social and Psychosocial History	
Include toileting (age at which daytime and nighttime control were achieved or current level of control, enuresis, encopresis, self-toileting abilities, terminology used); sleep (amount, time to bed, ease in falling asleep, whether child/adolescent stays asleep, bedtime rituals, security objects, fears, nightmares, snoring, daytime sleepiness, falling asleep at school); speech (lisping, stuttering, delays, intelligibility); sexuality (relationships with members of opposite sex, inquisitiveness about sexual information and activity, type of information given child); schooling (school grade level, academic achievement, adjustment to school); habits (thumb sucking, nail biting, pica, head banging); discipline (methods used, child's response to discipline); personality and temperament (congeniality, aggressiveness, temper tantrums, withdrawal, relationships with peers/family).	Behaviors, such as those related to toilet training or sleep patterns and habits, vary with culture. Open discussion of sexual matters might be restricted in some cultures (e.g., Hispanics). **Clinical Alert** Behavior and temperament might provide important diagnostic and intervention information. Children with hearing impairments and school-age children who experience recurrent abdominal pain are more likely to have difficult temperaments. Children with chronic cardiac disease are more intense, withdrawn, and more negative in mood than healthy children. Boys from violent home environments tend to bully, be argumentative, and have temper tantrums and short attention spans. Girls from violent homes tend to be anxious or depressed, to cling, and to be perfectionists. Infants born to mothers on cocaine exhibit sleep problems.
Children and adolescents should be asked if they ever feel sad or "down."	Daytime sleepiness, difficulties falling or staying asleep, and

Information	Comment

Social and Psychosocial History —cont'd

If yes, they should be asked if they have ever thought of killing themselves.

inadequate sleep might indicate sleep deprivation or an underlying sleep disorder, depression, sleep apnea, narcolepsy, or overuse of caffeinated drinks. If general aspects of the health history indicate concern with psychosocial functioning, include the more detailed assessments provided in Chapter 24.

Family History

Include the ages and health of immediate family members, familial diseases, presence and types of congenital anomalies, consanguinity of parents, occupations and education of parents, and family interactions, including who is primarily responsible for child care and for making decisions related to health care.

A genogram (Figure 2-1) is useful for showing the relationships, ages, health of family members, and who is in the household. (See Chapter 3 for a more detailed family assessment.) Needs of health care programs should be balanced with needs of families.

Parents identify their main needs as information about diagnosis, effect of diagnosis on development, information about treatment, and effect of condition on sexuality of child.

Clinical Alert

Be alert to symptoms of lead poisoning in children whose siblings or playmates are being treated for lead poisoning.

Information	Comment
Family History—cont'd	
	Parental age of less than 18 years at the time of child's birth might be a risk factor for maltreatment.
Systems Review	
1. General	Questions appropriate for each system are included in other chapters in this book, under the heading "Preparation."
2. Integument	
3. Head and neck	
4. Ears	
5. Eyes	
6. Face and nose	
7. Thorax and lungs	
8. Cardiovascular	
9. Abdominal	
10. Genitourinary/reproductive	
11. Musculoskeletal	
12. Neurologic	

A

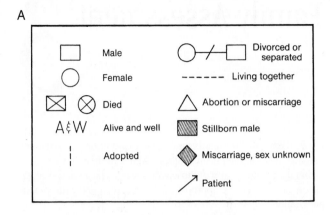

B

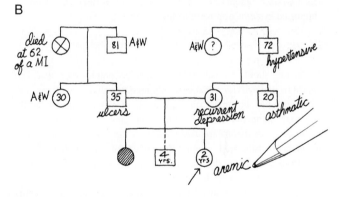

Figure 2-1
Constructing a genogram. **A,** Symbols used in genogram. **B,** Sample
genogram

Family Assessment

3

Assessment of the family includes exploration of structure, function, and developmental stage. Although family *therapy* is within the practice realm of those with special education and supervision, assessment is appropriate for practitioners with general preparation.

The assessment guidelines outlined in this chapter are adapted from those outlined by Wright and Leahey (2000) in the Calgary Family Assessment Model (CFAM) and reflect its strongly supported systems approach to family care.

Rationale

The family should be viewed as interacting, complex elements. The decisions and activities of one family member affect the others, and the family has an impact on the individual. Understanding family members' interactions and communications, family norms and expectations, how decisions are made, and how the family balances individual and family needs enables the nurse to understand the family's responses and needs during times of stress and well-being. This understanding can enrich the relationship between the nurse and family. The nurse's positive, proactive responses to family concerns and capabilities can help the family promote the development and well-being of its members.

General Concepts Related to Assessment

The primary premise in family systems assessment is that individuals are best understood in the context of their families. Studying a child and a parent as separate units does not constitute family assessment because it neglects observation of interactions. The parents and children are part of subsystems within a larger family system, which in turn is part of a larger subsystem. Changes in any one of these systems components affect the other components, a characteristic that has been likened to the impact of wind or motion on the pieces of a mobile.

The analogy of a mobile is useful for considering a second concept in family systems assessment. When piece A of the mobile strikes piece B, piece B might rebound and strike piece A with increased energy. Piece A affects piece B and piece B affects piece A. Circular causality assumes that behavior is reciprocal; each family member's behavior influences the others. If mother responds angrily to her toddler because he turned on the hot water tap while her infant was in the tub, the toddler reciprocates with a response that further influences the mother. It is important to remain open to the multiple interpretations of reality within a family, recognizing that family members might not fully realize how their behavior affects others or how others affect them.

All systems have boundaries. Knowledge of the family's boundaries can help the nurse predict the level of social support that the family might perceive and receive. Families with rigid, closed boundaries might have few contacts with the community suprasystem and might require tremendous assistance to network appropriately for help. Conversely, families with very loose, permeable boundaries might be caught between many opinions as they seek to make health-related decisions. Members within family systems might similarly experience extremely closed or permeable boundaries. In enmeshed families, boundaries between parent and child subsystems might be blurred to the extent that children adopt inappropriate parental roles. In more rigid families, the boundaries between adult and child subsystems might be so closed that the developing child is unable to assume more mature roles.

Families attempt to maintain balances between change and stability. The crisis of illness might temporarily produce a state of great change within a family. Efforts at stability, such as emphatic attempts at maintenance of usual feeding routines during the illness of an infant, might seem paradoxical to the period of change; however, both change and stability can and do coexist in family systems. Overwhelming change or rigid equilibrium can contribute to and be symptomatic of severe family dysfunction. Sustained change usually produces a new level of balance as the family regroups and reorganizes to cope with the change.

Stages in Family Development

Change and stability are integral concepts in development. Like individuals, families experience a developmental sequence, which can be divided into eight distinct stages.

Stage One: Marriage (Joining of Families)

Marriage involves the combining of families of origin as well as of individuals. The establishment of couple identity and the negotiation of new relationships with the families of origin is essential to the successful resolution of this stage. The new relationships will vary with the cultural context of the couple.

Stage Two: Families with Infants

This stage begins with the birth of the first child and involves integration of the infant into the family, design and acceptance of new roles, and maintenance of the spousal relationship. The birth of an infant brings about profound changes to the family and offers more challenges than any other stage in family development. A decrease in marital satisfaction is common during this stage, especially if the infant is ill or has a handicapping condition, and is influenced by individual characteristics of the parents, relationships within the nuclear and extended families, and division of labor.

Stage Three: Families with Preschoolers

Stage three begins when the eldest child is 3 years of age and involves socialization of the child(ren) and successful adjustment to separation by parents and child(ren).

Stage Four: Families with School-Age Children

This stage begins when the eldest child begins elementary or primary school (at about 6 years). Although all stages are perceived by some families as especially stressful, others report this as a particularly stressful stage. Tasks involve establishment of peer relationships by the children and adjustment to peer and other external influences by the parents.

Stage Five: Families with Teenagers

This stage begins when the eldest child is 13 years of age and is viewed by some as an intense period of turmoil. Stage five focuses on the increasing autonomy and individuation of the child, a return to midlife and career issues for parents, and increasing recognition by parents of their predicament as the "sandwich generation."

Stage Six: Families as Launching Centers

Stage six begins when the first child leaves home and continues until the youngest child departs. During this time, the couple realigns the marital relationship while they and the child(ren) adjust to new roles as parents and separate adults.

Stage Seven: Middle-Age Families

Stage seven begins when the last child leaves home and continues until a parent retires. (This is often a stage for maximum contact between the marriage partners.) Successful resolution depends on development of independent interests within a newly reconstituted couple identity, inclusion of new and extended family relationships, and coming to terms with disabilities and deaths in the older generation. Within some cultures, such as the Vietnamese culture, parents might be incorporated into a multigenerational household.

Stage Eight: Aging Families

This stage begins with retirement and ends with the death of the spouses. It is marked by concern with development of retirement roles, maintenance of individual/couple relationships, aging, and preparation for death.

Tasks and Characteristics of Stepfamilies

Stepfamilies face unique challenges as they attempt to build a new family unit from members who all bring a history of relationships, expectations, and life experiences. Intense conflict can arise as marriage partners attempt to cope with instant children without the benefit of instant affection. The parents move from a fantasy stage, in which they dream of fixing everything that went wrong in previous marriages, to a reality stage in which the challenges and losses of transition are realized.

Guidelines for Communicating with Families

- Display a sincere sense of warmth, caring, and encouragement.
- Demonstrate neutrality; perceptions of partiality toward particular family members can interfere with assessment and assistance.

- Use active and reflective listening.
- Convey a sense of cooperation and partnership with the family.
- Promote participatory decision making.
- Promote the competencies of the family.
- Encourage the family's use of natural support networks.

Assessment of the Family

Assessment of the family usually involves the entire family, except when the infant or child is too ill to participate.

Assessment	Findings
Internal Structure	
Use a genogram (see Chapter 2) to diagram family structure. The genogram is often useful in helping the family to clarify information related to family composition.	
Family Composition	
Refers to everyone in the household.	Extended families and multigenerational households are common among many cultures such as Vietnamese, Chinese, and South Asians.
Ask who is in the family.	**Clinical Alert**
	Losses or additions to families can result in crisis.
Rank Order	
Refers to the arrangement of children according to age and gender.	Family position is thought to influence relationships and even careers. Eldest children are considered more conscientious, perfectionistic; middle children are sometimes considered nonconformist, and to have many friends; and youngest children are sometimes seen as

Assessment	Findings
Rank Order—cont'd	precocious, less responsible with resources, and playful.
	Clinical Alert
	Frequent references to rank order ("She's the eldest") might signify a role assignment that is uncomfortable for the individual who is involved.
	The first child can be at increased risk for abuse in abusive families.
Subsystems	**Clinical Alert**
Smaller units in the family marked by sex, role, interests, or age.	A child acting as a parent surrogate might signify family dysfunction or abuse.
Ask if the family has special smaller groups.	Mothers who are highly involved with their infants and who form tight subsystems with the infants can unintentionally push the father to an outside position. This can exacerbate marital dissatisfaction and conflict.
Boundaries	Strength of boundaries might be influenced by culture. East Indian families, for example, tend to be close-knit and highly interdependent.
Refers to who is part of what system or subsystem.	
Need to consider if family boundaries and subsystems are closed, open, rigid, or permeable.	Cambodians and Laotians consider family problems very personal, private, and off limits to outsiders.

Assessment	Findings
Boundaries—cont'd	
	Clinical Alert
Ask who the family members approach with concerns.	A family with rigid boundaries might become distanced or disengaged from others. Disengagement might also occur within families; these families are characterized by little intrafamilial communication and highly autonomous members.
Can be visually represented with an ecomap (Figure 3-1).	Isolation or absent or poor social networks might indicate family dysfunction.
Culture	
Way of life for a group.	The internal and external
Ask if other languages are spoken.	structures of a family, as well as parenting practices,
Ask how long family has lived in area/country.	are affected by ethnicity. For example, Native
Ask if family identifies with a particular ethnic group.	American Indians discipline through observational
Ask how ethnic background influences their lifestyle.	learning rather than through coercive control.
Ask what they believe causes health/illness.	

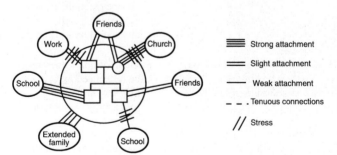

Figure 3-1
Ecomap.

Assessment	Findings
Culture—cont'd	
Ask what they do to prevent/treat illness.	
Might significantly affect care.	
Religion	
Influences family values and beliefs.	In families who are Jehovah's Witnesses, blood transfusions are not allowed. Christian Scientists believe that healing is a religious function and oppose drugs, blood transfusions, and extensive physical examinations.
Might affect care of the infant/child.	
Ask if family is involved in a church or if they identify with a particular religious group.	
Ask how religion is a part of their life.	
Observe for religious icons and artifacts in the home.	Buddhists might be reluctant to consent to treatments on holy days. Families who are Black Muslim prefer vegan diets and might refuse pork-base medicines. Islamic families might refuse narcotics and any other medicines that are deemed addictive or to have an alcohol base. Hindu families might refuse beef-based medical products.
Social Class Status and Mobility	
Mold family values.	**Clinical Alert**
Inquire about work moves, satisfaction, and aspirations.	Family dysfunction might be associated with job instability.
	Migrancy can result in social isolation and lack of health care.
Environment	
Refers to home, neighborhood, and community. Ask about living arrangements (house, apartment, other?), how long in current	**Clinical Alert**
	Chipped paint, heavy street traffic, uncertain water supplies, and sanitation can all affect family health.

Assessment	Findings
Environment—cont'd	
home. If transient, inquire about planned length of stay in community.	Temporary shelters or lack of dwelling might indicate homelessness of family, related to physical or substance abuse, job layoffs, domestic conflicts, parental illness, or other crisis.
Refers to adequacy and safety of home, school, recreation, and transportation.	
Can affect family's ability to visit and receive ongoing care.	
Extended Family	
Refers to families of origin and steprelatives.	Extended family might need to be involved in care if contact is significant. In some cultures (East Indian, Iranian, Japanese), extended family might be consulted about health care decisions.
Ask about contacts (who? frequency? significance?) with extended family members.	
Family Development	
Use age and school placement of oldest child to delineate stage.	**Clinical Alert**
	A family that resists change might become stuck in a stage. The adolescent, for example, might be treated as a young child, producing great distress.
Questions evolve from the developmental stage of the family. For stage two, the practitioner might inquire about the differences noticed since the birth of an infant.	
	Family breakdown and divorce affect the family differently depending on the timing in the family cycle.
Instrumental Functioning	
Refers to the routine mechanics of eating, dressing, sleeping.	**Clinical Alert**
	An ill or disabled child can significantly alter the family's pattern of activities and ability to carry out activities.
Inquire about concerns with accomplishment of daily tasks.	
In families with young infants, inquire about how child care and household tasks are shared.	Imbalances in the division of labor in families with young infants can be a

Assessment	Findings
Instrumental Functioning—cont'd	
Inquire about what families would like to change related to sharing of tasks and responsibilities, if anything.	significant source of stress and conflict.
Expressive Functioning	
Refers to the affective issues and is useful in delineating functional families and those families who are experiencing distress and who would benefit from intervention or referral.	**Clinical Alert** A family might refuse to show emotion appropriately or allow members to do so, which can suggest dysfunction. In alcoholic families, for example, members might show an unusually bland response to extremes in circumstances or behavior. Expression of emotions might be influenced by culture. In some cultures (e.g., Japanese), expression of emotions might be restrained.
Emotional Communication	
Range and type of emotions expressed in a family.	**Clinical Alert** Expression might be narrow, rigid, and inappropriate in dysfunctional families.
Inquire how intense emotions, such as anger and sadness, are expressed and who is most expressive.	
Ask who provides comfort in the family. When something new is to be tried, who provides support?	
Verbal Communication	
Verbal communication addresses the clarity, directness, openness, and direction of communication.	**Clinical Alert** Alcoholic and/or abusive families are frequently characterized by secrecy among family members and in relation to those
Can be observed during the interview. Indirect communication can be	

Assessment	Findings
Verbal Communication—cont'd	
clarified by asking questions such as, "What is your mom telling you?"	outside the family. Within dysfunctional families, verbal exchanges might evidence blaming, scapegoating, or derogatory remarks. Adolescents might be exposed to public ridicule, threats related to expulsion from the family or forced encounters with police, and intense criticism.
Observe congruence of verbal and nonverbal communications.	
Observe if family members wait to speak until others are through.	
Do parents or older siblings talk down to younger children?	
	Triangulation refers to an indirect communication pattern in which one member communicates with another through a third member.
Circular Communication	
Reciprocal communication that is adaptive or maladaptive.	
Useful in understanding communication in dyads.	
If a mother complains that her adolescent never listens to her, you might inquire: "So Susan ignores your. instruction What do you do then?"	
Problem Solving	
Refers to ability of family to solve own problems.	Decision making is culturally influenced. In many cultures (e.g., Hispanic, Vietnamese, Puerto Rican) the father is the main family decision maker.
Ask who first notices problems, how decisions are made, who makes decisions.	
	Clinical Alert
	Dysfunctional families might tend to employ a narrow range of strategies,

Assessment	Findings
Problem Solving—cont'd	consistently apply inappropriate strategies, or fail to adapt strategies to needs and stages of family members.
Roles	
Focuses on established behavior patterns.	**Clinical Alert**
Consider flexibility or rigidity of roles and whether certain idiosyncratic roles are applied to family members ("She's always been a problem" or "He's a good kid").	Dysfunctional families might assign narrowly prescriptive roles.
Consider the effect of culture on roles. Ask, "In your culture what do women do? What do men do?"	
Consider the influence of the multigenerational family on roles. "In your family, what did your father do? What did your mother do?"	
Control	
Refers to ways of influencing the behavior of others. Might be psychologic (use of communication and feelings), corporal (hugging or spanking), or instrumental (use of reinforcers such as privileges or objects).	**Clinical Alert** Excessive control or chaos in relation to rules can signify an abusive family.
Inquire about family rules and what occurs when rules are broken.	
Ask who enforces family rules. Do children have a say in rules?	
Consider the impact of culture on family expectations. Ask, "How are children expected	

Assessment	Findings

Control—cont'd
   to behave? What happens if
   they do not behave?"

Alliances/Coalitions

Refers to balance and intensity
   of relationships between or
   among family members.

Clinical Alert

In sexually abusive families,
   the father and daughter
   coalition can supplant the
   spousal relationship.

Related Nursing Diagnoses

Risk for trauma: related to neighborhood, home environment, lack
of safety measures, lack of safety education, insufficient resources
to purchase safety equipment or to make repairs.

Relocation stress syndrome: related to impaired psychosocial
health status, losses, moderate to high degree of environment
change, lack of adequate support system, feeling of powerless-
ness, little or no preparation for impending move.

Risk for altered growth: related to deprivation, poverty, violence,
natural disasters.

Altered growth and development: related to environmental and
stimulation deficiencies, inconsistent responsiveness.

Impaired home maintenance: related to family disease or injury,
unfamiliarity with neighborhood resources, inadequate support
systems, impaired emotional or cognitive functioning, insufficient family planning or organization.

Altered health maintenance: related to ineffective family coping,
lack of material resources.

Decisional conflict: related to support system deficit, lack of
experience with decision making.

Family coping, potential for growth: related to sufficient gratifica-
tion of needs, effective addressing of adaptive tasks.

Ineffective family coping, compromised: related to temporary
family disorganization, role changes, situational or developmental crises.

Ineffective family coping, disabling: related to highly ambivalent
family relationships.

Parental role conflict: related to change in marital status, interruptions of family life because of home care regimen.

Altered family processes: related to informal or formal interaction with community, modification in family social status or finances, developmental transition or crisis, shift in health status of family member, power shift of family members.

Risk for altered parenting: related to social factors, knowledge, psychologic factors, illness.

Risk for altered parent/infant/child attachment: related to physical barriers, anxiety associated with parent role, ill child, lack of privacy, separation, inability of parents to meet personal needs.

Home Visits and Assessments

4

Making home visits and delivering home-based nursing gives the nurse an excellent opportunity to observe and interact with families in an environment that is familiar to them. Further, by visiting the home, the nurse is able to assess safety, hygiene, support systems, and play stimulation within the environment that is closest and most familiar to the family.

Making Home Visits

In making home visits, it is essential that the nurse recognize his or her status as a visitor in the home with services that the family can accept or reject. The relationship is a negotiated one, and the nurse must recognize that successful negotiation entails gaining support and acceptance from the family.

To gain and maintain access to the home, the nurse needs to demonstrate flexibility, an understanding of the diversity present in homes, and an awareness of social rules that will affect the relationship between the family and nurse. In establishing initial contact with a family, some guidelines assist in ensuring that the contact is successful:

- With the first telephone call, identify affiliation, source of referral, purpose of referral, knowledge of situation, and how families can further contact the nurse.
- Demonstrate willingness to negotiate times for the visit.
- Ask for clear directions to the home. If the area is unfamiliar, check with a supervisor for more detailed directions and ensure that safety equipment, including a telephone, is included.
- Alert the family about when the visit will occur.
- Establish where to park and how to access the home.

Making the Initial Visit

When making the initial visit, family-centered actions will facilitate development of trust and rapport. The nurse must also be aware of variables that will affect assessment and the safety of the nurse:

- Maintain a respectful distance. Do not enter the family's space prematurely. Enter the home and less public areas within the home when verbally and nonverbally invited to do so.
- Respect customs. Place shoes and coat in areas comfortable to the family. Observe for and avoid special areas that certain family members claim for sitting.
- Suspend values. What works for a family might differ from the nurse's perception of what is acceptable.
- Be prepared to accept hospitality; professional boundaries are less secure in home settings, and the relationship might be less formal.
- Be prepared for the unpredictable. Homes can be more distracting than clinical settings; they have no common baseline, and variables are less controlled. Distractions and variations provide useful information for ongoing care and the relationship.
- Priorities need to remain fluid to accommodate differences between the family's perceptions and that of the nurse. Preset nurse agendas are often only a starting point. On the first visit, it is important to remember that it can take several visits to make a complete assessment and to avoid being excessively intrusive with questions and assessments. A family's perception of over-enthusiasm by the nurse in meeting assessment needs can destroy rapport and trust in a developing relationship with the family.
- Attend to personal safety. Keep car doors locked and park in a well-lighted area. Check surroundings before getting out of the car and for the presence of unfriendly animals or individuals; do not get out of the car if suspicious or aggressive behavior is occurring. Assess the safety of the interior environment of the home before entering.
- At the conclusion of the visit, establish dates and times for the next visit.

Assessment of the Home Environment
Safety

Observe the external home environment for presence of abandoned refrigerators, freezers, or automobiles; condition of steps and rails;

use of fuel-burning heaters; and condition and presence of play equipment. Observe within the home for condition of stairs, stairwells, doors, and windows; flaking or peeling paint or plaster; presence of unstored paints or lacquers; presence and condition of smoke and carbon monoxide detectors; source of heat and light; presence of infant gates and locks on cupboards; accessibility and storage of medications and of poisonous or corrosive substances; presence of hanging cords; presence of safety covers on electrical outlets; accessibility of cooking pot handles; delayed lighting of gas burner or oven; grease waste collected on stove; nonskid rugs; presence of poisonous plants; temperature of water; infant walkers; condition and design of crib and high chair; presence of needles and drug paraphernalia; presence and storage of firearms; proximity to pools; and age and condition of the dwelling. If a child in the home is technology dependent, observe for coverings, such as clear tape or panels over control knobs on equipment; disposal receptacles for sharps; and presence of intercom or monitoring systems. Observe for proximity of dwelling to smelters, battery recycling plants, or other industries likely to release lead and for proximity to major roadways or railway tracks. Ask about fire escape plans and plans for other emergencies (e.g., tornadoes, hurricanes, floods), where appropriate.

Hygiene

Observe for cleanliness, including storage and handling of perishable foodstuffs (especially meat), handling of pacifiers and bottles, unwashed cooking equipment or clothes, accumulations of dirt, disorderly surroundings, hand washing practices, odors, condition of water supply, type and adequacy of waste disposal, pests, pets, type and condition of clothing worn by family members, and hygiene of family members.

Availability of Transportation and Facilities

Observe for presence of vehicles; bus stops; condition of roads; driveways; distance to nearest neighbor; presence of telephone; and proximity to schools, shopping, recreation, and health care services.

Nutritional Practices

Observe for available snack foods, cooking odors, accessibility of food for children, availability of choice in menu, and ethnic or religious food observances.

Support Networks

Observe for family pictures and pictures of friends, presence of a telephone and type of calls received, and proximity to neighbors and other family members.

Family Interactions

Observe for spontaneous vocalization between parents and children, verbal responses of parents to vocalizations of children, use of praise with children, demonstrations of affection, use of scolding or shouting, attempts to explain or teach about objects or situations, attempts to look at children, teaching of culturally appropriate rules of behavior, display of children's art/crafts, introduction of children to nurse, and encouragement of age-appropriate independence.

Provision of Stimulation and Opportunities for Rest

Observe for presence of age-appropriate toys and toys with variety, recreational and exercise aids, books, pets, and television. Observe if children are playing with matches, candles, sharp-edged toys, or cigarettes. Observe for amount of time that children spend watching television and interaction of parents in relation to television, programs and games in which children are engaged, areas and space available in the home for privacy, amount of space or crowding evident in home, and adequacy of sleeping facilities (e.g., number, type, and safety of beds and cribs; presence of bed linens).

Religious and Cultural Influences

Observe for presence of religious icons, bibles, art, and cultural artifacts; ethnic cooking utensils; and type of clothing worn by family members.

Related Nursing Diagnoses

Impaired home maintenance: related to lack of knowledge, insufficient family planning or organization, inadequate support systems, insufficient finances, impaired cognitive or emotional functioning, family disease or injury, unfamiliarity with community resources.

Ineffective family coping: related to lack of knowledge of resources, isolation, family disorganization or role changes.

Effective family coping, potential for growth: related to priorities, health-promoting behaviors, enriching lifestyle that supports maturational processes, negotiation of treatment programs.

Knowledge deficit: home safety and hygiene, community and social supports: related to cognitive or emotional limitations, lack of interest in learning, lack of exposure or role modeling, unfamiliarity with resources.

Hopelessness: related to lack of social support, socioeconomic conditions.

Risk for injury: related to home environment, lack of knowledge of provider, pollutants.

Risk for suffocation: related to fuel-burning heaters, abandoned equipment and vehicles, cribs, clotheslines, inadequate supervision.

Risk for poisoning: related to unprotected medications or poisonous chemicals; flaking, peeling paint or plaster; contamination of food or water; atmospheric pollutants; lack of safety or drug education; cognitive or emotional difficulties.

Risk for trauma: related to neighborhood crime, high beds, unsecured weapons, inadequate home safety measures with infants and young children, defective or abandoned appliances, highly flammable toys and clothing, inadequately stored combustibles and corrosives.

Physical Assessment

5

Physical assessment skills include inspection, palpation, percussion, and auscultation. (The sequence in abdominal assessment is inspection, auscultation, percussion, and palpation.) The acquisition of these skills requires patience, practice, and continual refinement. A more detailed discussion of these skills can be found in a textbook of adult assessment skills.

Guidelines for Inspection

- Inspection is a simple but highly skilled technique.
- Inspection involves the use of sight, hearing, and smell in a systematic assessment of infants and children.
- Inspection is essential at the beginning of the health assessment to detect obvious health concerns and to establish priorities.
- Inspection should be thorough and should involve each area of the body.
- Body parts are assessed for shape, color, symmetry, odor (Table 5-1), and abnormalities.
- Careful inspection requires good lighting.

Guidelines for Palpation

- Palpation involves the use of fingers and palms to determine temperature, hydration, texture, shape, movement, and areas of tenderness. Palpation can be light or deep. Light palpation is used to assess skin temperature, texture, and hydration; overt, large, or superficial masses; fluid and muscle guarding; and superficial tenderness. Light palpation is performed with the dominant hand, fingers together. The fingerpads are placed on the skin in a plane parallel to the area and the skin is depressed gently and lightly (about 1 cm or 0.4 inches) in a circular motion. If the child

Table 5-1   **Significance of Common Body Odors**

Odor	Significance
Acetone or fruity odor	Might indicate diabetic acidosis
Ammonia	Might indicate urinary tract infection
Fecal odor (breath or diaper area)	Associated with soiled diapers, fecal incontinence, bowel obstruction
Foul-smelling stool	Might indicate gastroenteritis, cystic fibrosis, malabsorption syndromes
Halitosis	Associated with poor oral hygiene, dental caries or abscess, throat infection, sinusitis, constipation, foreign body in nasal passage
Musty odor	Associated with infection underneath a cast or dressing
Sweet, thick odor	Might indicate *Pseudomonas* infection

is ticklish, lift the hand fully off the skin before moving to another area. Deep palpation is used to assess the position of organs or masses, as well as their consistency, shape, mobility, and areas of discomfort. It is frequently used in abdominal and reproductive assessments. Deep palpation involves depressing the skin to a depth of approximately 4 to 5 cm (1.5 to 2 inches).

- Warm hands before beginning palpation.
- Keep fingernails short.
- Palpate areas of tenderness or vulnerability last. If pain is experienced during palpation, discontinue palpation in that area immediately.
- Palpate with fingertips for pulsation, size, shape, texture, hydration, and mobility and consistency of organs.
- Palpate with palms for vibration.
- Palpate with back of hand for temperature.

- Use conversation or games to relax child during palpation. Muscle guarding related to tension can obscure findings. Observe reactions to palpation rather than asking, "Does it hurt?"
- The nurse can assist the ticklish child by first placing the child's hands on the skin and gradually sliding hands over those of the child or by having the child keep his or her hands over the nurse's during examination.
- Move firmly and without hesitation.

Guidelines for Percussion

- Percussion involves the use of tapping to produce sound waves, which are characterized regarding intensity, pitch, duration, and quality (Table 5-2).
- Percussion can be *direct* or *indirect*.
  Direct percussion involves striking the body part directly with one or two fingers.
  Indirect percussion involves a pleximeter and a plexor.
  Place the middle finger (pleximeter) of the *nondominant hand* gently against child's skin.
  Strike the distal joint of the pleximeter with the tip of the middle finger (plexor) of the *dominant* hand (Figure 5-1).
  The blow to the pleximeter should be crisp, and the plexor must be perpendicular.
  The wrist movement is essential to percussion and must be a snapping motion.
  The nail of the plexor should be short.
- Percuss from resonance to dullness.

Guidelines for Auscultation

- Auscultation is the process of listening for body sounds.
- The bell (cupped portion) of the stethoscope is used for low-pitched sounds (e.g., cardiovascular sounds), and the diaphragm (flat portion) is used for high-pitched sounds (e.g., those found in the lung and bowel).
- The diaphragm of the stethoscope is placed firmly against the wall of the body part. The examiner must avoid pressing too firmly, causing the skin to flatten and vibrations to decrease. Resting the heel of the hand on the child will assist in avoiding

Table 5-2 Percussion Sounds

Percussion Sound	Intensity	Pitch	Duration	Quality	Body Region Where Sound Might Be Heard
Tympany	Loud	High	Moderate	Drumlike	Gastric bubble, air-filled intestine (simulate by tapping puffed-out cheeks)
Resonance	Moderate to loud	Low	Long	Hollow	Lungs
Hyperresonance	Very loud	Very low	Long	Booming	Lungs with trapped air, lungs of a young child
Dullness	Soft to moderate	High	Moderate	Thudlike	Liver, fluid-filled space (e.g., stomach)
Flatness	Soft	High	Short	Flat	Muscle

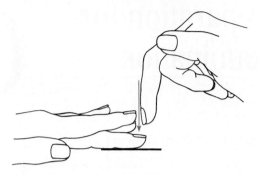

Figure 5-1
Percussion. Note position of fingers.

heavy pressure. Place the bell lightly on the skin surface. If it is placed too firmly, it stretches the skin, causing it to act like a diaphragm.
■ The examiner should practice identifying normal sounds before trying to identify abnormal ones.

Preparation for Examination

6

Preparation of Environment

- Try to perform assessments somewhere other than in the child's "safe areas," when possible. "Safe areas" include the child's bedside or play area.
- Place toys, bright posters, and motifs in the examination room or area to make it look less threatening to the child.
- Limit number of people in room and number of people entering and leaving the area.
- Set air conditioner on low because noisy fans can interfere with auscultation.
- Eliminate drafts from the examining area. Cold is uncomfortable for the infant or child who is minimally dressed and can alter findings. A child who is cold might appear mottled, which can also signify cardiac or respiratory disease.
- Provide privacy for school-age children and adolescents.

Preparation of Equipment

- Ensure that all equipment is readily available.
- Place threatening or strange equipment out of easy view before beginning examination of the young child.
- Warm hands and equipment before starting examination. Equipment can be warmed with hands or with warm water.

Equipment for Physical Assessment

Cotton-tipped applicators
Paper towels and tissue
Disposable pads
Drapes
Gown for child

Gloves
Lubricant
Scale for weight
Measuring board or measuring tray
Tape measure
Stethoscope
Pediatric blood pressure cuff
Sphygmomanometer
Thermometers (rectal and oral)
Tongue depressor
Flashlight
Otoscope
Ophthalmoscope
Eye chart
Percussion hammer
Safety pins
Wristwatch with second hand
Physical assessment forms
Denver II screening test (Denver Developmental Screening Test
  [DDST] or other tests/tools to assess development)

Guidelines for Physical Assessment of Infant or Child

- Perform a general head-to-toe assessment while collecting the health history and the vital signs. General assessment assists in establishing priorities. Note obvious areas of distress. For example, if a child is experiencing pronounced respiratory problems, assessment of this area is a priority.
- Physical assessment is an essential component of nursing care. Children often cannot tell the caregiver what is wrong. The caregiver must be able to assess and to communicate concerns of the child arising from the assessment.
- Some aspects of a complete physical examination might be omitted during the daily assessment, depending on the child's age, health status, and the reason for the health care contact. Examples of assessments that need not always be included are height, head circumference, weight, deep tendon reflexes, and neurologic tests.
- An orderly, systematic, head-to-toe approach to examination might not be possible; it is often necessary to vary the sequence to fit the child. *Flexibility is essential, especially with infants*

and toddlers; however, all necessary aspects of an examination must eventually be covered.

- Often several observations can be made at once because of the size of the area being examined. For example, while checking respiratory rate it is possible to observe the type and quality of respirations, the presence or absence of retractions, the color of the trunk, and whether there is a heave under the nipple.
- Perform as much of the examination as possible with the child in a sitting position, because lying down might cause the child to feel more vulnerable.
- Perform the least distressing and invasive aspects of the examination first. What is distressing for one age group might not be for another age group.
- When possible, use gaming, puppets, and dolls to ease the anxiety of younger children.
- Use a kind, firm, direct approach. Tell the child what to do rather than asking for cooperation. Demonstration assists with compliance.
- Examine painful areas last in sequence.
- Allow children to handle the equipment and provide time for play and anticipatory guidance before beginning the examination.
- Use both hands when possible. One hand or probing fingers might be construed as intrusive.
- Do not leave infants and children unattended on an examining room table.

Age-Related Approaches to Physical Assessment
Infant (1 to 12 Months)

- Approach the infant quietly and gently. Excessive smiling, loud voices, and rapid movements can frighten infants.
- Remove all clothes, except for the diaper of a male child.
- Allow the infant to be held by the parent for as much of the examination as possible.
- Distract the infant with bright toys, peek-a-boo games, and talking.
- Vary the sequence of the assessment with the infant's activity level. If the infant is quiet, obtain the pulse and respiratory rates and auscultate the lungs, heart, and abdomen at the beginning of the examination.
- Obtain the temperature and perform other intrusive examinations (throat, ear, blood pressure) at the end of the examination.

- The parent can assist, if willing, with assessment of the ears and mouth.

Toddler (12 Months to 3 Years)

- Approach the toddler gradually. Keep physical contact to a minimum until the toddler is acquainted with you.
- Allow the toddler to remain near the parent or to be held by the parent whenever possible.
- Introduce and use equipment gradually.
- Allow the child to handle the equipment.
- Use play to approach the child. If the child remains upset and apprehensive, carry out the assessment as quickly as possible.
- Expose the child minimally. Appropriate clothing should be removed immediately before specific assessments, and preferably by the parent.
- Sequencing of the assessment is similar to that recommended for the infant.
- Encourage use of comfort objects such as blankets and stuffed toys.
- Tell the child when the assessment is completed.
- Praise the child for cooperation.

Preschool-Age Child (3 to 6 Years)

- Allow the child to remain close to the parent.
- Allow the child to handle the equipment. Demonstrations of equipment are useful: "You can hear your own heartbeat."
- Expose the child minimally. Allow the child to take off own clothes. *This age group is particularly modest.*
- Use games to gain cooperation: "Let's see how far you can stick out your tongue."
- Tell a story or perform a simple trick to relieve apprehension.

School-Age Child (6 to 12 Years)

- Give the older child the choice about whether the parent is present during assessment.
- Allow the child to remove own clothing.
- Give the child a gown.
- Explain purposes of equipment: "The stethoscope is used to listen to your heartbeat."

Adolescent (12 Years and Older)

- Give the adolescent the choice about whether the parent is present.

- Allow the adolescent to undress in private.
- Give time for the adolescent to regain self-composure before beginning the examination.
- Explain the purposes of the equipment and of assessments.
- Emphasize normalcy of development.
- Give feedback about assessment findings during examination, if appropriate. If in doubt about whether the sharing of particular information is appropriate, check with a more experienced caregiver.
- Make comments about sexual development in a matter-of-fact fashion.

Dimensions of Nutritional Assessment

Nutritional assessment is an important initial step in nursing care and preventive health care. It aids in identifying eating practices, misconceptions, and symptoms that can lead to nutritional problems and eating disorders, including obesity, anorexia nervosa, and bulimia nervosa. Because the nurse often has continued contact with the parents and child, the nurse can often influence dietary practices.

Establishing Weight

Weight measurement is plotted on a growth chart (see Appendix B). Weight usually remains within the same percentile from measurement to measurement. Sudden increases or decreases should be noted. Average weight and height increases for each age are summarized in Table 7-1.

Measurements Related to Weight	Significance of Findings
Weight	
Infants (1 to 12 Months)	
Undress completely (including diaper) and lay on a balance infant scale. Protect the scale surface with a cloth or paper liner and zero the scale with the liner before weighing the infant.	Breastfed infants tend to display slower growth than bottle-fed infants, especially in the second half of the first year.
Place hand lightly above the infant for safety. If precise measurements are required, have a second nurse perform an independent measurement. If there is a	**Clinical Alert** Weight loss or failure to gain weight might be related to dehydration, acute infections, feeding disorders, malabsorption, chronic disease,

Table 7-1   Physical Growth During Infancy and Childhood

Age	Weight	Height
0 to 6 months	Average weekly gain 140-200 gm (5-7 oz) Birth weight doubles by 4-6 months	Average monthly gain 2.5 cm (1 in)
6 to 18 months	Average weekly gain 85-140 gm (3-5 oz) Birth weight triples by 1 year	Average monthly gain 1.25 cm (0.5 in)
18 months to 3 years	Average yearly gain 2-3 kg (4.4-6.6 lb)	Height at 2 years approximately half of adult height
1 to 2 years		Average gain 12 cm (4.8 in)
2 to 3 years		Average gain 6-8 cm (2.4-3.2 in)
3 to 6 years	Average yearly gain 1.8-2.7 kg (4-6 lb)	Yearly gain 6-8 cm (2.4-3.2 in)
6 to 12 years	Average yearly gain 1.8-2.7 kg (4-6 lb)	Yearly gain 5 cm (2 in)
Girl, 10 to 14 years	Average gain 17.5 kg (38.5 lb)	95% of adult height achieved by onset of menarche Average gain 20.5 cm (8.2 in)
Boy, 12 to 16 years	Average gain 23.7 kg (52.1 lb)	95% of adult height achieved by 15 years Average gain 27.5 cm (11 in)

Measurements Related to Weight	Significance of Findings

Infants (1 to 12 Months)—cont'd

difference between the two measurements, a third one should be performed. For reliability in making comparisons, it is important to use the same scale, at the same time of day, for subsequent weight measurements.

neglect, excessive ingestion of apple and pear juices, thyroid disorders, ectodermal dysplasias, diabetes, anorexia nervosa, cocaine use by mother in prenatal period, fetal alcohol syndrome, tuberculosis, or acquired immune deficiency syndrome (AIDS). A loss of 10% on a growth chart is indicative of severe weight loss. Excessive weight gain might be related to chronic renal, pulmonary, or cardiovascular disorders or to endocrine dysfunction. Children who are 120% or more of ideal body weight for height and age are considered obese.

Toddlers and Preschoolers (12 Months to 6 Years)
Undress, except for underpants, and weigh on a standing balance scale. (Children younger than 2 years are weighed on an infant or sitting scale unless they can stand well.)

Older Children (6 Years and Older)
Remove shoes. Weigh clothed, on a standing scale.

Clinical Alert
Marked weight loss is often an initial sign of Type I diabetes. A body weight of less than 85% of the expected norm in adolescents might signal anorexia nervosa, especially if bradycardia, cold intolerance, dry skin, brittle nails, body distortion, and

Measurements Related to Weight	Significance of Findings

Older Children (6 Years and Older)—cont'd

| | preoccupation with food are present. Weight loss can also accompany amphetamine use or changes in living conditions (e.g., homelessness). |

BMI

Body mass index (BMI) indicates body composition and is a valuable indicator of the degree of overweight or obesity and of underweight. BMI takes into account the child's height and weight and can be calculated through the following formula:

$$\frac{\text{weight in kilograms}}{(\text{height in meters})^2}$$

See Appendix B for BMI age charts.

Skinfold Thickness

Skinfold thickness is a more reliable indicator of body fat than weight because the majority of fat is stored in subcutaneous tissues. Measurements, as indicators of body fat, must be treated cautiously as findings will vary with experience and familiarity of assessor with technique. To measure skinfold thickness, use calipers such as Lange calipers. The most common sites for measurement are triceps and subscapular regions. For triceps, have

Clinical Alert

Obesity might be indicated by skinfold thickness greater than or equal to 85% for triceps measurement (see Appendix B).

Measurements Related to Weight	Significance of Findings

Skinfold Thickness—cont'd

child flex arm 90 degrees at elbow and mark midpoint between acromion and olecranon on the posterior aspect of the arm. *Gently* grasp fold of child's skin 1 cm (0.4 inch) above this midpoint. Gently pull fold away from muscle and continuing to hold, place caliper jaws over midpoint. Estimate reading to nearest 1.0 mm, 2 to 3 seconds after applying pressure. Take measurements until two agree within 1 mm.

Establishing Height

Measurement of Height/Length	Significance of Findings

Infants/Toddlers (1 to 24 Months)

Lay infant flat. Have parent hold infant's head as the infant's legs are extended and pushed *gently* toward the table. Measure the distance between marks made indicating heel tips (with toes pointing toward the deficiency, ceiling) and vertex of head. *Do not use a cloth tape* for measurement because it can stretch. If using a measuring board or tray, align the infant's head against the top bar and ask the parent to secure the infant's head there. Straighten the infant's body and, while holding the feet in a vertical position, bring the footboard snugly up against the bottoms of the feet.

Clinical Alert

Although short stature is usually genetically predetermined, it can also indicate chronic heart or renal disease, growth hormone deficiency, malnutrition, Kearns-Sayre syndrome, Turner's syndrome, dwarfism, methadone exposure, or fetal alcohol syndrome.

Measurement of Height/Length	Significance of Findings

Infants/Toddlers (1 to 24 Months)—cont'd

Use the same technique to obtain subsequent height measurements.

Children (24 Months and Older)

Have child, in stocking feet or bare feet, stand straight on a standard scale. Measure with the attached marker, to the nearest 0.1 cm (0.03 inch).

If a scale with a measuring bar is not available or if a child is afraid of standing on the scale's base, have the child stand erect against a wall. Place a flat object, such as a clipboard, on the child's head, at a right angle to the wall. Read the height at the point where the flat object touches the measuring tape or the wall-mounted unit (stadiometer).

Height is usually less in the afternoon than in the morning. Correct for this tendency by placing slight upward pressure under the jaw.

Assessment of Eating Practices

Assessment of nutrition, feeding, and eating practices requires sensitivity on the part of the nurse. Eating practices are highly personal, as well as cultural, and can be more accurately assessed after a rapport has been established. Guilt, apprehension, and the parent's desire to give the "right" responses can alter the accuracy of the assessment. Table 7-2 lists typical eating habits for various age groups. Table 7-3 lists assessment findings that are associated with anorexia nervosa and bulimia nervosa, and Table 7-4 describes physical assessments and findings associated with nutrition.

General Assessment

- Is your child on a special diet?
- Are there any suspected or known food allergies?

- Describe your child's typical intake over 24 hours (what child ate for each meal and between meals).
- Has your child lost or gained weight recently?
- Does your family eat together?
- Do any cultural, ethnic, or religious influences affect your child's diet? How?
- Do you have any concerns?

Assessment of Nutrition and Feeding Practices for Infants

- How much weight did you (mother) gain during pregnancy?
- What was your infant's birth weight? When did it double? Triple?
- What vitamin supplements does your infant receive?
- Do you give your infant extra fluids such as juice or water?
- How often does your infant wake at night? What kinds of things do you do to comfort at night (e.g., introduction of solid or table foods earlier than anticipated to help the infant sleep through the night)?
- At what age did you start cereals, vegetables, fruits, meat (or other sources of proteins), table foods, and finger foods?
- Does your infant spit up frequently? What are his or her stools like?
- Does your infant have any problems with feeding (e.g., lethargy, poor sucking, regurgitation, colic, irritability, rash, diarrhea)?
- Breastfed infants:
    How long does your infant feed at one time?
    Do you alternate breasts?
    How do you recognize that your infant is hungry? Full?
    Describe your infant's elimination and sleeping patterns.
    Describe your usual daily diet.
    Do you have concerns related to breastfeeding?
- Formula-fed infants:
    What type of formula is your infant taking?
    How do you prepare the formula?
    What type of bottle does your infant take?
    How many ounces (ml) of formula does your infant drink per day?
    Do you prop or hold your infant while feeding?
    Do you have concerns related to bottle feeding?

Assessment of Nutrition and Eating Practices of Toddlers and Children

- What foods does your child prefer? Dislike?
- Does the child snack? If so, when? What foods are given as snacks? When are sweet foods eaten? Are foods used as rewards (e.g., "If you eat your vegetables, you can have dessert")?
- What assistance does your child require with eating?
- What kinds of activities does your child enjoy? How many hours of television, video games, or computer usage does your child enjoy per day?

Assessment of Nutrition and Eating Practices of Adolescents

- What foods do you prefer? Dislike?
- What foods do you choose for a snack?
- Are you satisfied with the quantity and kinds of food you eat?
- Are you content with your weight? If not, have you tried to change your food intake? In what ways? Do you use skipping meals, diet pills, laxatives, or diuretics to lose weight? Have you ever eaten what others would regard as an unusually large amount of food? Have you ever made yourself vomit to get rid of food eaten?
- Have you started your menstrual periods (girls)? Are you taking an oral contraceptive?
- Are you active in sports or fitness activities? If so, are there any weight or food requirements (e.g., high protein intake, increased calories, weight restrictions or increases) associated with these activities?
- What exercise regimens do you follow?

Assessment of Physical Signs of Nutrition or Malnutrition

Many of the assessments related to nutritional status can be combined with other areas of the physical assessment. Table 7-4 outlines the head-to-toe observations that provide information about a child's nutritional status.

Related Nursing Diagnoses

Ineffective breastfeeding: related to knowledge deficit, nonsupportive partner, previous breast surgery, supplemental feeding, poor infant sucking reflex, maternal anxiety, interruption in breastfeeding, infant anomaly.

Ineffective infant feeding pattern: related to prematurity, anatomic abnormality, neurologic impairment.

Effective breastfeeding: related to gestational age greater than 34 weeks, normal oral structure, maternal confidence, basic breastfeeding knowledge, normal breast structure.

Altered nutrition, more than body requirements: related to early introduction of solids, reported or observed obesity in one or both parents, rapid transition across growth percentiles, use of food as reward or comfort measure, excessive intake.

Altered nutrition, less than body requirements: related to biologic, psychologic, or economic factors.

Risk for altered development: related to failure to thrive, inadequate nutrition.

Risk for altered growth: related to malnutrition, prematurity, maladaptive feeding behaviors, anorexia, insatiable appetite.

Altered parenting: related to lack of knowledge about child maintenance, unrealistic expectations for child, lack of knowledge about development, inability to recognize infant cues, illness.

Body image disturbance: related to psychosocial or biophysical factors, developmental changes.

Altered dentition: related to nutritional deficits, dietary habits, chronic vomiting.

Diarrhea: related to laxative abuse, malabsorption.

Constipation: related to insufficient fluid intake, insufficient fiber intake, poor eating habits, dehydration.

Perceived constipation: related to cultural or family beliefs, faulty appraisal.

Disorganized infant behavior: related to cue misreading, cue knowledge deficit, malnutrition.

Table 7-2 Eating Habits and Concerns Common to Various Age Groups

Age Group	Eating Practices	Concerns Arising from Eating Practices
Infants/toddlers (1 to 12 months)	Formula or breast milk forms major part of diet for first 6 months and is generally recommended until 1 year. Solid foods assume greater importance in second 6 months of life. By 1 year, infant is able to eat all solid foods unless food intolerance develops. White grape juice is a healthy form of juice. Juice intake should be limited to no more than 150 ml per day in infants.	Mothers might feed child in accordance with practices followed in their own upbringing. Early introduction of solid foods (before 5 or 6 months) can contribute to allergies. Sensitivity to cow's milk might be suggested by colic, sleeplessness, diarrhea, abdominal pain, chronic nasal discharge, recurrent respiratory ailments, eczema, pallor, or excessive crying. Colic, regurgitation, diarrhea, constipation, bottle mouth syndrome, and rashes are common concerns associated with infant feeding. Yellowish skin coloration might accompany persistent feeding of carrots. Excess milk intake in later infancy might lead to milk anemia.

| Toddlers/preschool-age children (12 months to 6 years) | Appetites tend to be erratic because of sporadic energy needs. Appetites of toddlers and preschoolers are smaller than those of infants because of slowed growth. Toddlers and preschoolers have definite likes and dislikes. Likes include foods such as yogurt, fruit drinks, fruit breads, and cookies that are easy to eat and to handle. Dislikes include casseroles, liver, and cooked vegetables. Food is often consumed "on the go." Children might go on "food jags," in which one food is preferred for a few days. | Excessive ingestion of pear and apple juices can be associated with failure to thrive, tooth decay, diarrhea, and obesity. Some children snack their way through the day and rarely consume a regular meal. Excessive intake of drinks (e.g., milk, juices, water, carbonated beverages) might result in reduced appetite for other foods. Mealtimes might become a battle between parents and toddlers over types and amounts of food eaten. Parents might express concern over toddlers' or preschoolers' diminished appetite. 80% of children with both parents obese are likely to be obese. It is recommended that children by 2 years of age receive baseline screening for cardiovascular |

Continued

Table 7-2 Eating Habits and Concerns Common to Various Age Groups—cont'd

Age Group	Eating Practices	Concerns Arising from Eating Practices
Toddlers/preschool-age children (12 months to 6 years)—cont'd	Variety is desirable, but not necessary as long as the child eats from all food groups during the course of a day.	disease factors such as parental obesity, age and weight, and blood pressure measurements.
School-age children (6 to 12 years)	Children generally have a good appetite and like variety. Plain foods still preferred. Increasing numbers of activities compete with mealtimes. Television and peers influence food choices.	Parents might express concern over table manners. A child is considered overweight when weight is equal to or exceeds the 85th percentile.
Adolescents (12 years and older)	Food habits include skipping meals (especially breakfast), consuming carbonated drinks and fast foods, snacking, and unusual food choices.	Alcohol might form a substantial portion of caloric intake. Preoccupation with food and feelings of guilt might be indicative of eating

Adolescents consume increasingly larger amounts of alcohol at younger ages.

Adolescent girls frequently are calorie conscious and might diet, thus severely restricting their calcium intake.

disorders. Anorexia nervosa and bulimia nervosa are serious disorders related to an obsession with losing weight (see Table 7-3 for assessment findings associated with common eating disorders).

Low calcium intake might place adolescent females at risk for osteoporosis.

Table 7-3 Assessment Findings Associated with Anorexia Nervosa and Bulimia Nervosa

Assessment Dimension	Anorexia Nervosa	Bulimia Nervosa
Personality	Introverted Avoids intimacy	Might be introverted
Behavioral and emotional functioning	Perfectionistic Obsessive compulsive High achieving Ultra responsible and well-behaved Marked preoccupation with food Might engage in compulsive exercising Denies existence of problem	Might engage in risky behaviors (e.g., shoplifting, alcohol abuse) Might lack impulse control Satiety control problematic; engages in binge eating Self-induced vomiting, fasting (purging type of bulimia), and misuse of laxatives, diuretics, enemas Fasting and excessive exercise (nonpurging type) Experiences frustration, fear, depression Is aware that eating pattern is abnormal
Family factors	Mothers might be over-involved, controlling, and overprotective Fathers might be emotionally distant Families often emotionally inexpressive and rigid	Parents might be disengaged and emotionally unavailable Might be family history of substance abuse, eating disorders, affective disorders

School performance	High achievement	Might aspire to athletic involvements or careers that emphasize low weight or weight control
Weight	Less than 85% of what is normally expected	Might be normal weight or even slightly above normal weight
Gender	Females	Primarily affects females
	Males make up approximately 10% of cases; half of these are homosexual or bisexual	Affected males tend to have history of involvement in sports activities
Clinical findings	Emaciation	Might have history of early menarche and weight gain
	Cold intolerance	Potassium depletion (especially if diuretics used), which can result in fatigue, abnormal reflexes, and cardiac arrhythmias
	Lethargy	
	Dryness of skin	Cramping, steatorrhea, gastrointestinal bleeding, and constipation associated with laxative use and malabsorption of fat, protein, and calories
	Bradycardia	
	Constipation	
	Amenorrhea (absence of 3 consecutive menstrual cycles)	Erosion of tooth enamel and increased dental caries (related to vomiting)
	Abdominal pain	Chronic sore throat and difficulty swallowing related to frequent vomiting
	Yellowing of skin	Spontaneous bleeding in eye
	Peripheral edema	
	Enlargement of salivary glands	

Table 7-4   Physical Assessment of Nutrition

Body Area	Signs of Adequate/Appropriate Nutrition	Signs of Inadequate/Inappropriate Nutrition	Possible Causes of Inadequate/Inappropriate Nutrition
General growth	Height, weight, head circumference within 5th and 95th percentiles	Height, weight, head circumference below or above 5th and 95th percentiles	Protein, fats, vitamin A, niacin, calcium, iodine, manganese, zinc deficiency/excess
	Sexual development age appropriate	Delayed sexual maturation	Less than expected growth possibly related to disease (especially endocrine dysfunction) or to genetic endowment
			Vitamin A or D excess
Skin	Elastic, firm, slightly dry; no lesions, rashes, hyperpigmentation	Dryness	Vitamin A deficiency
			Essential and unsaturated fatty acid deficiency
		Swollen red pigmentation (pellagrous dermatosis)	Niacin deficiency
		Hyperpigmentation	Vitamin B_{12}, folic acid, niacin deficiency
		Edema	Protein deficiency or sodium excess
		Poor skin turgor	Water, sodium deficiency

Hair	Shiny, firm, elastic	Petechiae	Ascorbic acid deficiency
		Delayed wound healing	Vitamin C deficiency
		Decreased subcutaneous tissue	Prolonged caloric deficiency
		Pallor	Iron, vitamin B_{12} or C, folic acid, pyridoxine deficiency
		Dull, dry, thin, brittle, sparse, easily plucked	Protein, caloric deficiency
		Alopecia	Protein, caloric, or zinc deficiency
Head	Head evenly molded, with occipital prominence; facial features symmetric	Skull flattened, frontal bones prominent	Vitamin D deficiency
	Sutures fused by 12 to 18 months	Suture fusion delayed	Vitamin D deficiency
		Hard, tender lumps in occipital region	Vitamin A excess
		Headache	Thiamine excess
Neck	Thyroid gland not obvious to inspection, palpable in midline	Thyroid gland enlarged, obvious to inspection	Iodine deficiency

Continued

Table 7-4   Physical Assessment of Nutrition—cont'd

Body Area	Signs of Adequate/Appropriate Nutrition	Signs of Inadequate/ Inappropriate Nutrition	Possible Causes of Inadequate/Inappropriate Nutrition
Eyes	Clear, bright, shiny	Dull, soft cornea; white or gray spots on cornea (Bitot's spots)	Vitamin A deficiency
	Membranes pink and moist	Pale membranes	Iron deficiency
		Burning, itching, photophobia	Riboflavin deficiency
	Night vision adequate	Night blindness	Vitamin A deficiency
		Redness, fissuring at corners of eyes	Riboflavin, niacin deficiency
Nose	Smooth, intact nasal angle	Cracks, irritation at nasal angle	Niacin deficiency, vitamin A excess
Lips	Smooth, moist, no edema	Angular fissures, redness, and edema	Riboflavin deficiency, vitamin A excess
Tongue	Deep pink, papillae visible, moist, taste sensation, no edema	Paleness	Iron deficiency
		Red, swollen, raw	Folic acid, niacin, vitamin B or B_{12} deficiency
		Magenta coloration	Riboflavin deficiency
		Diminished taste	Zinc deficiency

Gums	Firm, coral color	Spongy, bleed easily, receding	Ascorbic acid deficiency
Teeth	White, smooth, free of spots or pits	Mottled enamel, brown spots, pits	Fluoride excess, or discoloration from antibiotics
		Defective enamel	Vitamin A, C, or D, or calcium or phosphorus deficiency
		Caries	Carbohydrate excess, poor hygiene
Cardiovascular system	Pulse and blood pressure within normal limits for age	Palpitations	Thiamine deficiency
		Rapid pulse	Potassium deficiency
		Arrhythmia	Niacin, potassium excess; magnesium, potassium deficiency
		High blood pressure	Sodium excess
		Decreased blood pressure	Thiamine deficiency
Gastrointestinal system	Bowel habits normal for age	Constipation	Calcium excess, overrigid toilet training, inadequate intake of high-fiber foods or fluids
		Diarrhea	Niacin deficiency; vitamin C excess; high consumption of fresh fruit, other high-fiber foods, excessive consumption of juices

Continued

Table 7-4 Physical Assessment of Nutrition—cont'd

Body Area	Signs of Adequate/Appropriate Nutrition	Signs of Inadequate/Inappropriate Nutrition	Possible Causes of Inadequate/Inappropriate Nutrition
Musculoskeletal system	Muscles firm and well developed, joints flexible and pain free, extremities symmetric and straight, spinal nerves normal	Muscles atrophied, dependent edema	Protein, caloric deficiency
		Knock-knee, bowleg, epiphyseal enlargement	Vitamin D deficiency; disease processes
		Bleeding into joints, pain	Vitamin C deficiency
		Beading on ribs	Vitamins C and D deficiency
Neurologic system	Behavior alert and responsive, intact muscle innervation	Listlessness, irritability, lethargy	Thiamine, niacin, pyridoxine, iron, protein, caloric deficiency
		Tetany	Magnesium deficiency
		Convulsions	Thiamine, pyridoxine, vitamin D, calcium deficiency, phosphorus excess
		Unsteadiness, numbness in hands and feet	Pyridoxine excess
		Diminished reflexes	Thiamine deficiency

MEASUREMENT
OF VITAL SIGNS

II

Body Temperature, Pulse, and Respirations

8

Nursing fundamentals textbooks provide comprehensive discussions of measurement of vital signs. Only significant pediatric variations in the measurement of body temperature, pulse, and respirations are presented here.

Measurement of Body Temperature

Rationale

Environmental factors and relatively minor infections can produce a much higher temperature in infants and young children than would be expected in older children and adults. In most cases, an elevated temperature is the result of fever and is one of the most common manifestations of illness in young children. In very young infants, fever might be one of the few signs of an underlying disorder. In toddlers, febrile convulsions can parallel fever and are of particular concern. Ascertaining the absence or presence of fever and determining the cause of fever are important in planning nursing care. Body temperature should be measured on admission to the health care facility, before and after surgery or invasive diagnostic procedures, during the course of an unidentified infection, after fever-reduction measures have been taken, and any time that an infant or child looks flushed, feels warm, is lethargic, looks "glassy-eyed," or has increased pulse and respirations.

Anatomy and Physiology

Temperature is regulated from within the hypothalamus. During an infection, the body's normal set point is elevated, and the hypothalamus increases heat production until the body's core temperature is consistent with this new set point. Shivering and vasoconstriction during the chill phase help the body reach the new set point by conserving and generating heat.

The temperature-regulating mechanisms in infants and young children are not well developed, and dramatic fluctuations can occur. A young child's temperature can vary as much as 1.6° C (3° F) in a day. Infants and children are much more affected by environmental factors such as heat because of the immaturity of their thermoregulatory controls. Fluctuations are less apparent as these temperature-regulating mechanisms mature.

The control of body heat loss improves with age. The ability of muscles to shiver increases with maturity, and the child accumulates greater amounts of adipose tissue necessary for insulation against heat loss. Heat production decreases with age. The infant produces relatively more heat per unit of body weight than older children do, as reflected by the infant's higher average body temperature (Table 8-1). A variety of other factors also affect the body temperature of the child (Table 8-2).

Preparation

Ask the parent or child if the child has been febrile, and if so, when the fever began. Inquire whether the onset was abrupt or gradual and whether other symptoms or localizing signs accompany the fever. Most diseases have no particular fever pattern. However, although the rapidity of temperature elevation and response to antipyretics are not indicative of the severity of the disease, knowing the pattern of the fever (onset, magnitude, frequency, recurrence, defervescence or decrease) can be helpful, especially if there are no localizing signs with the fever (Table 8-3).

Table 8-1   **Body Temperature in Well Children**

	Temperature in Degrees	
Age	Celsius	Fahrenheit
3 mo	37.4	99.4
1 yr	37.6	99.7
3 yr	37.2	99.0
5 yr	37.0	98.6
7 yr	36.8	98.3
9 yr	36.7	98.1
13 yr	36.6	97.8

Modified from Lowrey GH: *Growth and development of children,* ed 8, St Louis, 1986, Mosby.

Table 8-2   Factors Influencing Body Temperature

Factor	Effect
Active exercise	Might temporarily raise temperature
Stress, crying	Raises body temperature
Diurnal variation	Body temperature is lowest between 0100 and 0400 hours (1:00 and 4:00 AM), highest between 1600 and 1800 hours (4:00 and 6:00 PM)
Environment, including clothing, swaddling, and nesting	Body temperature can vary with room temperature, amount and type of clothing
Pharmacologic agents (antipyretics, muscle relaxants, vasodilating anesthetic agents)	Decrease body temperature

Establish whether the parent has administered fever-reduction measures, and if so, how recently. Ask whether the child has had recent surgery, been in contact with persons with infectious or communicable diseases, or been immunized recently. If the child is a young infant, ask whether the infant has been anorexic or irritable (more obvious signs of fever such as shivering and diaphoresis are not usually seen in the young infant). If the child is 5 years or older, assess the child's ability to understand and to follow directions because oral temperature measurement might be desirable. If rectal temperature measurement is selected, the procedure might be left until near the end of the health assessment because preschoolers, in particular, find it intrusive.

Guidelines for Measurement of Body Temperature

- Select the site for temperature measurement based on the child's age and condition (Table 8-4), institutional policy, and what might be least traumatic for the child. The tympanic route, for example, has a high level of acceptability by children.
- Standard glass thermometers are not recommended for use because of risk of breakage and inhalation of toxic vapors.

Text continued on p. 103

Table 8-3   Fever Patterns for Selected Etiologies

Fever Pattern	Associated Etiologies	Additional Characteristics of Fever
Single spike: refers to a single increase or spike, usually within a 12-hour period or less	Transfusion of blood or blood products	
Double quotient: fever in which there are two distinct peaks in a day	Miliary tuberculosis	Fever with general symptoms such as weight loss, malaise, weakness, anemia, pallor, diminished breath sounds, crackles
Hectic: involves wide swings in fever, usually with chills and sweating	Bacterial pneumonia	Fever usually quite high, chills, abrupt onset, anorexia, headache, cough, meningeal symptoms
Intermittent: fever returns to normal at least once during the day	Bacterial (infective) endocarditis	Low-grade fever with nonspecific symptoms such as malaise, myalgia, headache, diaphoresis, weight loss
	Hodgkin's disease	Low-grade fever with enlargement of supra-clavicular or cervical nodes, weight loss, night sweats, pruritus, anorexia, nausea
Remittent: fever rises at least 0.6° C (1.0° F) in a 24-hour period and abates but does not return to normal	Viral upper respiratory tract infections	Fever with myalgia, malaise, headache, coryza; slow defervescence
Continuous or sustained: little or no variation in temperature	Roseola	Fever above 39° C (102° F) for 3 to 4 days without localizing signs

Scarlet fever	High fever with vomiting, headache, chills, malaise, abdominal pain in prodromal stage
Urinary tract infection (children younger than 5 years)	Fever of 39° C (102° F) or higher for 2 days or more, with no respiratory symptoms Diarrhea, vomiting, irritability, poor feeding, foul-smelling urine
Severe acute respiratory syndrome (SARS)	Fever at or above 38.5° C (101.5° F), cough, malaise, chills or rigor, coryza (younger than 12 years), headache, sputum, myalgia, sore throat, no crackles or wheezing
Acute rheumatic fever	Low-grade fever with late afternoon spike, polyarthritis, chorea, subcutaneous nodules, erythema marginatum, carditis
Infectious mononucleosis	Fever with malaise, sore throat, lymphadenopathy, splenomegaly that can persist for months
Noninfectious origin (neoplastic, trauma, heat stroke, drug fever) HIV	

Relapsing: recurrent over days and weeks; fever occurs at various intervals after initial episode

Extreme hyperthermia: fever above 41° C (106° F)

Table 8-4   Guidelines for Site Selection for Body Temperature Measurement

Site	Age Group	Special Considerations
Axilla	All age groups, but particularly preschoolers, who tend to fear invasive procedures. Can be used for children for whom the oral route is not possible and for those who would not tolerate the rectal route.	Measures shell temperature. Can be taken using standard glass (in rare use), electronic, digital, chemical dot, or infrared thermometers. Although some sources recommend the monitor mode for electronic thermometers, some evidence also suggests that the predictive mode be used for full-term infants. Wearable chemical dot thermometers enable continuous reading for as long as 48 hours (must be replaced after 48 hours). Reading might be increased for axillary route. Might be contraindicated when accuracy is especially critical or in the early stages of a fever when the axilla might not be sensitive to early changes. Accuracy can be affected by increased peripheral circulation.
Rectal	All age groups. Some sources recommend use in children older than 2 years because	Measures core temperature. Can be taken using standard glass (in rare use),

	of risks of breakage and perforation. Some evidence suggests that the rectal route is the most reliable route for measurement of temperature in infants and children, although others recommend its use only when no other route is appropriate (e.g., children who are too young or too agitated to cooperate or follow directions, children who have had oral or axillary surgery).	electronic, or chemical dot devices. Do not force insertion of thermometer. Do not use if child has diarrhea or rectal irritation, has had anal surgery, has had chemotherapy affecting the mucosa, or if it is possible to use oral or axillary sites. Presence of stool can decrease accuracy (reading might be increased).
Oral	Cooperative 5- and 6-year-old children, school-age children, and adolescents.	Reflects shell temperature (but might be less accurate in assessment of core temperature than rectal route). Can be taken using standard glass (rarely used), electronic, digital, or chemical dot thermometry. Do not use if child is uncooperative or unable to follow directions, is comatose, is seizure prone, has had oral surgery, mouth breathes, or is receiving oxygen therapy. Electronic thermometry produces acceptable results for the child who keeps mouth open during measurement.

Continued

Table 8-4   Guidelines for Site Selection for Body Temperature Measurement—cont'd

Site	Age Group	Special Considerations
Tympanic	All ages, although several sources suggest that the route is insufficiently sensitive and reliable for the detection of fever in children younger than 3 years and possibly even for children younger than 6 years.	Considered to measure core temperature. Easy to use, noninvasive, and quick for young children. Might be contraindicated in young children and infants because of their small ear canals. In children 3 years and younger, pull the ear down and back during temperature measurement (for ear-based temperature sensor). Tug not necessary for ear sensor type, which measures heat radiating from ear canal opening. For this type, insert hemispheric probe into opening. Might be advisable to select another method if precise measurements are necessary or if clinical symptoms suggest fever in the presence of a normal or lower than expected tympanic measurement.
Skin	All ages	Calibrated to oral or rectal routes. Measured using plastic strip thermometer. Variable accuracy. Beneficial for screening and for at-home use.

Temperature can be taken using electronic, tympanic, digital, and chemical indicator thermometers, as well as skin plastic strips (although these are recommended primarily for screening and at-home use).

- Position the child appropriately.

  For axillary temperature, hold the child quietly on your lap. Diversions, such as reading, are useful. Hold the child's arm firmly against the side.

  For oral temperature, have the child sit or lie quietly.

  For rectal temperature, place younger infants in a side-lying position. Large infants and children can be placed in prone or side-lying positions. If the parent is available, the child can wrap arms around the parent's neck and legs around the parent's waist or be placed prone across the parent's lap.

- Always record the route by which the temperature was taken, because the differences between routes cannot be assumed as constant. If possible, consistently use one route, because studies suggest variable differences among the routes. Normal peripheral temperature is usually considered to be 37° C (98.6° F).

- In addition to measurement of body temperature, all children should be assessed for:

  Signs and symptoms of dehydration, including sunken anterior fontanel (infants younger than 18 months), decreased or absent tearing (children older than 6 weeks), sunken eye orbits, dry or sticky mucous membranes, dry body creases, and poor skin turgor (tenting when pinched)

  Flushed appearance

  Chills, as evidenced by shivering and piloerection

  Restlessness

  Lethargy

  Skin mottling

  Increased pulse, respiratory rates, and blood pressure

  Twitching

  Seizure activity

  Young children might interpret "taking your temperature" as taking something away. Saying "let's see how warm you are" can avoid this interpretation.

Measurement of Pulse

Rationale

The measurement of pulse is a routine part of hospital procedure but should not be underestimated as an easily accessible indicator of the status of the cardiovascular system. Disorders of the cardiovascular system, the effects of fever, and the effects of drug therapies can be monitored through assessment of pulse. The pulse should be routinely monitored during disease processes, during fever, before and after surgery, and whenever a child's condition deteriorates. A decreased pulse rate is more ominous than tachycardia in a young child following trauma.

Anatomy and Physiology

Approximately 8.5% of the body weight in the neonate is blood volume, compared with 7% to 7.5% in the older child and adult. The heart size increases as the child grows, with a resultant decrease in heart rate. Variations in heart rate are much more dramatic in the child than in the adult. Table 8-5 lists normal pulse rates; Table 8-6, influences on pulse rate; and Table 8-7, deviations from normal pulse patterns.

Preparation

Ask the parent or child about a family history of arrhythmias, atherosclerosis, or myocardial infarction. Ask if the child has known heart disease or has experienced or is experiencing palpitations or arrhythmias. Determine if fever or pain is present, and ask if the child has recently taken medications or substances that might be expected to affect pulse rate.

Table 8-5   Pulse Rates in Children at Rest

Age	Resting (Awake)	Resting (Asleep)	Exercise and Fever
Birth	100-180	80-160	Up to 220
1-3 mo	100-220	80-180	Up to 220
3 mo to 2 yr	80-150	70-120	Up to 200
2 -10 yr	70-110	60-100	Up to 180
10 yr to adult	55-90	50-90	Up to 180

From Hockenberry MJ et al: *Wong's nursing care of infants and children*, ed 7, St Louis, 2003, Mosby.

Table 8-6   Influences on Pulse Rate

Influence	Effect
Medications	Aminophylline, racemic epinephrine, atropine sulfate increase pulse rate. Digoxin decreases pulse rate.
Activity	Activity increases pulse rate. Sustained, regular exercise eventually decreases rate. Pulse varies if a child is sleeping, increasing during inspiration and decreasing during expiration (sinus arrhythmia). Crying and feeding increase pulse rate in an infant.
Fever	Increases pulse rate by about 10 to 15 beats per degree (in Celsius) temperature increase. High fever accompanied by low pulse and respiratory rates can signal a drug reaction. Low fever with high pulse and respiratory rates can signal septic shock. Tachypnea in children younger than 2 years, with a fever, might be the most sensitive predictor of pneumonia.
Apprehension, acute pain	Increases pulse rate.
Hemorrhage	Increases pulse rate.
Increased intra-cranial pressure	Decreases pulse rate.
Respiratory distress	Pulse rate increases in early distress and decreases in late distress.

Guidelines for Measurement of Pulse

- Measure the pulse when the infant or child is quiet or, preferably, asleep. Because of lability of the pulse, carefully document the child's activity or anxiety level when the pulse is recorded.
- Select the appropriate site. The apical pulse is measured in children younger than 2 years of age because the radial pulse is difficult to locate. The apical pulse should be measured at any age when the radial pulse is difficult to locate, when cardiac disease has been identified, or when the radial pulse is irregular.

Table 8-7 Deviations from Normal Pulse Patterns

Pulse	Characteristics and Significance
Bradycardia	Slowed pulse rate.
Tachycardia	Increased pulse rate. In the absence of apprehension, crying, increased activity, or fever, tachycardia can indicate cardiac disease.
Sinus arrhythmia	Pulse rate increases during inspiration, decreases during expiration. Sinus arrhythmia is a normal variation in children, especially during sleep.
Alternating pulse (pulsus alternans)	Alteration of weak and strong beats. Might indicate heart failure.
Bigeminal pulse	Coupled beats related to premature beats.
Paradoxical pulse	Strength of pulse diminishes with inspiration.
Thready pulse	Weak, rapid pulse. Might be indicative of shock. Pulse is difficult to palpate; seems to appear and disappear.
Corrigan's pulse (water-hammer pulse)	Forceful, jerky beat caused by wide variation in pulse pressure.

Radial, femoral, and popliteal pulses should be compared at least once in the young child to detect circulatory impairment.
- Listen for the apical pulse at the point of maximal impulse (PMI). This will be found in the *fourth intercostal space* in children *younger than 7 years*. In children *older than 7 years* the apical pulse will be found in the *fifth interspace* and will be more lateral.
- Take radial and apical pulses for 1 full minute because of possible alterations in rhythm. If frequent apical pulses are required, use shorter counting times.
- Pulses can be graded (Table 8-8).

Measurement of Respirations
Rationale

Assessment of respiration involves external assessment of ventilation. Because the quality and rate of respirations can be affected by

Table 8-8   Grading of Pulses

Grade	Meaning
0	Not palpable.
+1	Thready, weak. Difficult to find. Easily obliterated.
+2	Difficult to find. Pressure might obliterate.
+3	Easy to find. Difficult to obliterate (normal).
+4	Bounding, strong. Cannot be obliterated.

disorders in every body system, the character of respirations must be carefully assessed and reported.

Anatomy and Physiology

Infants and young children inhale a relatively small amount of air and exhale a relatively large amount of oxygen. Young children and infants have fewer alveoli and therefore less alveolar surface through which gas exchange can occur. These factors, together with a higher metabolic rate, are influential in increasing respiratory rates in infants and children. Table 8-9 outlines normal respiratory rates, and Table 8-10 outlines influences on respiratory rates.

Preparation

Ask the parent or child about the use of medications; whether there is difficulty breathing, or apnea (infants); and about the presence of respiratory infections or fever. Inquire about a family history of cardiac or respiratory disorders.

Guidelines for Measurement of Respirations

■ Assess the infant's or child's respirations before beginning more intrusive procedures. If the infant or child is already crying, wait for calmer behavior before assessing respiratory rates.

Table 8-9   Variations in Respiration with Age

Age	Rate (breaths/min)	Average
1 yr	20-40	30
3 yr	20-30	25
6 yr	16-22	19
10 yr	16-20	18
Adult	12-20	16

Modified from Zator Estes ME: *Health assessment & physical examination*, ed 2, New York, 2002, Delmar Learning.

Table 8-10   Influences on Respiration

Influencing Factor	Effect
Age	Respiratory rate decreases as the child grows older.
	The rate tends to increase dramatically in infants and young children relative to anxiety, crying, fever, disease.
	The rhythm is irregular in young infants, who experience sharp increases in rate and apneic spells. (Apneic spells of 15-20 seconds or longer are considered pathologic.)
Medications	Narcotic analgesics decrease respiratory rate. Xanthine derivatives can cause an increase in rate.
Position	Slumping impedes ventilatory movements.
Fever	Respirations increase in rate and depth.
Increased activity	Respirations increase in rate or depth.
Anxiety or fear	Respirations increase in rate and depth.
Pathologic states	Respiratory rate, rhythm, and depth alter as a result of cerebral trauma, respiratory disorders, hemorrhage, anemia, meningitis, cardiac disorders, infectious disorders, and tetanus.
Pain	Respiratory rate can decrease or increase.

■ Avoid letting the child know that respirations are being counted; self-consciousness can alter the respiratory rate and depth. Assess the respirations when counting the pulse or performing an assessment of the thorax and lungs. Table 8-11 gives a description of respiratory rhythms.

■ When assessing the respirations of *infants and younger children,* the nurse places fingers or a hand just below the child's xiphoid process so that the inspiratory rises can be felt. Alternatively, the respirations can be assessed by listening to breath sounds through the stethoscope. In infants, respirations can also be assessed by observing abdominal movements because respirations are diaphragmatic.

Table 8-11   Altered Respiratory Patterns

Pattern	Description
Dyspnea	Difficult or labored breathing; indicated by presence of retractions.
Bradypnea	Abnormally slow rate of breathing; rhythm regular.
Tachypnea	Abnormally fast rate of breathing.
Hyperpnea	Rapid, deep respirations.
Apnea	Absence of respirations.
Cheyne-Stokes respiration (periodic breathing)	Periods of deep, rapid breathing alternating with periods of apnea. Commonly seen in infants, and can be seen normally in children during deep sleep. Abnormal causes include drug-induced depression and brain damage.
Kussmaul's respiration	Abnormally deep breathing. Can be rapid, normal, or slow. Commonly associated with metabolic acidosis.
Biot's respiration (ataxic breathing)	Unpredictable, irregular breathing. Seen with lower brain damage and respiratory depression.

- Observe a complete respiratory cycle (inspiration plus expiration).
   Count respirations for *1 full minute.* Respirations of infants and
   young children can be quite irregular.
   While counting, note the depth and rhythm of breathing. Depth
   is a subjective estimation and is usually noted as shallow,
   normal, or deep. If unable to label a rhythm, describe it.
- Observe the child for:
   Cyanosis of the nailbeds, hands, and feet, which might indicate
   central or *peripheral cyanosis.* Peripheral cyanosis can be
   caused by vasoconstriction and is common in the young
   infant.
   Cyanosis of the lips, oral mucosa, and generalized body cyanosis
   are indicative of *central cyanosis.* Central cyanosis indicates a
   significant drop in the oxygen-carrying capacity of the blood.
   Restlessness, anxiety, and decreasing levels of consciousness,
   which can be related to hypoxia.

Related Nursing Diagnoses

Anxiety: related to threat to health status.

Hypothermia: related to cool environment, medication, inadequate
   clothing, malnutrition, decreased metabolic rate, inactivity.

Hyperthermia: related to illness or trauma, increased metabolic
   rate, medications or anesthesia, hot environment, dehydration,
   inappropriate clothing.

Altered tissue perfusion, cardiopulmonary and peripheral: related
   to hypovolemia, hypoventilation; interruption of flow, venous or
   arterial; impaired transport of oxygen; exchange problems.

Decreased cardiac output: related to illness or trauma.

Impaired gas exchange: related to alveolar-capillary membrane
   exchanges, ventilation perfusion imbalance.

Ineffective airway clearance: related to smoking, second-hand smoke,
   smoke inhalation, airway spasm, retained or excessive secretions,
   foreign body in airway, infection, allergic airways, asthma.

Altered family processes: related to shift in health status, situational
   crisis.

Risk for activity tolerance: related to imbalance between oxygen
   supply and demand.

Knowledge deficit: related to unfamiliarity with information
   resources.

Blood Pressure

9

Rationale

Blood pressure readings provide significant information about the child's health status. Until recently, children younger than 3 years were commonly not screened for blood pressure because of the extra skill and patience required to obtain a blood pressure reading in such young patients. Most children with hypertension have renal disease; many fewer have coarctation of the aorta or pheochromocytoma. Screening of blood pressure in young children permits early detection of serious disorders and should be performed at least yearly on children from 3 years of age to adolescence. Blood pressure determination is routine on admission to health care facilities and in postoperative procedures. It should also be performed after invasive diagnostic procedures and before and after administration of drugs known to alter blood pressure. Blood pressure is taken whenever a child "feels funny" or when a child's condition deteriorates.

Anatomy and Physiology

Blood pressure is a product of cardiac output and increased peripheral resistance. In the neonate, systolic blood pressure is low, reflecting the weaker ability of the left ventricle. As the child grows, the size of the heart and of the left ventricle also increases, resulting in steadily increasing blood pressure values. At adolescence the heart enlarges abruptly, which also results in an increase in blood pressure values, comparable to those of the adult (Table 9-1).

An increase in cardiac output or in peripheral resistance will raise blood pressure. Decrease in cardiac output or in peripheral resistance will lower blood pressure. Overall maintenance of blood pressure reflects an intimate relationship among cardiac output,

Table 9-1   Blood Pressure Values for 90th and 95th Percentiles of Blood Pressure at Various Ages*

Age	Girls Systole (mmHg)	Girls Diastole (mmHg)	Boys Systole (mmHg)	Boys Diastole (mmHg)
1 yr	97-107	53-60	94-106	50-59
3 yr	100-110	61-68	100-113	59-67
6 yr	104-114	67-75	105-117	67-76
8 yr	108-118	70-78	107-120	71-80
10 yr	112-122	73-80	110-123	73-82
12 yr	116-126	75-82	115-127	75-83
14 yr	119-130	77-85	120-132	76-84
16 yr	122-132	79-86	125-138	79-87

Modified from Hockenberry MJ et al: *Wong's nursing care of infants and children*, ed 7, St Louis, 2003, Mosby.

*Values that fall at or below the lower number in each range are considered normotensive. Values that fall above the higher number in each range might be indicative of hypertension.

peripheral resistance, and blood volume, which can be influenced by several other factors (Table 9-2).

Equipment for Measuring Blood Pressure

- Pediatric stethoscope
- Sphygmomanometer with either a mercury or an aneroid manometer or electronic blood pressure devices (oscillometer, Doppler ultrasound)
- Ace or tensor bandage (flush technique)

Preparation

Ask the parent or child about family history of hypertension or cardiac or kidney disease. Ask if the child has or has had headaches, nosebleeds, swelling, alterations in voiding patterns, or clotting disorder or whether the child is on anticoagulant therapy.

Table 9-2   **Influences on Blood Pressure**

Influence	Effect
Medications	Narcotic analgesics, general anesthetics, diuretics decrease blood pressure.
	Aminophylline increases blood pressure.
Conditions	Blood pressure decreases during hemorrhage.
	Blood pressure increases with renal disease, increased intracranial pressure, coarctation of aorta (blood pressure in arms), pheochromocytoma, hyperthyroidism, diabetes mellitus, and acute pain.
	Pulse pressure widens with increased intracranial pressure.
Diurnal variation	Blood pressure usually is higher during morning and afternoon than during evening and night.
Apprehension and anxiety	Increases blood pressure.
Increased activity	Increases blood pressure.

Guidelines for Measurement of Blood Pressure

■ Select appropriate method. Palpation rather than auscultation can be performed if the child has a narrow or deep brachial artery. The flush technique can be selected if it is impossible to obtain blood pressure readings in young children or infants by other means. Oscillometric devices yield readings that correlate better with direct radial artery values than methods using auscultation and avoid problems associated with auscultation such as too rapid deflation of the cuff. Doppler ultrasound is accurate for systolic blood pressure but unreliable for diastolic pressure measurement. Limbs must be stabilized during measurement with oscillometric devices if accurate readings are to be obtained. Electronic or automatic cuffs must be used cautiously if the child is receiving anticoagulant therapy and has a disorder that affects clotting. The maximal inflation pressure on the automatic blood pressure machine should be adjusted to the child's last systolic blood pressure. Once the child's blood pressure is stable, the intervals between measurement should be increased to avoid too frequent inflation of the cuff.

■ Select appropriate site (Figure 9-1). Extremities in casts, those in which intravenous fluids are being infused, or those that are traumatized should not be used. Thighs can be selected if only large cuffs are available.

■ Select appropriate cuff size. The cuff should cover at least 75% of the upper arm or thigh in children and adolescents (Table 9-3), leaving enough room to place the bell of the stethoscope at the antecubital fossa and to avoid obstruction of the axilla. An overly large cuff might produce low readings. A cuff that is too narrow might produce high readings. If a correctly fitting cuff is not available, a wider cuff can be used. (Wider cuffs do not create the low readings in infants and young children that are produced in adults.) The cuff bladder should be long enough to encircle the arm without overlapping. In children who are overweight or who have thick arms, measuring limb circumference can be a more accurate method for determining cuff size. When considering limb circumference, the cuff should be 40% to 50% of the limb circumference when measuring at the upper arm, midway between the top of the shoulder and the olecranon. Limb circumference guidelines should be used when using an area other than the upper arms for blood pressure measurement.

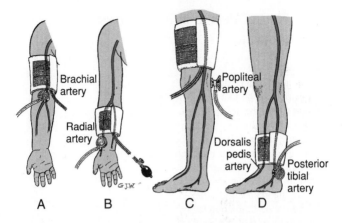

Figure 9-1
Sites for blood pressure measurement. **A,** Upper arm. **B,** Lower arm or forearm. **C,** Thigh. **D,** Calf or ankle.
(From Hockenberry MJ et al: *Wong's nursing care of infants and children,* ed 7, St Louis, 2003, Mosby.)

- Check bulb and pressure valve. Valve should adjust smoothly.
- Check needle of aneroid manometer. It should be at zero.
- Check mercury column of mercury-gravity manometer. It should be at zero.
- Blood pressure readings should be performed before other anxiety-producing procedures. The infant or child should be sitting quietly or lying down. The very young child might be most comfortable cradled in the parent's arms or lap.

Table 9-3   Guidelines for Selecting Age-Appropriate Cuff Sizes

Age	Bladder Width (cm)	Bladder Length (cm)
Infant	5	8
Child	8	13
Adult	13	24

Modified from Frohlich ED et al: Recommendations for human blood pressure determination by sphygmomanometers: report of a special task force appointed by the Steering Committee, American Heart Association, *Circulation* 77:501A, 1988.

Auscultation Method of Blood Pressure Measurement

Assessment	Findings
Select appropriate site and cuff. Position the child's limb. The arm should be at heart level. If positioned below the heart, falsely high reading might be obtained. If obtaining a thigh reading, the child can be positioned on the abdomen or with the knee slightly flexed. Expose the limb completely. Compression of the limb by rolled-up clothing can give a low reading. If the child is upset by removal of clothing, it is best to apply the cuff over the sleeve rather than rolling it up. Rolling produces a tight band.	
Palpate the brachial artery if using the arm, or the popliteal artery if using the thigh. Ensure that the cuff is fully deflated. Center the arrows on the cuff over the brachial artery of the arm, or position the bladder over the posterior aspect of the thigh. Position the manometer at eye level.	Viewing the manometer from above or below gives inaccurate readings.
Palpate the radial or popliteal artery, and inflate the cuff to 20 mmHg above the point at which the pulse disappears.	
Deflate the cuff; wait 15 to 30 seconds.	Inadequate release of venous congestion gives falsely high readings.

Assessment	Findings
Place the earpieces of the stethoscope in your ears. Earpieces should point forward to be inserted correctly. A pediatric stethoscope and bell should be used for infants and small children.	Incorrect placement of earpieces produces muffling or no sound at all.
Relocate the brachial or the popliteal artery. Place the bell or the diaphragm over the artery. Turn the valve of the pressure bulb clockwise until tight, and inflate cuff to 20 mmHg above the child's systolic reading.	Improper placement of the stethoscope produces low systolic and high diastolic readings.
Gradually release the valve to reduce pressure at a rate of 2 to 3 mmHg/sec.	Rapid release can cause inaccurate reading of the systolic pressure.
Observe the point at which the first clear reading (first Korotkoff sound) is obtained (systolic pressure) and at which the first muffling occurs (fourth Korotkoff sound) for the diastolic pressure in children younger than 13 years. Record the point at which all sound disappears (fifth Korotkoff sound) as the diastolic pressure in children 13 years and older.	In children younger than 1 year, thigh pressures should equal arm pressures; in children older than 1 year, thigh pressure is approximately 20 mmHg higher. Blood pressure will tend to be higher in children who are large for age than in children who are small. Korotkoff sounds might not be audible in early childhood because of a narrow or deeply placed artery.

Clinical Alert

A thigh pressure reading that is the same or lower than upper arm readings in infants might indicate coarctation of the aorta.

Assessment	Findings
Deflate the cuff rapidly after readings have been obtained. Wait 30 seconds before obtaining further readings.	**Clinical Alert** Repeat blood pressure readings if lower or higher than expected.
Record limb, position, cuff size, and how reading was obtained.	Document and report persistently elevated or lowered blood pressure readings. Consistently elevated serial readings can indicate hypertension. Persistently low diastolic pressure can indicate a patent ductus arteriosus. *Pulse pressure* (difference between systolic and diastolic pressures) of more than 50 mmHg can indicate congestive heart failure. Pulse pressure of less than 10 mmHg can indicate aortic stenosis.

Palpation Method of Blood Pressure Measurement

Assessment	Findings
Select appropriate site and cuff. Position child's limb, and prepare the cuff as though determining blood pressure by auscultation method.	
Palpate the brachial or the radial artery (arm) or the popliteal artery (thigh), and inflate the cuff 20 mmHg above point at which pulse disappears.	

Assessment	Findings
Slowly deflate the cuff, at a rate of 2 to 3 mmHg/sec.	
Determine point at which the pulse is first felt. This is the *systolic* pressure. The diastolic pressure cannot be determined by this method.	The systolic pressure obtained by radial palpation is approximately 10 mmHg lower than arm pressure.

Flush Method of Blood Pressure Measurement

Assessment	Findings
Wrap cuff around the limb. Elevate the limb. Wrap an elastic bandage from the fingers toward the antecubital space (or from the toes toward the knee).	
Inflate the cuff above the expected systolic pressure. Remove bandage. Place the child's arm at his or her side.	The limb will appear pale.
Slowly deflate the cuff until color suddenly returns. The reading is taken when color appears.	The value (flush pressure) obtained is the mean blood pressure (average of the diastolic and systolic pressures).

Related Nursing Diagnoses

Decreased cardiac output: related to arrhythmias, congenital anomalies, medications.

Fluid volume deficit: related to active volume loss.

Fluid volume excess: related to excess fluid intake.

Altered tissue perfusion, cardiopulmonary and peripheral: related to hypovolemia, interrupted arterial or venous blood flow, blood pressure changes in extremities.

ASSESSMENT OF BODY SYSTEMS

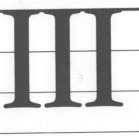

Integument

10

Assessment of the integument involves inspection and palpation of skin, nails, hair, and scalp and can be combined with assessment of other areas of the body.

Rationale

Assessment of the integument, or skin, should be an integral part of every health assessment, regardless of setting or situation. Many common pathophysiologic disorders have associated integumentary disorders. For example, many contagious childhood diseases have associated characteristic rashes. Rashes of all sorts are common in childhood. The integument yields much information about the physical care that a child receives and about the nutritional, circulatory, and hydration status of the child, which is valuable in planning health teaching interventions.

Anatomy and Physiology

The skin, which begins to develop during the eleventh week of gestation, consists of three layers (Figure 10-1). The *epidermis* is the outermost layer and is further divided into four layers. The top layer, or horny layer (stratum corneum), is of primary importance in protecting the internal homeostasis of the body. Melanin, produced by the regeneration layer of the epidermis, is the main pigment of the skin. The *dermis* underlies the epidermis and contains blood vessels, lymphatic vessels, hair follicles, and nerves. *Subcutaneous tissue* underlies the dermis and helps cushion, contour, and insulate the body. This final layer contains sweat and sebaceous glands. The sebaceous glands produce sebum, which can have some bactericidal effect.

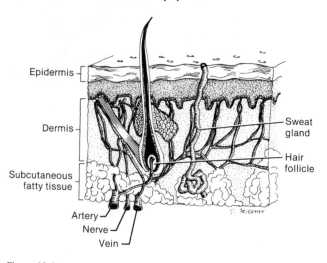

Figure 10-1
Normal skin layers.
(From Potter PA, Weilitz PB: *Pocket guide to health assessment,* ed 5, St Louis, 2003, Mosby.)

The skin has four main functions: protection against injury; thermoregulation; impermeability; and sensor of touch, pain, heat, and cold.

The normal pH of the skin is acidic, which is thought to protect the skin from bacterial invasion. In infants the pH of the skin is higher, the skin is thinner, and the secretion of sweat and sebum is minimal. As a result, infants are more prone to skin infections and conditions than older children and adults. Further, because of loose attachment between the dermis and epidermis, infants and children tend to blister easily.

Preparation

Inquire about a family history of skin disorders, the lifestyle of the family (diet, bathing, use of soaps and perfumes, sun exposure), recent changes in lifestyle, and use of jewelry and medications. Ask when lesions began and whether other symptoms accompanied the lesions. Ask the parent to describe the size, configuration, distribution, type, and color of the lesions. Inquire about home remedies.

A well-illuminated room with white walls is essential for proper visualization of the skin. (Yellow walls can give the appearance of jaundice and blue walls the appearance of cyanosis.) Daylight is preferable for assessment, especially for assessment of skin color, but if daylight is unavailable, add overhead fluorescent lights. The room should also be warm.

Assessment of Skin

Assessment of the skin is usually performed during assessment of each body system.

Assessment	Findings
Observe the skin for odor.	**Clinical Alert** The presence of odor can indicate poor hygiene or infection.
Observe the color and pigmentation of the skin. If a color change is suspected, carefully inspect the areas of the body where there is less melanin (nailbeds, earlobes, sclerae, conjunctivae, lips, mouth). Inspect the abdomen (an area less exposed to sunlight) and the trunk. Use natural daylight for assessment if *jaundice* is suspected. Pressing a finger against a skin area produces blanching, which supplies contrast and enables closer assessment of the presence of jaundice. Note location, distribution, and pattern of color changes. If a child has a different	Overall skin color normally varies between and within races and affects assessment findings. **Clinical Alert** A brown color to the skin can indicate Addison's disease or some pituitary tumors. A reddish-blue skin tone suggests polycythemia in light-skinned children. Red skin color can result from exposure to cold, hyperthermia, blushing, alcohol, or inflammation (if localized). Skin redness is more difficult to detect in dark-skinned children and assessment needs to be augmented by palpation and assessment of skin temperature.

Assessment	Findings
pigmentation from that of the accompanying parent, ask about the absent parent for hereditary trait recognition.	Blue (cyanosis) coloration of nails, soles, and palms can indicate *peripheral* or *central* cyanosis. Peripheral cyanosis can arise from anxiety or cold; central cyanosis is indicative of a marked drop in the oxygen-carrying capacity of the blood and is best identified in the lips, tongue, and oral mucosa. Generalized body cyanosis can be evident in central cyanosis. Dark-skinned children might appear ashen-gray or pale with cyanosis, and lips and tongue might appear ashen-gray or pale. Yellow-green to orange skin color can indicate jaundice (which accompanies liver disease, hepatitis, red cell hemolysis, biliary obstruction, or severe infection in infants) and is best observed in the sclerae, mucous membranes, fingernails, soles, palms, and on the abdomen. In dark-skinned children, jaundice can appear as yellow staining on the palate, palmar surfaces, or sclerae. Yellowing of the palms, soles, and face (and not of the sclerae or mucous membranes) can indicate carotenemia, produced from ingestion of carrots, squash, and sweet potatoes.

Assessment	Findings
	Yellowing of the exposed skin areas (and not of the sclerae and mucous membranes) can indicate chronic renal disease.
	Bruising in soft tissue areas (e.g., buttocks) rather than on shins, knees, or elbows can indicate child abuse or cultural practices such as spooning that are used to heal.
	A generalized lack of color involving the skin, hair, and eyes indicates albinism.
	Symmetric white patches indicate vitiligo.
	Café-au-lait or light brown spots and axillary or inguinal freckling that develops in infancy or early childhood can indicate neurofibromatosis.
	Pallor (lack of pink tones in fair-skinned children; ash-gray or yellow-brown color in dark-skinned children), suggestive of syncope, fever, shock, edema, or anemia, is best observed in the face, mouth, conjunctivae, and nails.
Observe the moistness of exposed skin areas and mucous membranes.	The skin is normally slightly dry. Exposed areas normally feel dryer than body creases. Mucous membranes should be moist.
Lightly stroke body creases. Compare body creases to one another.	**Clinical Alert**
	Dry skin on the lips, hands, or genitalia suggests contact dermatitis.

Assessment	Findings
	Generalized dryness, accompanied by moist body creases and moist mucous membranes, indicates overexposure to the sun, overbathing, or poor nutrition. Dry arm creases and mucous membranes suggest dehydration. Clamminess can indicate shock or perspiration.
Palpate the skin with the back of the hand to determine *temperature.* Compare each side of the body with the other, and the upper with the lower extremities.	**Clinical Alert** Generalized hyperthermia can indicate fever, sunburn, or a brain disorder. Localized hyperthermia can indicate burn or infection. Generalized hypothermia can indicate shock. Local hyperthermia can indicate exposure to cold. Coolness in hands and feet with pallor and cyanosis might suggest Raynaud's phenomenon.
Inspect and palpate the texture of the skin. Note the presence of thickening, scars, and excessive scar tissue (keloid).	An infant's or child's skin is normally smooth and even. **Clinical Alert** Rough, dry skin can indicate overbathing, poor nutrition, exposure to weather, or an endocrine disorder and is associated with Down syndrome. Flaking or scaling between the fingers or toes can be related to eczema, dermatitis, or a fungal infection. Thin, dry, wrinkled skin can indicate ectodermal hypoplasia. Oily scales on the scalp indicate seborrheic dermatitis (cradle cap).

Assessment	Findings
	Scaly, hypopigmented patches on the face and upper body, or scattered papules (Table 10-1) over the arms, thighs, and buttocks, and fine, superficial scales can indicate eczema.
	Malar butterfly rash of cheeks (excluding the nasolabial folds) and maculopapular rashes occurring on sun-exposed skin, especially in an adolescent, can be indicative of lupus erythematosus.
	Thickened and enfolded areas of the skin can suggest neurofibromatosis.
	Moist, warm, flushed skin occurs with hyperthyroidism.
	A crackling sensation on palpation can indicate subcutaneous emphysema.
Palpate for *turgor* by grasping a fold on the upper arm or abdomen between the fingers and quickly releasing. Note the ease with which the skin moves (mobility) and returns to place (turgor) without residual marks.	Skin normally returns quickly to place with no residual marks. **Clinical Alert** A skinfold that returns slowly to place or retains marks commonly indicates dehydration or malnutrition. Other possible causes are chronic disease and muscle disorders.
Palpate for *edema* by pressing a thumb into areas that look swollen.	**Clinical Alert** Thumb indentations that remain after the thumb is removed indicate pitting edema. Edema in the periorbital areas can indicate crying, allergies, recent sleep, renal disease, or juvenile hypothyroidism.

Assessment	Findings
	Edema (dependent) of the lower extremities and buttocks can indicate renal or cardiac disorders.
Inspect and palpate the skin for *lesions* (see Table 10-1). Note the distribution or arrangement of lesions (Figure 10-2), shape, color, size, and consistency of the lesions and birthmarks (Table 10-3).	**Clinical Alert** Rashes are associated with several childhood disorders (Table 10-2). Petechiae and ecchymoses can indicate a bleeding tendency. A painful, nonpruritic, maculopapular rash over the trunk is found in some instances of West Nile virus.
Enquire about pruritus.	**Clinical Alert** Itching can indicate the onset of an asthmatic attack or can occur with hepatitis A or renal disorders or with some skin disorders (itching is particularly associated with eczema or atopic dermatitis, head lice, or scabies).

Table 10-1   Common Skin Lesions

Lesion		Description
Primary Lesions (arise from normal skin)		
Macule	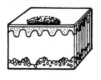	Small (less than 1 cm or 0.4 in), flat mass; differs from surrounding skin. Example: freckle.
Papule		Small (less than 1 cm or 0.4 in), raised, solid mass. Example: small nevus.

Table 10-1   Common Skin Lesions—cont'd

Lesion		Description
Primary Lesions (arise from normal skin)—cont'd		
Nodule		Solid, raised mass; slightly larger (1-2 cm or 0.4-0.8 in) and deeper than a papule.
Tumor		Solid, raised mass; larger than a nodule; can be hard or soft.
Wheal		Irregularly shaped, transient area of skin edema. Example: hive, insect bite, allergic reaction.
Vesicle		Small (less than 1 cm or 0.4 in), raised, fluid-filled mass. Example: herpes simplex, varicella.
Bulla		Raised, fluid-filled mass; larger than a vesicle. Example: second-degree burn.
Pustule		Vesicle containing purulent exudate. Example: acne, impetigo, staphylococcal infections.

Continued

Table 10-1   Common Skin Lesions—cont'd

Lesion		Description
Secondary Lesions (arise from changes in primary lesions)		
Scale	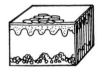	Thin flake of exfoliated epidermis. Example: psoriasis, dandruff.
Crust		Dried residue of serum, blood, or purulent exudate. Example: eczema.
Erosion	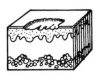	Moist lesion resulting from loss of superficial epidermis. Example: rupture of lesion in varicella.
Ulcer		Deep loss of skin surface; can extend to dermis and subcutaneous tissue. Example: syphilitic chancre, decubitus ulcer.
Fissure		Deep, linear crack in skin. Example: athlete's foot.

Table 10-1   Common Skin Lesions—cont'd

Lesion		Description
Secondary Lesions (arise from changes in primary lesions)—cont'd		
Lichenification		Thickened skin with accentuated skin furrows. Example: sequela of eczema.
Striae		Thin white or purple stripes, commonly found on abdomen. Can result from pregnancy or weight gain.
Purpuric Lesions Petechia		Flat, round, deep red or purplish mass (less than 3 mm or 0.1 in).
Ecchymosis		Mass of variable size and shape; initially purplish, fading to green, yellow, then brown.

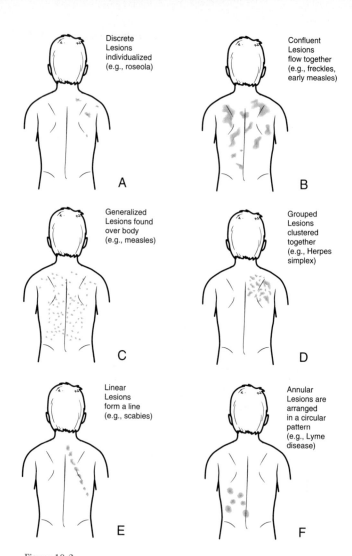

Figure 10-2

Arrangement of lesions. **A,** Discrete: lesions individualized (e.g., roseola). **B,** Confluent: lesions flow together (e.g., freckles, early measles). **C,** Generalized: lesions found over body (e.g., measles). **D,** Grouped: lesions clustered together (e.g., herpes simplex). **E,** Linear: lesions form a line (e.g., scabies). **F,** Annular: lesions are arranged in a circular pattern (e.g., Lyme disease). (Adapted from Zator Estes ME: *Health assessment & physical examination,* ed 2, New York, 2002, Delmar Learning.)

Table 10-2   Distribution and Characteristics of Lesions Associated with Common Childhood Disorders

Disorder	Accompanying Lesions	Typical Location of Lesions
Allergic Disorders		
Allergic reaction	Almost any type of lesion possible. Common manifestations are urticaria (hives), eczema, and contact dermatitis. Lesions can be intensely pruritic.	
Urticaria	Wheals can be small or large, discrete or confluent, sparse or profuse. Wheals tend to come in crops and fade in a few hours.	
Eczema (atopic dermatitis)	Acute: erythema, vesicles, exudate, and crusts. Chronic: pruritic, dry, scaly, and thickened rash.	Infantile form found on cheeks, forehead, scalp, and extensor surfaces. Childhood form found on wrists, ankles, and flexor surfaces. Adolescent form found on face, sides of neck, hands, feet, and flexor surfaces.

Continued

Table 10-2   Distribution and Characteristics of Lesions Associated with Common Childhood Disorders—cont'd

Disorder	Accompanying Lesions	Typical Location of Lesions
Allergic Disorders—cont'd		
Contact dermatitis	Pruritic red swelling that can be well demarcated from normal skin. Papules and bullae can be present.	
Contagious Diseases		
Molluscum contagiosum	Sharply circumscribed or multiple pearly umbilicated papules.	Located on any area of the body.
Mumps	Painful swelling of parotid glands.	Can be unilateral or bilateral.
Measles (rubeola)	Red maculopapular rash. Confluent at early sites of involvement, discrete at later sites. Becomes brownish in 3-4 days and desquamates.	Begins on face.
Rubella (German measles)	Pinkish red maculopapular rash. Discrete lesions. Rash disappears within 3 days.	Begins on face and spreads downward.
Roseola (baby measles)	Rose-pink macules or maculopapules. Discrete lesions fade on pressure. Nonpruritic. Rash disappears in 1-2 days.	Rash appears first on trunk before spreading.

Chickenpox (varicella zoster)	Rash progresses from macule to papule to vesicle to crust. Pruritic.	Begins on trunk and spreads primarily to face and proximal extremities.
Scarlet fever	Tiny red lesions. Desquamation begins in 1 week. Tongue initially is white and swollen (first 1-2 days), then becomes red and swollen.	Involves all but the face; more intense in joint areas.
Erythema infectiosum (fifth disease or slapped cheek disease)	Erythema for 1-4 days. Approximately 1 day after erythema, a maculopapular rash appears. After rash disappears, it can reappear with heat, cold, or sun.	Erythema involves cheeks. Maculopapular rash is symmetrically distributed on all limbs and progresses from proximal to distal surfaces.
Bacterial Infections		
Impetigo contagiosa	Rash begins with reddish macule, then vesicle appears. Vesicle ruptures, producing a moist erosion. Exudate dries, producing a honey-colored crust. Pruritic.	
Cellulitis	Skin red, swollen, warm to touch, firmly infiltrated. "Streaking" can be present.	

Continued

Table 10-2   Distribution and Characteristics of Lesions Associated with Common Childhood Disorders—cont'd

Disorder	Accompanying Lesions	Typical Location of Lesions
Viral Infections		
Herpes simplex (cold sore)	Grouped vesicles on an erythematous base. Vesicles dry, leaving a crust.	Found near lips, nose, genitalia, buttocks.
Herpes zoster (shingles)	Appears in crops of vesicles. Pain and itching are common.	Follows dermatome of affected nerve.
West Nile virus	Morbilliform, erythematous, maculopapular rash is painful but not pruritic and blanches with pressure. Occurs with approximately 25% of West Nile infections.	Found on trunk.
Fungi		
Candidiasis	Eruptions have sharp borders and include red papules, pustules, and satellite lesions.	Commonly occur in skin creases and can be associated with oral thrush.
Tinea capitis	Pruritic circumscribed areas of scaling. Alopecia present.	Found on the scalp.
Tinea corporis	Pruritic red, round, or oval scaly areas. Central area clear.	

Tinea pedis (athlete's foot)	Maceration and fissuring. Pruritic.	Found between toes or vesicles on plantar surface.
Infestations		
Scabies	Linear, brownish-gray burrows are produced by the female mite. Sarcoptic infestations produce papules, pustules, vesicles, and hives.	In infants, lesions are primarily found on face, palms, and soles. In children, lesions are commonly found on apposed surfaces of skin and interdigital areas, on the extensor surfaces of joints and wrists, lower back, abdomen, genitalia, and buttocks.
Pediculosis corporis (body lice)	Lesions appear as red macules, wheals, excoriated papules. Pruritic.	Found on the back and on areas that have close contact with clothing.
Lyme disease	Erythema chronicum migrans (ECM) appears 4-20 days after bite by a tick. Presents as a red macule or papule at the bite site and can be painless and nonitchy or warm, tender, and stinging. If untreated, ECM can have central clearing and can progress to ulceration.	ECM commonly found on groin, axilla, and/or proximal thigh.

Continued

Table 10-2 Distribution and Characteristics of Lesions Associated with Common Childhood Disorders—cont'd

Disorder	Accompanying Lesions	Typical Location of Lesions
Miscellaneous		
Psoriasis	Thick, dry, red lesions covered with silvery scales. More common in children 5 years of age and older.	Lesions appear on scalp, ears, forehead, eyebrows, trunk, elbows, knees, and genitalia.
Seborrheic dermatitis (cradle cap)	Oily, scaly patches.	Found on the scalp or along the hairline.
Henoch-Schönlein purpura (HSP)	Systemic purpura as well as maculopapular lesions, erythema, and urticaria.	Primarily involves buttocks and lower extremities.
Acne vulgaris	Lesions can be noninflamed (comedones) or inflamed. Comedones can be closed and are compact masses (commonly called *whiteheads*). Open comedones, or *blackheads*, have visible openings that are discolored through exposure of fatty acids to air. Inflamed lesions can lead to scarring and appear as papules, pustules, nodules, and cysts.	Lesions appear on the face, neck, shoulders, upper chest, and back in about 85% of adolescents.

Table 10-3   **Common Birthmarks**

Birthmark	Description
Vascular nevi	
Salmon patch ("stork beak" mark)	Flat, light pink mark found on the eyelids, in nasolabial region, or at the nape of the neck. Most disappear by the end of the first year of life.
Nevus flammeus (port-wine stain)	Flat, deep red or purplish-red patches. Enlarge as child grows.
Strawberry nevus (raised hemangioma)	Begins as circumscribed grayish-white area; becomes red, raised, well defined. Might not be present at birth; resolves spontaneously by 9 years of age.
Hyperpigmented nevi	
Mongolian spot	Large; flat; blue-, black-, or slate-colored area found on the buttocks and in the lumbosacral region.

Assessment of Nails

Assessment	Findings
Inspect nails for color, shape, and condition.	**Clinical Alert** Clubbing can indicate chronic respiratory or cardiac disease. Convex or concave curving nails can be hereditary or related to injury, iron deficiency, or infection.

Assessment	Findings
	Yellow or white coloration in a thickened nailbed can indicate a fungal infection of the nail (onychomycosis), which can occur with cosmetic nail applications.
	A transverse furrow in the nail can indicate acute infection, anemia, or malnutrition.
	Splinter hemorrhages (small, dark linear formations) in nailbeds can indicate subacute bacterial endocarditis or mitral stenosis.
Inspect nails for nail biting, skin picking, infection.	

Assessment of Hair

Assessment	Findings
Assess hair for distribution, color, texture, amount, and quality. Hair distribution is useful in estimating sexual maturity.	Hair normally covers all but the palms, soles, inner labial surfaces (girls), and prepuce and glans penis (boys).
Assess hair for dandruff and nits. If nits are suspected, use a fine-toothed metal or electronic comb on the hair to differentiate between nits, dandruff, and lint.	Scalp hair is normally shiny, silky, strong. **Clinical Alert** Dry, brittle, or depigmented hair can indicate nutritional deficiency or thyroid disorder. A hairline that extends to mid-forehead can be normal or can indicate cretinism. Delayed or absent hair growth can indicate an ectodermal dysplasia.

Assessment	Findings
	Unusually fine hair that is unable to hold a wave can indicate hyperthyroidism.
	Alopecia (loss of hair) can be related to tinea capitis, compulsive hair pulling, tight hairstyles (e.g., ponytails, corn braids), abuse, or persistent positioning on one side (in infants).
	Hair tufts on the spine or buttocks can indicate spina bifida.
	White eggs that are firmly attached to hair shafts indicate head lice. Dandruff can be removed.

Related Nursing Diagnoses

Pain: related to itching, loss of skin surface.

Hyperthermia: secondary to illness.

Knowledge deficit (hygienic needs, prevention of infection, prevention of scarring): related to cognitive limitations, lack of exposure, lack of interest in learning, information misinterpretation.

Sleep deprivation: related to discomfort.

Risk for infection: related to broken skin, exposure to pathogens.

Altered oral mucous membrane: secondary to infection, dehydration, medication side effects, malnutrition or vitamin deficiency.

Altered parenting: related to lack of knowledge about child maintenance.

Chronic low self-esteem: related to presence of acne, birthmarks, scarring.

Impaired tissue integrity: related to injury, infection, nutritional disorders, altered pigmentation, alterations in turgor.

Impaired tissue integrity: related to mechanical injury, infection, nutritional deficit, chemical factors, developmental factors, fluid volume deficit or excess, impaired physical mobility, infection, altered circulation, knowledge deficit, irritants.

Head and Neck

11

Assessment of the neck includes evaluation of the trachea and the thyroid gland. The head is assessed for size, shape, and symmetry. The fontanels and sutures are examined, and head control is noted. Proceeding downward from the head to the neck provides a smooth progression of assessment.

Rationale

Examination of the head and neck is important in screening pediatric clients for acute disorders and long-term disabilities. The determination of disorders such as skull asymmetry can also signal the need for parent teaching.

Anatomy and Physiology

The head accounts for one fourth of the body length and one third of the body weight in the newborn infant, in comparison with one eighth of the body length and one tenth of the body weight in the adult. Head size, which is 32 to 38 cm (12.6 to 14.9 inches) at birth, normally exceeds chest circumference by 1 to 2 cm (0.4 to 0.8 inches) until 18 months of age. After 18 months, chest growth exceeds head size by 5 to 7 cm (2 to 2.76 inches) (see Appendix B for charts of head circumference norms). The newborn skull consists of separate bones that fuse when brain growth is complete. Soft, fibrous tissue joints, called *sutures,* separate the bones (Figure 11-1). Sutures begin to unite by 6 months of age but can be separated by increased intracranial pressure until 12 years of age.

Fontanels are formed by the juncture of three or more skull bones (see Figure 11-1) and are felt as soft concavities. Although there are several fontanels (sagittal or parietal, sphenoidal, mastoid, anterior, and posterior), normally only the posterior and anterior

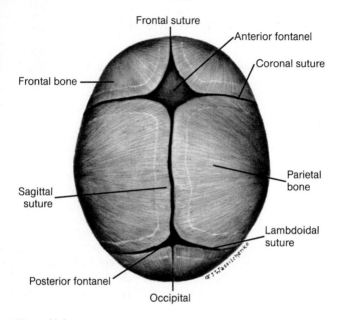

Figure 11-1
Location of sutures and fontanels.
(From Hockenberry MJ et al: *Wong's nursing care of infants and children,* ed 7, St Louis, 2003, Mosby.)

fontanels can be palpated. The sagittal fontanel, located between the anterior and posterior fontanels and along the sagittal suture, can be palpated in some neonates and in some infants with Down syndrome. The posterior fontanel might be closed at birth and should always be closed by the second month. The anterior fontanel closes between 9 and 26 months of age; 90% close between 7 and 19 months.

By 4 months of age the infant should be able to hold the head erect and in midline. By 6 months no significant head lag should be noted when the child is pulled to a sitting position.

The neck in the infant and toddler is short, but by 4 years of age it assumes adult proportions. Although the thyroid gland is fully active at birth, it might not be palpable in infants and young children.

Equipment for Measurement of Head Circumference

- Paper or narrow flexible metal tape (not cloth tape, which can stretch)

Measurement	Findings
Measure head circumference if the child is 2 years of age or younger, if the size of the child's head warrants concern, or if there is possible concern about neurologic or developmental health issues. Place the tape around the head at points just above the eyebrows and the pinna and around the occipital prominence (Figure 11-2). If head circumference is measured daily, the head should be marked at key	Head circumference provides an estimate of cranial volume, which reflects brain size and correlates with neurologic and developmental functions. The head can appear disproportionately large (but normal) in infants born prematurely or in children whose familial pattern exhibits large heads. **Clinical Alert** If an infant's head circumference is above or below growth norms for the infant's established percentile, further evaluation is indicated. An abnormally

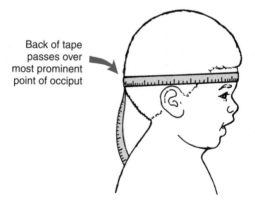

Back of tape passes over most prominent point of occiput

Figure 11-2
Measurement of head circumference.

Measurement	Findings
points to ensure consistency of measurement. Head circumference should be plotted on gender-specific charts. If the infant is premature, then the age of the infant should be corrected for prematurity and the head circumference plotted by conceptual rather than chronologic age.	large head circumference can indicate hydrocephalus, brain tumor, cerebral gigantism, neurofibromatosis, hemorrhage, or autism. A small head circumference can indicate craniostenosis or microcephaly. Infants born to mothers who use cocaine or alcohol or who experienced intrauterine infection can have smaller head circumferences.

Preparation

Sit or lay the child in a comfortable position. The infant or young child might be most at ease on the parent's lap.

Assessment of Head

Assessment	Findings
Observe the shape and symmetry of the child's head from different angles. If possible, also note the shape and symmetry of the parents' heads. Part the hair of the child and inspect for lesions or masses.	Minor asymmetry in infants younger than 4 months is common and is related to molding. A head might be longer, narrower, or flatter than expected, as a result of genetic influences.
	Clinical Alert
	A markedly flattened occiput can be the result of persistent placement of the child in the supine position. If flattening is observed, ask the parents about the child's preferred sleep or play position.
	Parent teaching might be indicated. A flattened occiput and a small, rounded head are found with Down syndrome.
	Head asymmetry can reflect premature closure of suture lines and requires further evaluation.

Assessment	Findings
	A gaping skull wound can be indicative of a compound skull fracture.
Palpate the skull, using the fingerpads. Palpate the suture lines in infants.	Sutures are felt as prominent ridges or like cracks between the cranial bones. In a newborn infant the suture lines override as a result of molding, but usually flatten by 6 months.
	Palpation of the suture lines can occasionally lead to slight give in the underlying bone due to osteoporosis of the outer table of bone. This is known as *craniotabes*. Craniotabes is sometimes found in normal infants.

Clinical Alert

A separated sagittal suture is one of the most common findings in Down syndrome.

Craniotabes can suggest increased intracranial pressure as in hydrocephaly, infection as in syphilis, and metabolic disturbances such as rickets.

A localized, easily moveable accumulation of blood in subcutaneous tissue is indicative of a hematoma, which can result from trauma to the skull.

Single, round, nontender, moveable masses can indicate sebaceous cysts.

Observe and palpate the fontanels, if open, while the infant is sitting.	The anterior fontanel should be soft, flat, and pulsatile. The fontanel bulges slightly when the infant is crying.

Clinical Alert

A bulging fontanel can indicate increased intracranial pressure and is found in conditions such as head injury, meningitis, or neoplasm.

Assessment	Findings
	A depressed fontanel can indicate dehydration.
	An enlarged anterior fontanel or the presence of a sagittal fontanel can indicate Down syndrome.
	An enlarged posterior fontanel can suggest congenital hypothyroidism.
Measure the width and length of an open anterior fontanel.	Until 9 to 12 months the anterior fontanel measures from 1 to 5 cm (0.4 to 2 in) in length and width. **Clinical Alert** An abnormally small or large fontanel can suggest a bone growth disorder.
Percuss the parietal bone on each side by tapping the index finger against the surface.	Percussion produces a "cracked pot" sound (Macewen's sign) in normal infants before closure of sutures. **Clinical Alert** Presence of Macewen's sign in older infants and children can indicate separation of sutures because of increased intracranial pressure as a result of conditions such as lead encephalopathy and brain tumor.

Assessment of Neck

Assessment	Findings
Pull the infant to a sitting position while observing head control.	The infant younger than 4 months might show some head lag when pulled to a sitting position. **Clinical Alert** Significant head lag after 6 months can indicate cerebral palsy.
Put the child's head and neck through a full range of motion. The older child should be asked to look up, down, and sideways.	The child should exhibit no pain or limitation of movement in any direction. **Clinical Alert** Pain and resistance to flexion can indicate meningeal irritation.

Assessment	Findings
	Lateral resistance to motion can indicate torticollis as a result of injury to the sternocleidomastoid muscle.
Inspect the neck for lymph nodes, masses, cysts, webbing, extra folds of skin, and vein distention.	**Clinical Alert**
	Webbing and extra neck folds can indicate Turner's syndrome.
	Excessive and lax skin is found in children with Down syndrome.
	Small, round, firm swelling felt at midline just above the thyroid cartilage in a young infant suggests a thyroglossal duct cyst.
	Cervical lymphadenopathy can suggest viral or bacterial infections. General lymphadenopathy is associated with HIV infection in infants and with infectious mononucleosis in older children and adolescents. Bilateral tonsillar lymph node enlargement can indicate acute tonsillitis.
	Parotid swelling and tenderness can indicate mumps, bacterial infection, or presence of a stone.
	Enlarged occipital nodes can indicate rubella or roseola infantum.
	Vein distention might be present with labored respirations.
Palpate the trachea by placing the thumb on one of the trachea and the index finger on the other. Slide the fingers up and down while the child's neck is slightly hyperextended.	The trachea should be at midline or slightly to the right.
	Clinical Alert
	Any shift in the position of the trachea should be noted because serious lung problems might be present.
Palpate the thyroid gland by standing behind the	In normal children the thyroid gland might not be felt.

Assessment	Findings
child and placing your fingers or hands gently over the area of the gland (at the base the neck). The gland rises as a mass as the child swallows. Palpation of the thyroid gland in the infant and young child is difficult because of the shortness of the neck. Infants are best examined while lying supine across a parent's lap.	**Clinical Alert** An enlarged thyroid gland can indicate goiter, lymphatic thyroiditis.

Related Nursing Diagnoses

Pain: related to physical factors.

Anxiety: related to uncertainty of diagnoses, possibility of disability.

Risk for trauma: related to balancing difficulties, cognitive difficulties, reduced coordination.

Altered tissue perfusion: related to mechanical reduction in blood flow, interruption in arterial or venous flow.

Altered health maintenance: related to perceptual or cognitive impairment.

Impaired verbal communication: related to decrease in circulation to brain, anatomic defect.

Altered family processes: related to situation transition and/or crisis, developmental crisis.

Risk for altered parenting: related to handicapping condition, developmental delay.

Risk for altered growth and development: related to effects of physical disabilities.

Hyperthermia: related to illness, trauma, increased metabolic rate.

Hypothermia: related to illness, decreased metabolic rate.

Altered comfort: pain secondary to infection, meningeal irritation.

Compromised family coping: related to situational crisis.

Fear: related to rapid onset of illness.

Hyperthermia: related to altered metabolic rates secondary to altered thyroid function.

Hypothermia: related to altered metabolic rates secondary to altered thyroid function.

Impaired physical mobility: related to neuromuscular deficits.

Self-care deficit: related to inability or interruption in performing age-appropriate activities of daily living.

Impaired swallowing: secondary to enlarged thyroid gland, altered level of consciousness, infection, alcohol exposure.

Ears

12

Assessment of the ears involves inspection of the external and internal ear, testing of hearing acuity, and otoscopic examination. The nurse also focuses on the child's health history in an effort to identify factors that could place the child at risk for hearing problems.

Rationale

Ear disorders are disruptive to language, speech, and social development. Early screening and detection can assist in minimizing or eliminating hearing deficiencies and their effects. Temporary and correctable conditions such as otitis media are common in young children but might go undetected. Abnormalities of the external ear can be important in alerting health professionals to the presence of syndromes and should be reported. Assessment of the ear is performed in conjunction with the eye examination, because eye problems are nearly twice as common in children with hearing deficiencies.

Anatomy and Physiology

The ear consists of the external ear, middle ear, and inner ear. The outer ear consists of the auricle, cartilaginous shell, and external ear canal. In children younger than 3 years the canal points upward; in older children it is directed downward and forward. The lining of the external ear canal secretes cerumen, which protects the ear.

The middle ear consists of the tympanum (eardrum) and three bones (ossicles) that touch the tympanum on one side and the membrane covering the opening to the inner ear on the other side. Vibrations of the tympanum are transmitted through the ossicles to the inner ear. The middle ear also contains an opening to the eustachian tube. The eustachian tube allows secretions to pass from the middle ear to the nasopharynx and enables air to enter the middle ear from the throat. Equalization of air pressure between the external ear canal and middle ear is essential for proper functioning of the tympanic membrane. The shorter and less angled eustachian tube in infants and young children permits secretions from the nose and throat to readily enter the middle ear, predisposing this age group to more frequent ear infections.

The inner ear contains auditory nerve endings, which pick up sound waves from the middle ear and transmit them along the eighth cranial nerve, or auditory nerve, to the brain. Sound waves that contact the skull directly can also be picked up by the inner ear. The inner ear contains the structures for balance and hearing.

The three divisions of the ear develop in the embryo at the same time as other vital organs are developing, which is why deformities of the ears can provide clues to developmental aberrations elsewhere in the body. External ear development begins at about the fifth week of gestation, and middle ear development begins at around the sixth week. The ears are particularly vulnerable to developmental aberration in the ninth week of gestation.

Neonates are capable of sound discrimination at birth and respond more readily to high-pitched voices. The presence of mucus in the eustachian tube can limit hearing when the neonate is first born but clears shortly after birth. Vernix caseosa in the external ear canal can make visualization of the tympanic membrane difficult.

The young infant responds to loud noises with the startle reflex, blinking, or cessation of movement. Infants 6 months of age or older attempt to locate the source of the sound.

Equipment for Ear Assessment

- Otoscope
- Ear speculum

Preparation

Ask about family history of hearing problems, prenatal influences (infection, alcohol use), postnatal factors (mechanical ventilation, neonatal jaundice, asphyxia at birth), childhood infections (mumps, measles, ear and respiratory tract infections), surgery to the ear, use of ototoxic drugs, head trauma, and exposure to loud noises (e.g., music).

If an otoscopic examination is to be performed in a young child or infant, it is safer to restrain the child. Explain and demonstrate to the parent how to hold the child. The child can be placed on the side or abdomen, with the hands at the side and the head turned so that the ear to be examined points toward the ceiling. The parent can assist by placing one hand on the child's head above the ear and the other on the child's trunk. Alternatively, the child can sit on the parent's lap with one arm tucked behind the parent's back. The parent holds the child's head against his or her shoulder and the child's other, free arm (Figure 12-1).

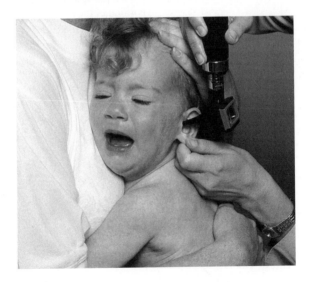

Figure 12-1
Position for restraining infant or child during otoscopic examination.
(From Hockenberry MJ et al: *Wong's nursing care of infants and children,* ed 7, St Louis, 2003, Mosby.)

Assessment of External Ear

Assessment	Findings
Examine the ear for placement and position.	The top of the ear should cross an imaginary line from the inner eye to the occiput. The pinna should deviate no more than 10 degrees from a line perpendicular to the horizontal line. (Use of a pen or tongue blade can provide more concrete estimations of where the ear is positioned in relation to a vertical line.) Figure 12-2 illustrates normal placement and position of the ear.

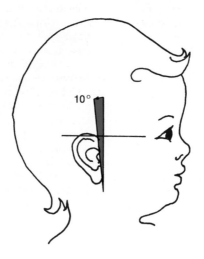

Figure 12-2
Ear placement and position.
(From Whaley LF, Wong DL: *Nursing care of infants and children,* ed 4, St Louis, 1991, Mosby.)

Assessment	Findings
	Clinical Alert
	Low or obliquely set ears are sometimes seen in children with genitourinary or chromosomal abnormalities and in many syndromes.
Observe the ears for protrusion or flattening.	The ears of neonates are flat against the head.
	Clinical Alert
	Flattened ears in older infants can suggest persistent side lying.
	Protruding ears can indicate swelling related to insect bites or to conditions such as mastoiditis, postauricular abscess, or mumps.
Inspect the external ear for unusual structure and markings and the skin around the ear for sinuses and small openings. Figure 12-3 illustrates usual markings.	Markings and structure of the external ear vary little from child to child. Variations can be normal but should be recorded. For example, a small skin tag on the tragus is a remnant of embryonic development and suggests no pathologic process. Skinfolds can be absent from the helix. Parents and children might be sensitive about this abnormality.
	Clinical Alert
Inspect the external ear canal for general hygiene, discharge, and excoriations.	A sinus can indicate a fistula that drains into the ear or neck.
	The skin of the external auditory meatus (see Figure 12-3) is normally flesh colored. Soft yellow-brown wax is normal. If cerumen is hard, it will appear dark, crusted, and dry.

Assessment	Findings
	Absence of wax in the external ear can indicate overly vigorous cleaning. Hygienic measures can best be determined by commenting on how clean the ears are and then asking how the ears are cleaned. Parents might need teaching about the dangers of using sharp objects. Advise use of a soft washcloth.
	Absence of wax can also be related to acute otitis media. If cleaning practices are acceptable, ask about ear pulling, irritability, and fever.

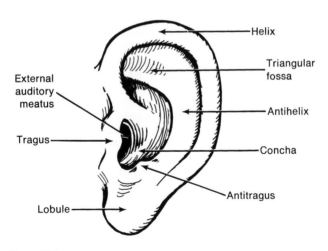

Figure 12-3
Usual landmarks of pinna.
(From Hockenberry MJ et al: *Wong's nursing care of infants and children,* ed 7, St Louis, 2003, Mosby.

Assessment	Findings
	Foul-smelling yellow or green discharge can indicate rupture of a tympanic membrane or recent insertion of myringotomy tubes.
	Bloody discharge can indicate foreign body irritation, scratching, or trauma or rupture of tympanic membrane.
	Serous discharge can indicate allergies.
	Clear discharge can indicate a CSF leak from skull fracture.
Pull on the auricle.	Pulling normally produces no pain and does not produce pain in purulent otitis media.
	Clinical Alert
	Pain produced by pulling on the auricle can indicate otitis externa. Pain will not be produced in purulent otitis media.
Palpate the bony protuberance behind the ear (mastoid) for tenderness.	No pain or tenderness should be experienced when the mastoid is palpated.
	Clinical Alert
	Pain and tenderness over the mastoid process can indicate mastoiditis.

Assessment of Hearing Acuity

Hearing loss is the most common disability. The three types of hearing loss are conduction hearing loss, sensorineural loss, and mixed loss. *Conduction hearing loss* results from disruption of sound transmission through the outer and middle ear, most often as the result of serous otitis media. *Sensorineural loss* is a result of damage to the inner ear or auditory nerve. *Mixed loss* reflects both conduction and sensorineural hearing loss.

Hearing loss is found in approximately 11% of infants with syndromes associated with hearing effects (Pierre Robin syndrome, CHARGE syndrome, choanal atresia, Rubinstein-Taybi syndrome, and oculoauriculovertebral spectrum) and with some neurodegenerative disorders (Hunter's syndrome, sensory motor neuropathies). Progressive hearing loss is associated with neurofibromatosis, osteopetrosis, and Usher's syndrome. Hearing loss is also found in infants and children with craniofacial anomalies.

Assessment and detection of hearing impairments are critical components of a health evaluation. Assessment involves identifying children who are at risk for hearing impairments by virtue of their history, observing for behaviors that would suggest a hearing loss, and screening for hearing acuity.

Preparation

Inquire about weight at birth and presence of hyperbilirubinemia as a neonate. Ask if child was on prolonged mechanical ventilation as a neonate or required admission to neonatal intensive care for 48 hours or more, or if child has had meningitis, mumps, frequent ear infections, or experienced head trauma. Inquire about family history of hearing disorders or hearing loss. Ask about use of alcohol during pregnancy. Ask if parents have concerns about their child's hearing, speech, or language. Inquire about use of hearing aids.

Equipment for Assessment of Hearing Acuity

- Noisemakers (squeeze toy, rattle, bell, paper)
- Tuning fork
- Tympanometer
- Audiometer

Assessment	Findings
Infant	
Assume that parents' impressions of their infant's hearing difficulties are correct unless otherwise proven.	

Assessment	Findings

Infant—cont'd

Ask if infant wakes in response to loud noises, if infant turns to an interesting sound, or if infant is beginning to repeat some of the sounds that parents make.

Stand behind the infant and ring a small bell, move a rattle, snap fingers, clap hands, or rustle paper.

Be careful not to bump the examining table or to cause an air stream because this evokes a false response from the infant.

The infant younger than 4 months evidences a startle reflex. Infants 6 months of age or older try to locate the sound by shifting their eyes or turning their heads. The infant might also cease sucking or other movement in response to sound. Infants older than 12 months will localize to all sounds beside, below, and above.

Clinical Alert

Suspect hearing loss in a young infant who does not startle or cease movement or who has been premature and in intensive care.

Suspect hearing loss in an older infant who does not attempt to localize sound.

Preschool-Age Child

Stand 0.6 to 0.9 m (2 to 3 ft) in front of the child and give commands, such as "Please give me the doll."

School-Age Child or Adolescent

Stand about 0.3 m (1 ft) behind the child. Instruct the child to cover one ear.

Assessment	Findings

School-Age Child or
Adolescent—cont'd

Ask the child to repeat what
is heard while you whisper
numbers in random order.
Repeat the process with
the other ear.

*Rinne's Test (to compare air and
bone conduction)*

Strike the tuning fork against
your palm, then hold the
stem to the child's mastoid
process. When the child
indicates that the sound is
no longer audible, hold the
prongs near the external
meatus of one ear and ask
the child if the sound can
be heard.

Repeat the process with
the other ear.

Normally the child can hear the
sound of the tuning fork
at the external meatus after it
is no longer audible at the
mastoid process (positive test
result) because air conduction
is better than bone
conduction.

Sound should be heard equally
well in both ears
(positive test result).

Clinical Alert

Not useful in toddlers because
the test requires the
cooperation and ability of
the child to signal when
the sound is no longer
audible.

Interference with conduction of
air through the external
and middle chambers causes
the child to experience
sound better through bone
conduction.

*Weber's Test (to differentiate
conduction from sensorineural
deafness)*

Strike the tuning fork against
the palm and hold the stem
in the midline of the child's
head. Ask the child where
sound is heard best.

Not useful for young children
because of difficulty
discriminating among
"better, more, less."

Clinical Alert

With air conduction loss the
sound is heard best in the
affected ear. The sound is
heard best in the *unaffected*
ear if loss is sensorineural.

Assessment	Findings

Tympanometry

Tympanometry is used to evaluate middle ear infection in children older than 7 months, although some sources suggest that it is not useful as a screening tool in a health examination. Tympanometry provides information about the presence of fluid in the middle ear, mobility of the tympanic membrane, and ear canal volume. It is quick, painless, and is not influenced by environmental noise. Some sources recommend training by an audiologist in this procedure.

Before placing the tympanometer, examine the ear with the otoscope to ensure that the path to the drum is clear. If child is older, warn that a noise will be heard after the tympanometer is placed, but that the test is not uncomfortable. Place the portable tympanometer in the ear. A soft tone will be transmitted through the probe while pressure is changed in the outer canal. Results will be recorded on a graph or tympanogram.

An A curve is considered normal in a tympanogram.

Clinical Alert

If the tympanogram shows an As curve, the stapes might be partially immobilized.

If the tympanogram shows an Ad curve, this indicates flaccidity of the tympanic membrane and separation of middle ear bones.

If the tympanogram shows a B (flat) curve, this indicates fluid in the eardrum.

If the tympanogram shows a C curve, this indicates a retracted eardrum and decreased pressure in the eardrum.

Assessment	Findings
Audiometry	
Audiometry is used to assess the threshold of hearing for pure tone frequencies (measured in hertz or Hz) at varying levels of loudness (measured in decibels or dB). In threshold acuity, the child is presented with a sound that is easily heard. The sound is gradually reduced in loudness until it is no longer audible to the child. The child usually wears headphones and is instructed to hold up a hand or push a button when the sound is heard. Audiometry is not considered reliable for children younger than 5 years, although young children might be able to respond if they practice with the equipment.	

Otoscopic Examination

The apprehension many children feel about the otoscopic examination can be lessened by letting them see and handle the otoscope and to turn the light on and off. Reassure that the examination might tickle but does not hurt. Playing a game such as "let's look for the elephant in your ear" can help allay fear (after the examination, it is important to explain that "the elephant" was only pretend). Demonstrating on a doll can also reduce apprehension. It is helpful to move the speculum around the outer rim of the meatus to allow the child to adjust to the feel of the speculum. Restrain infants to prevent sudden movement.

Assessment	Findings
Select the largest speculum that fits comfortably into the ear canal. Hold the otoscope in an inverted position.	The ear canal is normally pink, but can be more pigmented in dark-skinned children, and has minute hairs.
Check the canal opening for foreign bodies and scratches.	The tympanic membrane is translucent and pearly pink or gray. Slight redness is normal in newborns and can be normal in older children and infants who have been crying. The tenseness of the membrane causes the otoscopic light to reflect at the 5 o'clock (right ear) or 7 o'clock (left ear) position. The light reflex is a cone-shaped reflection pointing away from the face. The umbo (tip of the malleus) appears as a small, round, concave spot near the middle of the eardrum. The manubrium (handle of the malleus) appears as a whitish line up from the umbo to the membrane margin. A sharp, knoblike protrusion at the 1 o'clock position represents the short process of the malleus (Figure 12-4).
Straighten the ear canal. In children younger than 3 years, pull the earlobe gently down and out. In children older than 3 years, pull the pinna up and back.	
Place the speculum in the canal. In children younger than 3 years, direct the speculum upward; in children older than 3 years, direct it downward and forward.	
Avoid sudden movement. In otoscopes with a pneumonic attachment, air can be introduced and removed from the ear canal by squeezing a rubber bulb during otoscopic examination.	
Inspect the ear canal for lesions, discharge, cerumen, and foreign bodies. Inspect the tympanic membrane for bony landmarks, color, fluid level, bubbles, scarring, holes, and vesicles.	

Clinical Alert

A red, bulging tympanic membrane, dull or absent light reflex, and obscured bony landmarks can indicate acute otitis media (erythema itself does not indicate acute otitis media).

Assessment	Findings
	A dull yellow or gray tympanic membrane can indicate serous otitis media.
	An ashen-gray membrane can suggest scarring from a previous rupture or perforation.
	A black area on the tympanic membrane suggests a perforation that has not yet healed. An area of thin-appearing membrane suggests a healed perforation.
	Absence of movement of the tympanic membrane with the introduction of air can indicate chronic ear infection.

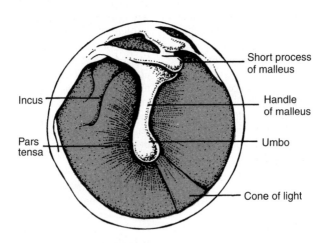

Figure 12-4

Usual landmarks of tympanic membrane.

(From Potter PA, Weilitz PB: *Pocket guide to health assessment,* ed 5, St Louis, 2003, Mosby.)

Assessment	Findings
	An apparent line that changes position with movement suggests fluid is present. Circles or rings behind the membrane suggest bubbles in the fluid. Vesicles on the membrane are suggestive of viral infections.

Related Nursing Diagnoses

Pain: related to infection.

Impaired social interaction: related to communication barriers.

Social isolation: related to inability to engage in satisfying personal relationships.

Impaired verbal communication: related to physical barrier, anatomic defect, alteration of central nervous system.

Impaired parenting: related to lack of resources, lack of knowledge about health maintenance, physical illness.

Altered family processes: related to shift in health status of family member.

Disorganized infant behavior: related to illness, congenital or genetic disorders, teratogenic exposure, sensory deprivation, cue misreading.

Sensory/perceptual alterations (visual, auditory): related to altered sensory perception, altered sensory reception.

Hyperthermia: related to illness affecting temperature regulation.

Chronic low self-esteem: related to perception of disability.

Risk for altered development: related to hearing impairment or frequent otitis media.

Eyes

13

Assessment of the eye involves examination of the external and internal eye, visual acuity, extraocular movement, position, alignment, and color vision.

Rationale

Disorders of vision can interfere with a child's ability to respond to stimuli, learn, and independently perform activities of daily living. The American Academy of Pediatrics recommends that assessment of the eye for children younger than 3 years include ocular history; vision, external eye, and ocular mobility assessments; and pupil and red reflex examinations. For children older than 3 years, the assessment also needs to include age-appropriate visual acuity measurement and ophthalmoscopy (if possible). Early detection and referral can minimize the effects of deficiencies in vision and prevent lifelong impairment. Vision disturbances can alert health practitioners to underlying congenital and acquired disorders.

Anatomy and Physiology

The eye is composed of three layers. The first, outermost layer consists of the sclera, or white of the eye, which is opaque, and the cornea, which is transparent (Figure 13-1). Underlying the cornea is the iris, which is colored and muscular. At its center is the pupil. The lens lies posterior to the pupil, which is suspended by ciliary muscles. A final layer, the retina, contains rods and cones, which receive visual stimuli and send them to the brain via the optic nerve. The fovea centralis, which appears as a small depression at the back of the retina, contains the most cones. The macula immediately surrounds the fovea centralis. The optic nerve enters the orb through the optic disk. Six muscles hold the eyes in position in their sockets. Coordinated movement of the muscles produces binocular vision.

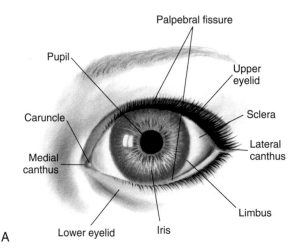

A

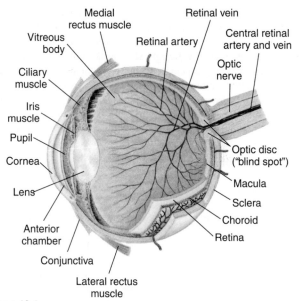

B

Figure 13-1

Normal structure of the eye. **A,** Anterior view. **B,** Cross-sectional view.

(**A** from Hockenberry MJ et al: *Wong's nursing care of infants and children,* ed 7, St Louis, 2003, Mosby; **B** from Seidel HM et al: *Mosby's guide to physical examination,* ed 5, St Louis, 2003, Mosby.)

The eyelid, which protects the eye, is lined with the conjunctiva, which is vascular.

At 22 days of gestation the eye appears, and by 8 weeks assumes its familiar form. Its structure and form continue to evolve until the child reaches school age. At birth, myelinization of the nerve fibers is complete and a pupillary response can be elicited. The newborn infant, however, has limited vision.

The neonate is able to identify the mother's form and is aware of light and motion, as evidenced by the blink reflex. Searching nystagmus is common. The definitive ability to follow objects is not developed until about 4 weeks of life, when the infant is able to follow light and objects to midline. By 8 weeks the infant is able to follow light past midline, although strabismus might be evident.

Intermittent convergent strabismus is common until 6 months of age, then disappears. The muscles assume completely mature function by 1 year. The macula and fovea centralis are structurally differentiated by 4 months. Macular maturation is achieved by 6 years of age. Color discrimination is present between 3 and 5 months. The infant is normally farsighted at birth. Like small children, infants see well at close range. Visual acuity in infants ranges from 20/300 to 20/50 (Table 13-1). The iris usually assumes permanent color by 6 months, but in some children not until 1 year. Lacrimation is present by 6 to 12 weeks of age.

Equipment for Eye Assessment

- Penlight
- Nonstretchable measuring tape
- Tape
- Visual acuity chart or system (choice of chart or system based on age of child)

Table 13-1   Visual Acuity in Infants and Children

Age	Visual Acuity
Birth	Infant fixates on objects 0.2 to 0.3 m (8 to 12 in) away (such as mother's face)
4 mo	20/300 to 20/50
3 yr	± 20/40
5 yr	20/30 to 20/20

- Snellen Letter chart
- Snellen E chart
- Blackbird Preschool Vision Screening System
- HOTV
- Allen cards
- Ishihara's test (for color vision)
- Occluder
- Pirate eye patches
- Stereoscopic glasses
- Ophthalmoscope

Preparation

Ask the parent or child if the child seems to see well or if the child seems clumsy, holds books close to eyes, rubs eyes excessively, sits close to the television, has difficulty seeing the board (school-age child), or responds to approaching objects without blinking (infant). Ask if the parents think that the child's eyes appear unusual or if they have noticed the child's eyelids drooping or tending to close in an unusual way. Inquire about school performance; the presence of pain, headache, dizziness, or nausea while doing close work; discharge; excessive tearing; squinting; blurred or double vision; burning; itching; and light sensitivity. Alert the physician to any of these symptoms. Inquire about history of eye injuries. Inquire whether there is a family history of vision problems (use of glasses in parents or siblings, glaucoma, color blindness) and whether the child wears glasses, contact lenses, or a prosthesis.

Assessment of External Eye

Assessment	Findings
Position and Placement	
Note whether the eyes are wide set (hypertelorism) or close set (hypotelorism). Measure the distance between the inner canthi, if in doubt (Figure 13-2).	Inner canthal distance averages 2.5 cm (1 in). Wide spaced eyes can be a normal variant in some children.
	Clinical Alert
	Hypertelorism is present in Down syndrome.

Assessment	Findings
Position and Placement—cont'd	
Observe for vertical folds that partially or completely cover the inner canthi.	Epicanthal folds are normally seen in Asian children and in some non-Asian children. **Clinical Alert** Epicanthal folds can indicate Down syndrome, renal agenesis, glycogen storage disease, or fetal alcohol syndrome.
Observe the slant of the eyes by drawing an imaginary line across the inner canthi (Figure 13-3).	The palpebral fissures lie horizontally along the imaginary line. Asian children normally have an upward slant to their eyes. **Clinical Alert** Upward slant of the eyes is present in Down syndrome and can be associated with infants exposed to AIDS/HIV. Short palpebral fissures can indicate fetal alcohol syndrome.

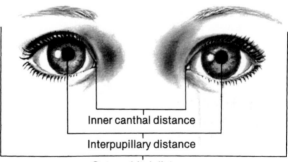

Inner canthal distance

Interpupillary distance

Outer orbital distance

Figure 13-2
Anatomic landmarks of the eye.
(From Hockenberry MJ et al: *Wong's nursing care of infants and children*, ed 7, St Louis, 2003, Mosby.)

Assessment	Findings
Position and Placement—cont'd	
Observe the eyelids for proper placement.	The eyelid falls between the upper border of the iris and the upper border of the pupil.
	Entropion, or turning-in of the eyelid, is a normal variant in Asian children.
	Clinical Alert
	Appearance of sclera between the upper lid and iris (sunset sign) is present in hydrocephalus, although it can be a normal variant.
	Drooping of the eyelid over the pupil (ptosis) can be a normal variant or can signal a variety of disorders, such as paralysis of the oculomotor cranial nerve or myasthenia.
	If the eyelids turn inward (entropion), the corners can become irritated by the eyelashes.
	If the eyelids turn outward (ectropion), the conjunctiva is exposed.

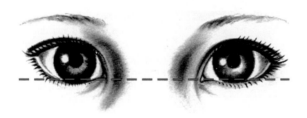

Figure 13-3
Upward palpebral slant.
(From Hockenberry MJ et al: *Wong's nursing care of infants and children,* ed 7, St Louis, 2003, Mosby.)

Assessment	Findings
Position and Placement—cont'd	
	Lid lag and incomplete closure of the eyelid can indicate hyperthyroidism.
Eyebrows	
Inspect the eyebrows for symmetry and hair growth.	Eyebrows normally are shaped and move symmetrically. They do not meet in midline.
Eyelids	
Observe distribution and condition of eyelashes.	Eyelashes curl outward.
Inspect eyelids for color, swelling, discharge (amount, type), and lesions.	Eyelids normally are the same color as the surrounding skin. **Clinical Alert** Flat, pink areas on eyelids can be telangiectatic nevi or "stork bite marks," which disappear by 1 year of age. A painful, red, swollen eyelid can indicate a stye. A nodular nontender area can be a chalazion (cyst). Puffiness can be related to thyroid or renal disorders. Swelling, redness, and purulent discharge can be related to inflammation of the lacrimal sac (dacryocystitis), often the result of a blocked tear duct, which can disappear as an infant reaches 6 months of age. If the area around the eyelids appears sunken, the child might be dehydrated. Shadow under the eyes can indicate fatigue or allergy. Persistent tearing or discharge can indicate infection, allergy, lacrimal duct obstruction, or glaucoma.

Assessment	Findings
Conjunctivae	
Inspect the lower lid by pulling down as the child looks up. Inspect the upper lid by holding the upper lashes and pulling down and forward gently as the child looks up.	The conjunctivae should be pink and glossy. Yellow striations along the edge are sebaceous glands near the hair follicle. The lacrimal punctum appears as a tiny opening in the medial canthus.
	Clinical Alert
	Redness of the conjunctivae can be related to bacterial or viral infection (including gonorrhea and chlamydia), allergy, or irritation.
	Redness and discharge can be indicative of avian flu, if there is also fever, cough, sore throat, myalgia, respiratory distress, and history of direct or indirect contact with chickens or pigs.
	A cobblestone appearance of the conjunctivae can accompany severe allergy.
	Excessive pallor of the conjunctivae can accompany anemia.
Inspect the bulbar conjunctivae for color.	The bulbar conjunctivae should be clear and transparent, allowing the white of the sclerae to be clearly visible.
	Clinical Alert
	Redness can indicate fatigue, eyestrain, irritation, or bleeding disorders.
	Overgrowth of conjunctival tissue (pterygium) can cover the cornea.
Inspect the sclerae for color.	The sclerae should be white and clear. Tiny black marks in dark-skinned children are normal.

Assessment	Findings
Conjunctivae—cont'd	
	Clinical Alert
	Yellow appearance can indicate jaundice.
	Bluish discoloration can indicate osteogenesis imperfecta, glaucoma, later stages of increased bilirubin, or prenatal exposure to AIDS/HIV.
Pupils and Irises	
Inspect the irises for color, shape, and inflammation.	Irises of different colors can be normal.
	Irises should be round and clear.
	The cornea covering the iris and pupil should be clear.
	Clinical Alert
	A notch at the outer edge of the iris (coloboma) can indicate a visual field defect and should be reported.
	White or light speckling of the iris (Brushfield's spots) can indicate Down syndrome.
	Absence of color and a pinkish glow can indicate albinism.
	Dome-shaped, clear to yellow or brown elevations (Lisch nodules) on the iris develop near the onset of puberty in children with neurofibromatosis.
Inspect the pupils for size, equality, and response to light. Observe and record the pupil size in normal room light.	Pupils are normally round and equal in size, although inequality is not uncommon and can be nonpathologic if other findings are normal.

Assessment	Findings
Pupils and Irises—cont'd	
Darken the room and observe the response of each pupil when light is directly shone into it (direct light reflex) and quickly removed. Assess the response of the pupils to light as the light is moved toward the face (accommodation). Assess the consensual light reflex by placing your nondominant hand down the midline of the eye and observing what happens when light is shone into the opposite eye. In infants younger than 5 months, check pupillary reaction by covering each eye with a hand and then uncovering the eye. Pupils that are equal, round, and react to light and accommodation are recorded as PERRLA.	Pupils should respond briskly to light. In the consensual reaction the pupil should constrict when light is shone in the contralateral eye. In infants younger than 5 months, pupil inequality is common but should be considered significant if it persists and is accompanied by other central nervous system findings. **Clinical Alert** Constriction of the pupils (miosis) can occur with iritis and with morphine administration. Dilation of pupils (mydriasis) can be related to emotional factors, acute glaucoma, some drugs, trauma, circulatory arrest, and anesthesia. Fixed unilateral dilation of a pupil can indicate local eye trauma or head injury. White or grayish spots in the pupils can indicate cataracts.

Assessment of Extraocular Movement

Two tests are commonly used to test binocular vision: the corneal light reflex test and the cover test. The random-dot-E stereoscopic test can be used to test depth perception in older children, which can indicate lesser degrees of imbalance in the eye muscles. The eyes are also assessed for nystagmus (rapid, jerky movements of the eye) through field-of-vision testing.

Assessment	Findings
Corneal Light Reflex Test (Red reflex gemini or Hirschberg test)	
Assess for strabismus by shining a light directly into the eyes from a distance of about 40 cm (16 in). Observe the site of the reflection in each pupil.	Normally the light falls symmetrically on each pupil. Epicanthal folds, often found in Asian children, can give an impression of malalignment.
	Intermittent alternating convergent strabismus is normal during the first 6 months of life.
	Clinical Alert
	Report any malalignment. If malalignment is present, the light falls off center in one eye and neither eye deviates.
	Infants with a birth weight of less than 1500 gm (3.3 lb) are more prone to muscle imbalance and warrant early, periodic screening.
Cover Test	
Ask the child to look at your nose; then cover one of the child's eyes. Observe whether the uncovered eye moves. Uncover the occluded eye and inspect for movement.	**Clinical Alert**
	Movement can indicate strabismus. Record the direction of any eye movement. Refer for further testing.
Random-dot-E Stereoscopic Test	
Test cards are held 40 cm (16 in) from the child's eyes. The child wears stereoscopic glasses while looking directly at cards that are presented randomly and from different angles. The cards consist of a blank card, a card with a raised E, and one with a	**Clinical Alert**
	Failure to identify the E card correctly may indicate lesser degrees of muscle imbalance.

Assessment	Findings

Random-dot-E Stereoscopic Test—cont'd

recessed E. The child must correctly identify the E card on four out of six attempts.

Field of Vision

Ask the child to follow a finger or shiny object through the six cardinal fields of gaze (Figure 13-4). Children younger than 2 or 3 years of age might not be able to cooperate with this test. Observe the eye movements of the younger child as the examination progresses.

A few beats of nystagmus in the far lateral gaze are normal.

Clinical Alert

Report easily elicited nystagmus.

Assessment of Color Vision

Color vision can be assessed by using Ishihara's test, which is composed of a set of cards with a series of round dots in the shape of a figure or number. The figures or numbers are not discernible by persons with impaired color vision. Color vision deficits and

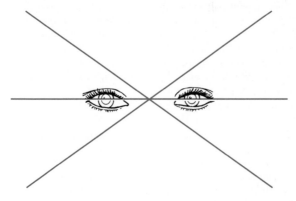

Figure 13-4
Six cardinal fields of gaze.

blindness can be indicated in younger children who have difficulty coordinating clothes colors or who have difficulty discerning their colors in school activities.

Assessment of Visual Acuity

Testing of visual acuity in children is not simple and can be directly affected by the child, nurse, and environment. There is no simple method to accurately test visual acuity in children younger than 3 years.

Assessment	Findings
Observe whether the infant blinks and exhibits dorsiflexion in response to light.	**Clinical Alert** Report absence of blink reflex.
Observe whether the infant of 4 weeks or older is able to fixate on a brightly colored object, maintain fixation, and follow the object through various gaze positions.	Drowsiness can interfere with the infant's interest in the object and ability to cooperate. **Clinical Alert** Report inability to follow an object, and reassess when older.
Snellen Letter Chart	
Hang the Snellen chart so that it lies smoothly and firmly on a light-colored wall and so that there is no glare on the chart. The chart should be placed so that the 20 to 30 foot lines are at the eye level of 6 to 12 year old children who are seated. Mark the correct distance from the chart with tape or with footprints. Have the child stand so that heels are touching the distance line or seated so that the back of the chair is on the line. Although most charts are designed to test from a distance of 6.2 m (20 ft.), a distance of 3.1m (10 ft.)	**Clinical Alert** Refer children with a two-line difference between eyes, even within pass range. Refer children, three years of age who have vision in either eye of 20/50 or less. Refer children of all other ages who have vision in either eye of 20/40 or less. Refer all children who show signs of possible visual disturbances (for example, squinting,

Assessment	Findings

Snellen Letter Chart—cont'd

is recommended for children as this distance enhances focus and cooperation. Test both eyes first, then the right eye, then the left eye by having the child cover each eye with an occluder, or with young children, a pirate patch. Unless the child has very poor vision, begin with the line on the chart that corresponds to a distance of 12.2 m (40 ft). If the child is unable to read this line, move up the chart until a line is found that the child can read and then begin to move down the chart again, until the child is unable to read the line. The child must be able to see four of six symbols or three out of four symbols on a line to correctly visualize the line. Record the results as a fraction, with the numerator representing the distance from the chart and the denominator the last line read correctly (hence 20/20 means that the child read the 20-foot line correctly from a distance of 20 feet or 6.2 m.) If testing from a distance of 3.1 m (10 ft), convert fractions to the standard 20-foot scale by multiplying the numerator by 2. Test with glasses or contact lenses if the child wears them. (A Snellen number chart is available for children who know their numbers.)

excessive tearing, or excessive blinking).

Assessment	Findings

Snellen Letter Chart—cont'd

If using the Snellen E or tumbling E chart, have the child indicate the direction of the E's "legs" with his or her fingers or with a cardboard E. Use the 20/100 E to determine whether the child understands what to do. Proceed as for regular Snellen testing. The tumbling E is useful for children 4 years and older who are unable to read numbers and letters.

HOTV Test

The HOTV test involves a wall chart composed of Hs, Os, Ts, and Vs. The child is asked to match the symbol to which the examiner is pointing on the chart with the correct letter on a board that the child holds.

Blackbird Preschool Vision Screening System

Using either the wall-mounted chart or flashcards, ask the child to indicate direction of the bird's flight. This system is useful for nonreaders and children whose first language is not English.

Allen Cards

Show the child the cards at close range and have the child name the pictures from a distance of 4.6 m (15 ft). Test each eye, if possible. The Allen cards are useful for young children (2 to 4 years) who are unable to perform the HOTV or tumbling E tests.

The child should be able to name three of seven cards in a maximum of five tries.

Assessment	Findings

Visual Acuity in Young Infants

Assessment	Findings
Assess for visual acuity in young infants by shining a light into the eyes and noting blinking, pupil constriction, and following of light to midline.	**Clinical Alert** Fixed pupils, constant nystagmus, and slow lateral movements can indicate visual loss in young infants.

Ophthalmoscopic Examination

Ophthalmoscopic examination requires practice and patience, as well as a cooperative child. In young infants and children it might be possible to elicit only the red reflex. The retina, choroid, optic nerve disk, macula, fovea centralis, and retinal vessels are visualized with the ophthalmoscope.

Darken the room. Sit the child on the parent's lap or examination table or lay the child on the table. Have the child remove glasses unless glasses are worn to correct astigmatism, which can distort images. Use your right hand and eye to examine the child's right eye and your left hand and eye for the left eye. Ask the child to gaze straight ahead, or use your nondominant hand to attract the child's gaze away from the light source of the ophthalmoscope.

Assessment	Findings
Perform the examination in a dimly lit room and have the child remove glasses, unless glasses are worn to correct astigmatism, which can cause distortion of images. Set the dial of the ophthalmoscope at +8 to +2. Approach from a distance of 30.5 cm (12 in), centering the light in the eye. The pupil glows red (red reflex). Gradually move closer and change the dial of the ophthalmoscope	In infants the optic disk is pale and the peripheral vessels are not well developed. The red reflex appears lighter in infants. In children the red reflex appears as a brilliant, reddish-yellow (or light gray in dark-skinned, brown-eyed children) uniform glow. The optic disk is creamy white to pinkish, with clear margins. At the center of the optic disk is a small depression (the physiologic cup). Arteries are smaller and

Assessment	Findings
to plus or minus diopters to focus. Move the ophthalmoscope up and down and from side to side to visualize eye structures.	brighter than veins. The macula is the same size as the optic disk and located to the right of the disk. The fovea is a glistening spot in the center of the macula.

Clinical Alert

Report a partial or white reflex, dark spots in the red reflex, blurring of the disk margins, bulging of the disk, and hemorrhage.

Blockage of the red reflex can indicate cataract.

Papilledema in an older child can indicate acute head injury. Retinal hemorrhage is also associated with acute head injury and Shaken Baby syndrome.

Related Nursing Diagnoses

Risk for injury: related to sensory dysfunction.

Risk for trauma: related to reduced eye-hand coordination, poor vision.

Altered health maintenance: related to significant alteration or lack of communication skills.

Social isolation: related to factors contributing to the absence of satisfying personal relationships.

Impaired social interactions: related to communication barriers.

Altered parenting: related to lack of knowledge about child health maintenance, illness.

Altered family processes: related to shift in health status of a member, situation transition.

Sensory/perceptual alterations (visual): related to altered sensory perception.

Disorganized infant behavior: related to sensory deprivation.

Risk for altered development: related to vision impairment.

Impaired tissue integrity: related to irritants, mechanical factors, chemical factors, lack of knowledge.

Impaired comfort: related to infection, irritation, trauma, strain.

Face, Nose, and Oral Cavity

14

Rationale

The face provides a map of the child's emotional status and clues to neurologic, congenital, and allergic conditions. The nose provides entry to the respiratory tract, and the mouth provides entry to the digestive tract. Examination of the nose, mouth, and sinuses provides information about the functioning of the respiratory and digestive tracts and about the overall health of the child.

The common occurrence of tonsillitis provides reason enough for inspection of the oropharynx; however, examination of the nose, oral cavity, and oropharynx also yields valuable information about congenital anomalies, nutritional status, feeding practices, hydration, hygienic practices, and overall health. The information obtained can be used in the prevention, early detection, and nursing management of such disorders.

Anatomy and Physiology

The face of the newborn infant and child is noticeably different from that of the adult. Typically the neonate appears to have a slightly receding chin. By 6 years of age the mandible and maxilla have grown significantly in length and width and the chin shows greater development. A 6-year-old child has approximately 80% of the facial dimensions of the adult.

Sinuses are air pockets adjacent to the nasal passage. Only the ethmoid and maxillary sinuses are present at birth (Figure 14-1). The frontal sinus develops at around 7 years of age, and the sphenoid sinus develops in adolescence. Development of the sinuses is assisted by enlarging skull bones.

The nose warms, filters, and moistens air entering the respiratory tract and is the organ of smell. Infants have a narrow bridge and are obligate nose breathers, which readily predisposes them to

185

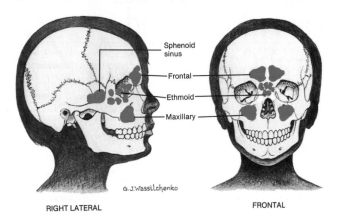

Figure 14-1
Location of sinuses.
(From Hockenberry MJ et al: *Wong's nursing care of infants and children,* ed 7, St Louis, 2003, Mosby.)

compromise of the upper airway. The sense of smell is poor at birth but develops with age.

The mouth of the young infant is short, smooth, and has a relatively long, soft palate. The tongue appears large in the shorter oral cavity and tends to press into the concavity of the roof of the mouth, which allows milk to flow back to the pharynx. By 6 months of age the mouth is proportioned like that of the adult. Until approximately 4 months of age the infant demonstrates an active tongue thrust, or extrusion reflex, in which the tongue is pressed under the nipple. This reflex is of concern to some parents, who think that the infant is rejecting solid foods by thrusting them out as soon as they are placed on the tongue. By approximately 6 months of age the rhythmic up-and-down sucking motions of the tongue become the more adult forward-backward tongue movement. The rooting reflex, in which the infant turns the mouth in the direction that the cheek is touched, assists in food attainment and is seen in the infant younger than 3 or 4 months.

Typically the infant of 3 months begins to drool as salivation increases. The increased saliva production, together with an inappropriate swallowing reflex and lack of lower teeth, allows saliva to flow outward.

The sense of taste is immature at birth but becomes acute by 2 to 3 months as taste buds mature; however, the sense of taste is not fully functional until approximately 2 years of age, as evidenced by the strange things that young children ingest.

In newborn infants the gingivae (gums) are smooth, with a raised fringe of tissue along the gum line. Pearlike areas might be seen along the gingivae. These are often mistaken for teeth but are retention cysts and disappear in 1 to 2 months. True dentition begins at approximately 6 months of age, when the lower central incisors appear. By 30 months the child has 20 teeth and primary dentition is complete (Figure 14-2). During middle childhood the permanent

	Age of eruption (mo)	Average age of shedding (yr)
Maxilla	9.6	7.5
	12.4	8
	18.3	11.5
	15.7	10.5
	26.2	10.5
	26.0	11
	15.1	10
	18.2	9.5
Mandible	11.5	7
A	7.8	6

Figure 14-2
Primary and secondary dentition. **A,** Sequence of eruption and shedding of teeth.

Continued

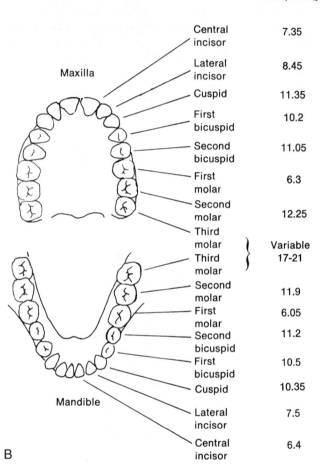

Average age
of eruption (yr)

Maxilla	
Central incisor	7.35
Lateral incisor	8.45
Cuspid	11.35
First bicuspid	10.2
Second bicuspid	11.05
First molar	6.3
Second molar	12.25
Third molar	Variable 17-21

Mandible	
Third molar	Variable 17-21
Second molar	11.9
First molar	6.05
Second bicuspid	11.2
First bicuspid	10.5
Cuspid	10.35
Lateral incisor	7.5
Central incisor	6.4

B

Figure 14-2—cont'd
B, Sequence of eruption of secondary teeth.
(From Wong DL: Whaley & Wong's essentials of pediatric nursing, ed 4, St Louis, 1993, Mosby.)

molars erupt and the primary teeth are lost. The typical 6 year old appears toothless because of the loss of the middle teeth. Tooth eruptions and losses are genetically predetermined.

Tonsils are found in the pharyngeal cavity and are part of the lymphatic system. Several pairs of tonsils make up Waldeyer's tonsillar ring, which encircles the pharynx; but only the palatine, or faucial, tonsil is readily visible behind the faucial pillars in the oropharynx (Figure 14-3). The pharyngeal tonsils and adenoids are located on the posterior wall of the oropharynx. Although tonsillar tissue begins to shrink by approximately 7 years of age, the child normally has larger tonsils and adenoids than either the adolescent or adult.

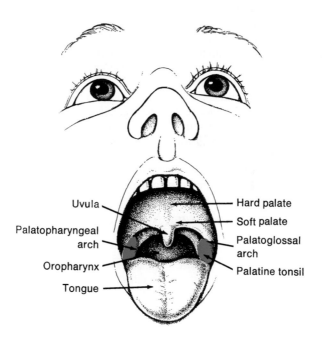

Figure 14-3
Interior structures of mouth.
(From Hockenberry MJ et al: *Wong's nursing care of infants and children*, ed 7, St Louis, 2003, Mosby.)

Equipment for Face, Nose, and Oral Cavity Assessment

- Tongue blade (flavored, if available)
- Penlight
- Glove

Preparation

Inquire whether the child is a mouth breather or has or has had frequent sore throats; epistaxis; allergies; hay fever; fever; difficulty swallowing; vocal changes (e.g., hoarseness, nasality); or recent contact with persons with communicable disease. Ask about oral hygiene practices and date of last dental visit (if 1 year or older). Ask if the child is receiving medications.

Infants and children find examination of the mouth intrusive, and it is best left until the end of the examination. The nurse often has an opportunity to visualize the oral cavity without a tongue blade when the infant or child cries, laughs, or yawns. Infants and young children are often more comfortable on the parent's lap during this part of the examination and can be reclined slightly for a better view. Letting the child examine the parent's mouth or that of a puppet can assist in relieving apprehension about the examination. Having the child tilt the head slightly and breathe deeply can eliminate the need for use of the tongue blade as this will lower the tongue to the floor of the mouth. Infants and young children might need restraining.

Assessment of Face and Nose

Assessment	Findings
Observe the spacing and size of facial features.	Infants who were premature might have a narrow forehead.
	Clinical Alert
	Coarse features combined with a low hairline and large tongue can indicate cretinism.
	An enlarged forehead can indicate hydrocephalus or ectodermal dysplasia.

Assessment	Findings
	A long, narrow face with prominent jaw can suggest fragile X syndrome, especially if there are developmental and language delays.
	A flat midface, thin upper lip, smooth philtrum, and micrognathia can be suggestive of fetal alcohol syndrome.
Carefully observe the facial expression, especially around the eyes and mouth.	**Clinical Alert**
	A child with a persistently sad and forlorn expression might be abused, particularly if bruises can be detected on the body.
	A child who demonstrates an open mouth and facial contortions might be suffering from allergic rhinitis.
	Shadows under the eyes can indicate fatigue or allergy.
Observe the symmetry of the nasolabial folds as the child cries and smiles.	Normal nasolabial folds are symmetric.
	Clinical Alert
	Asymmetry of the nasolabial folds can indicate facial nerve impairment or Bell's palsy.
Tilt the head backward and push the tip of the nose upward to visualize the internal nasal cavity. Use a penlight for better illumination. Observe the integrity, color, and consistency of the mucosa, the position of the septum, and for perforation of the septum. Perforation will be indicated by light showing through the perforation to the other nostril.	The nasal mucosa should be firm and pink.
	Clinical Alert
	A pale, boggy nasal mucosa, with or without pink-grape polyps, indicates allergic rhinitis.
	A red mucosa indicates infection.
	Excoriation of the nasal mucosa can indicate nose picking, a common cause of epistaxis in children, or cocaine or amphetamine use.

Assessment	Findings
Usually inspection without a speculum is adequate; however, if closer examination is warranted, a short-barreled speculum, attached to the otoscope, can be used. Explain beforehand what will happen and insert the speculum into the nasal passageway, avoiding the septum. Tilt the otoscope upward to straighten the passageway toward the posterior wall.	Grayish soft outgrowths of mucosa are polyps that can partially obstruct the nares. Report any deviation of the nasal septum. Diminished nasal hair can suggest cocaine or amphetamine use.
Observe the size and shape of the nose. Draw an imaginary line down the center of the face between the eyes and down the notch of the upper lip.	The nose should be symmetric and in the center of the face. A flattened bridge is sometimes seen in Asian and black children.
	Clinical Alert
	A flattened nose can indicate congenital anomalies and should be reported. Fissures associated with cleft lip can extend to the nostril and involve one or both nostrils.
	Clinical Alert
Observe the external nares for flaring, discharge, excoriation, and odor.	Flaring external nares can indicate respiratory distress or crying. The skin of the external nares should be intact. No discharge should be seen, although a clear, watery discharge might be present if the child has been crying.

Assessment	Findings
	Excoriation of the external nares can indicate the presence of an irritating discharge and frequent nose wiping.
	A clear, thin, nasal discharge is often present with allergic rhinitis. Purulent yellow or green discharge accompanies infection.
	Clear nasal discharge that tests positive for glucose after a head injury or dental or nose surgery can suggest leakage of spinal fluid.
	A foul odor and discharge from one nostril can indicate the presence of a foreign body.
Test the patency of the nares by placing the diaphragm of the stethoscope under one nostril while blocking the other. A film appears on the diaphragm if the naris is patent. While assessing patency, the sense of smell can also be assessed. While each nostril is blocked, ask the child to close his or her eyes and to identify distinctive odors such as coffee and lemon. The child should be able to correctly identify each.	Both nares should be patent. **Clinical Alert** Diminished smell can indicate olfactory nerve impairment or upper respiratory infection. Occlusion of the nostrils can indicate upper respiratory infection, presence of a foreign body, deviated septum, allergies, or nasal polyps.
Palpate above the eyebrows and on each side of the nose to determine whether pain and tenderness are present.	**Clinical Alert** Pain and tenderness in these regions can indicate sinusitis.

Assessment of Oral Cavity

Assessment	Findings
Inspect the lips for color, symmetry, moisture, swelling, sores, and fissures.	The lips should be intact, pink, and firm. **Clinical Alert** Blueness of the lips is a reliable sign of cyanosis in fair-skinned children; ashen coloration can indicate cyanosis in dark-skinned children. Deep red coloration can be present during an asthmatic attack. Pallor can indicate anemia. Cherry red coloration is seen with acidosis. Cracked lips are usually the result of harsh climate, lip biting, mouth breathing, or fever. Fissures at the corners of the mouth can indicate deficiency of riboflavin or niacin. Notching of the vermillion border of the lip indicates cleft lip. Drooping of one side of the lips indicates facial nerve impairment. A thin upper lip and long philtrum can suggest fetal alcohol syndrome, if other features of the syndrome are present.
Inspect the buccal margins, gingivae, tongue, and palate for moisture, color, intactness, and bleeding.	The oral membranes are normally pink, firm, smooth, and moist. The buccal cavity, tongue margins, and gums appear bluish in black children.

Assessment	Findings
To inspect the buccal mucosa, ask the child to use his or her fingers to move the outer lip and cheek to one side. With toddlers and infants, it is necessary to use a tongue blade, unless a good view is possible while the child is crying. When using the tongue blade, slide it along the side of the tongue.	**Clinical Alert** Clefts or notches in the hard or soft palate should be noted. An abnormally high, narrow arch can cause problems with sucking in the infant and with speech in the older child. White ulcerated sores on the oral mucosa are cankers, related to mild trauma, viral infection, or local irritants. Saltlike areas rimmed with red and found on the inner cheek opposite the second molar are Koplik's spots and indicate the onset of measles.
Use a glove and penlight for clearer visualization of any suspected abnormalities.	White curdy patches on the gum margins, inner cheeks, tongue, or palate usually indicate thrush (oral moniliasis).
Observe for the presence of odor or halitosis.	Thrush is common in infants (particularly during or following antibiotic therapy), but in children could indicate a deficient immune system disorder such as AIDS or HIV infection. These patches can be distinguished from milk curds in that they cannot be easily scraped away. Petechiae on oral mucous membranes can indicate presence of emboli, accidental biting, or infection. Hyperplasic gum tissue can be related to anticonvulsant therapy.

Assessment	Findings
	Reddened, swollen, bleeding gums can indicate infection, poor nutrition, or poor oral hygiene.
	A red tongue is related to vitamin deficiencies and to scarlet fever ("strawberry tongue").
	A gray, furrowed tongue can be normal or can indicate drug ingestion, allergy, or fever.
	Odor or halitosis can indicate poor oral hygiene, tooth decay, constipation, dehydration, sinusitis, food trapped in tonsillar crypts, diabetic ketoacidosis or other systemic illness.
	Drooling accompanied by fever and respiratory distress is indicative of epiglottitis.
	Dry, sticky mucous membranes suggest dehydration or mouth breathing.
Inspect the tongue for movement and size. The older child can be asked to reach the tip of the tongue to the roof of the mouth.	The frenulum attaches to the undersurface of the tongue or near its tip, allowing the child to reach the areolar ridge with the tip of the tongue.
	Clinical Alert
Observe the movement of the tongue in infants and younger children as they vocalize or cry.	Inability to touch the tongue to the areolar ridge can signify tongue tie and later speech problems.
	Glossoptosis, or tongue protrusion, is seen in mental retardation and cerebral palsy.

Assessment	Findings
Inspect the teeth for number, type, condition, and occlusion. To estimate the number of teeth that should be present in a child 2 years of age or younger, subtract 6 months from the child's age in months. Ask the child who is 5 years or older if teeth are loose. To assess malocclusion, ask the child to bite teeth together. Observe for fillings and braces.	A normal 30-month-old child has 20 temporary teeth. A child with full permanent dentition has 32 teeth. The upper teeth should slightly override the lower teeth. **Clinical Alert** Brown and black spots usually indicate caries. Mottling can indicate excessive fluoride intake. Green and black staining can accompany oral iron intake. Extensive decay of the maxillary or upper incisors and molars in infants and young children suggests bottle or nursing caries. An increase in dental caries in adolescents can indicate frequent, self-induced vomiting. Absent, delayed, or peg teeth can indicate ectodermal dysplasia. Protrusion of the lower teeth or marked protrusion of the upper teeth should be noted.
Tonsils can be inspected in the older child by asking the child to say "Ahh" or to yawn. Asking the child to tilt the head slightly back, to breathe deeply, and to hold the breath can also aid in visualization.	Tonsils, if present, are normally the same color as the buccal mucosa. They are large in the preschool-age and young school-age child and appear larger as they move toward the uvula. Crypts might be present on their surface.

Assessment	Findings
If the child has difficulty holding the tongue down, the tongue can be *lightly* depressed with the tongue blade on either side. Playing games and demonstrating what is expected of the child through the use of a parent or doll can be very useful. If the nurse is unable to observe the tonsil bed while the infant or older child is crying, the tongue blade can be slid between the lips, along the side of the gum, then quickly slipped between the gums along the side of the tongue. *Any inspection of the pharynx that involves use of the tongue blade and that might elicit the gag reflex must not be performed on a child who is suspected to have any of the croup syndromes.*	**Clinical Alert** Reddened tonsils covered with white exudate suggest group A hemolytic streptococcal infection or infectious mononucleosis. Thick, gray exudate can indicate diphtheric tonsillitis. Visualization of adenoids suggests that they are enlarged. If adenoids are visualized during gagging or saying "Ahh," they appear as grapelike structures.
Observe movement of the uvula during examination of the tonsils.	The uvula remains in midline. Upon gagging the uvula moves upward.
Movement of the uvula can be assessed by producing a gag reflex.	**Clinical Alert** Deviation of the uvula or absence of movement can signal involvement of the glossopharyngeal or vagus nerves. Producing the gag reflex in a child with epiglottitis could produce total obstruction.

Assessment	Findings
Observe the quality of the voice.	**Clinical Alert** A nasal quality to the voice suggests enlarged adenoids. A hoarse cry or voice can indicate croup, cretinism, tetany, or congenital hypothyroidism. A shrill, high-pitched cry can indicate increased intracranial pressure.

Related Nursing Diagnoses

Ineffective airway clearance: related to retained secretions, excessive mucus, foreign body in airway, infection, asthma, allergic airways.

Altered oral mucous membrane: related to barriers to professional care, immunosuppression, cleft lip or palate, medication side effects, trauma, NPO status, mouth breathing, malnutrition or vitamin deficiency, dehydration, infection, ineffective oral hygiene, mechanical factors, impaired salivation.

Impaired skin integrity: related to altered nutritional state, altered fluid status.

Altered dentition: related to ineffective oral hygiene, barriers to self-care, barriers to professional care, nutritional deficits, dietary habits, genetic predisposition, selected prescription drugs, premature loss of primary teeth, excessive intake of fluorides, chronic vomiting, lack of knowledge regarding dental health, bruxism.

Risk for infection: related to inadequate primary defenses, inadequate secondary defenses, malnutrition, insufficient knowledge to avoid exposure to pathogens, immunosuppression.

Impaired verbal communication: related to anatomic defect.

Impaired swallowing: related to congenital deficits, neurologic problems.

Ineffective infant feeding pattern: related to anatomic abnormality.

Sensory/perceptual alterations (gustatory, olfactory): related to altered sensory perception.

Risk for fluid volume deficit: related to deviations affecting intake.

Altered nutrition, less than body requirements: related to inability to ingest food because of biologic factors.

Altered family processes: related to shift in health status of a family member.

Thorax and Lungs

15

Assessment of the respiratory system includes close observation of the child's behavior and assessment of the thorax and the anterior and posterior chest.

Rationale

Respiratory disorders are common in infancy and childhood and can be acute, life threatening, or chronic. Early screening and detection are essential to being able to refer children for medical treatment. Knowledgeable assessment also assists in monitoring the progress of treatment.

Anatomy and Physiology

Lungs have two main functions: to supply the body with oxygen and eliminate carbon dioxide and to maintain the body's acid-base balance. The lungs are paired and symmetric. The right lung has three lobes, and the left lung has two lobes. Air enters the lungs via the trachea and larynx from the mouth or nose. The trachea branches into two major bronchi. The right bronchus is shorter, wider, and angled less sharply to the side than the left.

Fetal lung buds arise in the first lunar month of gestation, along with nasal pits, the trachea, and the larynx. Subsequent budding and branching create the mainstem bronchi pulmonary lobules in the second month. Branching continues into early childhood, although it is less proliferative. By the third month, elementary respiratory-like movements are observed. From the sixth month on, the lobules have developed alveolar ducts, and the ducts have developed alveoli.

As the alveolar sacs develop, the epithelium lining the sacs thins. Pulmonary capillaries press into the walls of the sacs as the lungs are prepared for the exchange of oxygen and carbon dioxide, near the end of the sixth month of gestation. During the final weeks of gestation the lungs secrete surfactants that reduce the surface tension of the alveolar sacs and prevent the alveoli from collapsing and producing atelectasis. At birth, the lungs are fluid filled. This fluid is rapidly dispelled and absorbed as the lungs fill with air.

The newborn infant's thoracic cage is nearly round. Gradually the transverse diameter increases until the chest assumes the elliptic shape of the adult, at about 6 years of age. The infant's thoracic cage is also relatively soft, which allows the cage to pull in during labored breathing. Infants have relatively less tissue and cartilage in the trachea and bronchi, which allows these structures to collapse more readily.

Airways tend to grow faster than the vertebral column. In infancy the bifurcation of the trachea is at the level of the third thoracic vertebra. By adulthood the bifurcation is at the level of the fourth thoracic vertebra. Smaller airways in young children and infants tend to narrow more readily from edema and secretions than in older children and adolescents. Shorter distances between structures in the young child also contribute to rapid transmission of organisms and widespread involvement.

Young infants (younger than 6 months) are obligatory nose breathers, and their nasal passages are narrower. Breathing is less rhythmic than in the child. In infants and children younger than 6 or 7 years, respirations are chiefly diaphragmatic or abdominal; in older children and especially females, respirations are chiefly thoracic. The volume of oxygen expired by the infant and the child is greater than that expired by the adult. The volume of air that is inspired increases as the child grows. At the age of 12 years the child has approximately nine times the number of alveoli that were present at birth.

As with heart rate, the respiratory rate in infants and children responds more dramatically than in adults to emotion, illness, and exercise. The rate tends to show greater variability and wider range than in adults.

Equipment for Assessment of Thorax and Lungs

- Stethoscope
- Pulse oximeter

Preparation

Ask the parent or child about cough (onset, progress, pattern, secretions), fever, shortness of breath, difficulty breathing, chest pain (or pain at the base of the neck), wheezing, easy fatigability, meningeal signs, abdominal pain, vomiting, sore throat, past respiratory tract infections, frequent colds, family history of respiratory disorders and smoking, history of allergies, immunization status, and type of child care setting (e.g., home, daycare) and environment (e.g., animals, birds, second-hand smoke).

Allow the young child to play with the stethoscope before you perform the assessment. Children often enjoy listening to the sounds in their chests and in their parents' or the nurse's chest. Remove the child's shirt or blouse for best visualization of the chest. Infants and toddlers are often best assessed while held by their parents.

Assessment of Thorax and Lungs

Assessment	Findings
Assess for stridor (high-pitched crowing sound), grunting, hoarseness, snoring, labored breathing, audible wheezing, and cough (Table 15-1). Precisely describe the sounds and their occurrence.	**Clinical Alert** Stridor, hoarseness, and a barking cough accompany croup syndromes. Inspiratory stridor and expiratory snoring are indicative of epiglottitis. Audible wheezing can indicate asthma, respiratory syncytial virus, or foreign body aspiration. Short, rapid coughs followed by a crowing sound or whoop indicate whooping cough. Snoring can indicate enlargement of the adenoids, polyps, or presence of a foreign body. A persistent dry cough that later becomes productive, hoarseness, and gasping and grunting respirations are found with congestive heart failure.

Assessment	Findings
Observe the external nares for flaring.	**Clinical Alert** Flaring is a significant sign of respiratory distress in infants (although this can also be observed in the crying infant).
Observe the nailbeds for color and for clubbing (widening and l engthening) of the terminal phalanges (Figure 15-1).	**Clinical Alert** Cyanosis (bluish coloration of nailbeds) is sometimes indicative of respiratory failure. Cyanosis can also be related to vasoconstriction or polycythemia. Clubbing usually indicates chronic hypoxemia, as in cystic fibrosis and bronchiectasis.
Evaluate oxygen saturation (Sao_2) levels through pulse oximetry. If using fingers for sensor placement, remove nail polish because it can distort readings. Placement distal to a blood pressure cuff can also distort readings. Observe the color of the child's trunk.	The normal reference range for Sao_2 for infants, children, and adolescents is 75% to 100%. **Clinical Alert** Mottling and cyanosis of the trunk indicate severe hypoxemia and usually are indicative of cardiopulmonary disease.
Inspect the thorax for configuration, symmetry, and abnormalities. Measure the size of the chest by placing a tape around the chest at the nipple line. For greatest accuracy, record measurement during inspiration and expiration and average the two. Chest size is largely important in relation to head circumference in infants.	The chest is rounder in young children. By 6 years of age the ratio of anteroposterior diameter to transverse diameter is about 1:35. In some infants the sternum is so pliant that the chest appears to cave in with each breath. The thorax should move symmetrically. **Clinical Alert** A round chest in an older child usually indicates a chronic lung disorder.

Assessment	Findings
	A protuberant sternum (pectus carinatum, or pigeon breast) or depressed sternum (pectus excavatum) should be noted. Either can compromise lung expansion.
	Decreased movement of one side of the thorax can indicate pneumonia, pneumothorax, or a foreign body.
	Enlargement of one side of the thorax can indicate a diaphragmatic hernia. Enlargement of the left side can indicate an enlarged heart.
Note the size of the breasts in relation to the age of the child.	Enlarged breasts can be seen in the young infant as a result of maternal hormonal influences.
	Clinical Alert
	Enlarged breasts (gynecomastia) in older male children can indicate obesity or hormonal or systemic problems.
Observe the chest for retractions, or indrawings, in the clavicular (above the clavicles), suprasternal (in the sternal notch), substernal (below the sternum), subcostal (anterior lower rib margins) and intercostal (between the ribs) areas (Figure 15-2).	**Clinical Alert**
	Retractions indicate labored breathing in infants and children.
	Puffiness accompanies severe air trapping.
	Head bobbing in an exhausted or sleeping infant on inspiration can indicate use of accessory muscles and severe respiratory disease.
Puffiness or bulging of these areas can also be present.	In children younger than 7 years respirations are diaphragmatic, and the abdomen rises with inspiration. In girls older than 7 years breathing becomes thoracic. Abdomen and chest should move together regardless of type of breathing.
Observe the child for type of breathing.	

Assessment	Findings
	Clinical Alert
	Abdominal breathing in an older child can indicate a respiratory disorder or fractured rib.
	In labored abdominal breathing the abdomen pushes out abruptly.
Observe the depth and regularity of respirations and the duration of inspiration in relation to expiration.	**Clinical Alert**
	A prolonged expiratory phase can indicate an obstructive respiratory problem, such as asthma.
	Deep respirations (hyperpnea) can indicate fever (the respiratory rate increases four breaths per minute for every degree increase in Fahrenheit temperature), respiratory acidosis associated with diabetes or diarrhea, or central nervous system involvements.
	Shallow respirations (hypopnea) can indicate respiratory acidosis that is associated with central nervous system depression or pleural irritation.

Palpation

Assessment	Findings
To assess respiratory excursion, place your hands, thumbs together, along the costal margins of the child's chest or back while the child is sitting.	Movement is symmetric with each breath.
	Posterior base descends approximately 6 cm (2.3 in) during deep inspiration.
Palpate for tactile fremitus by using either the fingertips or the palmar surfaces of your hands. Move symmetrically while the child says "99" or "blue moon."	Fremitus is normally less at the base of the lung.
	Clinical Alert
	Decreased fremitus can indicate asthma, pneumothorax, or a foreign body.

Assessment	Findings
Palpation—cont'd	
In the infant, fremitus can be felt as the infant cries. Note other vibrations, as well, during palpation.	Increased fremitus occurs with pneumonia and atelectasis.
	A pleural friction rub (felt as grating during respiratory movements) occurs with pneumonia and tuberculosis.
	Crepitation (coarse, crackling sensation as fingers press against the skin) indicates escaped air from the lungs in the tissues, associated with injury or surgery.
Percussion	
Percussion is more useful in older children.	Resonance (a low, long sound) is heard over all lung surfaces.
Using the indirect method, percuss the anterior and posterior chest.	Dullness can be heard over the fifth right intercostal space, because of the liver, and over the second to fifth left intercostal space, because of the heart.
Percuss over the intercostal spaces, moving symmetrically and systematically. The child can sit or lie while the anterior chest is percussed, and sit while the posterior chest is percussed.	Tympany (a loud, musical sound) can be heard over the sixth left intercostal space.
	Clinical Alert
	The percussion note is dull if fluid or a mass is present in the lungs.
	Hyperresonance occurs during an asthmatic episode.
Auscultation	
Using the warmed diaphragm and bell of the stethoscope, auscultate the lung fields systematically and symmetrically from apex to base. The bell is used for low-pitched sounds and	Breath sounds (Table 15-2) normally seem louder and harsher in the infant and young child because of the thinness of the chest wall.
	Vocal sounds are normally heard as indistinct syllables.

Assessment	Findings

Auscultation—cont'd

the diaphragm for high-pitched sounds.

Use a pediatric diaphragm or the bell for infants and small children. Children can be encouraged to breathe deeply by pretending to blow up balloons or blow out candles, or by blowing away a piece of tissue or cotton ball.

Auscultate the axillae of children with pneumonia. Rales or crackles can be easily heard in these areas.

Auscultate for vocal resonance by asking the child to say "99" or count from 1.

Sounds can be referred from the upper respiratory tract if a child has mucus in the nose or throat. To determine if sounds are referred, place the diaphragm near the child's mouth. Referred sounds are loudest near their origin and are symmetric.

Clinical Alert

Report any adventitious sounds (Table 15-3) or breath sounds heard in other than expected areas. If unable to name the sound heard, describe it. Asymmetric rhonchi or wheezes can signal presence of a foreign body. Unilaterally absent breath sounds can indicate pneumothorax. In infants, breath sounds can be diminished, and not absent, in pneumothorax. Inaudible breath sounds and crackles can indicate severe spasm or obstruction during an asthmatic episode.

Decreased or absent vocal sounds are found with asthma, pneumothorax, or a foreign body.

Whispered pectoriloquy (words are heard on whispering), bronchophony (words are not distinguishable but sounds are clear and loud), and egophony ("ee" is heard as "ay") can be indicative of lung consolidation.

Table 15-1   Characteristics and Common Etiologies of Cough in Infants and Children

Characteristics of Cough	Pattern and Progression of Cough	Fever	Common Age Group Affected	Associated Symptoms	Possible Etiology
Dry, hacking	Can become productive of mucoid or blood-streaked sputum.	Low-grade to high	Any	■ Headache ■ Malaise ■ Dyspnea ■ Fine rales	Viral pneumonia
Dry, hacking, harsh	More pronounced than with common cold. Tends to become more persistent and annoying by end of second week. Can progress to paroxysmal stage, in which cough involves explosive bursts on expiration, followed by an inspiratory "whoop."	None to low-grade	Any but primarily in children younger than 4 years, who have not been immunized	■ Copious lacrimation and coryza ■ Looks distressed while coughing; face becomes red or cyanotic ■ Eyes prominent while coughing ■ Can have retinal hemorrhages ■ Vomits thick, tenacious material with coughing	Pertussis (whooping cough)

Congestive heart failure			
Dry, hacking, persistent	Coughing can be precipitated by eating or drinking, especially milk. Can progress to a productive cough.	Absent	Any; frequently secondary to congenital health defects in which structural defects lead to increased volume load or pressure on the ventricles	<ul><li>Tachypnea</li><li>Dyspnea</li><li>Rales</li><li>Orthopnea</li><li>Hoarseness</li><li>Gasping/grunting respirations</li><li>Wheezing</li><li>Cyanosis</li><li>Fatigue</li><li>Restlessness</li><li>Anorexia</li><li>Pale, cool extremities</li><li>Decreased pulse</li><li>Gallup rhythm</li><li>Poor weight gain (infants)</li></ul>

Continued

Table 15-1   Characteristics and Common Etiologies of Cough in Infants and Children—cont'd

Characteristics of Cough	Pattern and Progression of Cough	Fever	Common Age Group Affected	Associated Symptoms	Possible Etiology
				■ Peripheral edema with periorbital involvement (in infants, edema is generalized and can be difficult to detect) ■ Neck vein distention (usually observed only in older children) ■ Developmental delays (particularly in infants)	
Dry, irritated	Persistent	Absent	Can accompany allergic manifestations or be present in child with family	■ Clear nasal discharge ■ Sneezing ■ Conjunctivitis	Allergic cough

Dry, hacking	Worse at night; productive in 2 to 3 days.	Moderate	history of allergies First 4 years of life; can also be found in teens using marijuana.	▪ Upper respiratory infection	Bronchitis
Dry, nonproductive	Becomes paroxysmal with mucus production.	None, unless infection present	Onset before 3 years	▪ Chronic rhinitis ▪ Chronic sinusitis ▪ Chronic respiratory infections ▪ Failure to thrive ▪ Clubbing of fingers and toes ▪ Increasing dyspnea and wheezing ▪ Barrel chest ▪ Numerous other symptoms associated with involvement of gastrointestinal and other systems	Cystic fibrosis

Continued

Table 15-1 Characteristics and Common Etiologies of Cough in Infants and Children—cont'd

Characteristics of Cough	Pattern and Progression of Cough	Fever	Common Age Group Affected	Associated Symptoms	Possible Etiology
Brassy	Slowly progressive.	Low-grade	3 months to 8 years	■ Hoarseness ■ Dyspnea ■ Restlessness	Acute laryngotracheo-bronchitis
Croupy	Sudden onset; common at night. Symptoms disappear in daytime.	High	3 months to 3 years	■ Stridor ■ Hoarseness ■ Restlessness ■ Retractions ■ Rapid, labored respirations ■ Pallor ■ Upper respiratory infection ■ Recurs	Acute spasmodic laryngitis (spasmodic croup)
Croupy	Moderately progressive with purulent secretions.	High	1 month to 6 years	■ Stridor ■ Upper respiratory infection	Acute tracheitis

Paroxysmal, nonproductive	Mild symptoms at first, progressing to paroxysmal cough and sometimes wheezing.	High	2 to 12 months	■ Rhinorrhea ■ Pharyngitis ■ Air hunger ■ Tachypnea ■ Cyanosis ■ Apneic spells	Respiratory syncytial virus (RSV)
Hacking, wheezing, productive	Cough can produce frothy, clear, gelatinous sputum.	Absent	Onset 1 to 5 years	■ Audible wheeze ■ Prolonged expiratory phase ■ Malar flush and red ears ■ Chest hyper-resonant ■ Older children might sit upright, shoulders forward ■ Exhaustion	Asthma

Continued

Table 15-1   Characteristics and Common Etiologies of Cough in Infants and Children—cont'd

Characteristics of Cough	Pattern and Progression of Cough	Fever	Common Age Group Affected	Associated Symptoms	Possible Etiology
Productive cough	Progressive; productive of mucoid, purulent, blood-streaked, or rusty sputum.	High	Any	■ Abrupt onset ■ Chills ■ Neck stiffness ■ Chest pain exaggerated by deep breathing ■ Abdominal discomfort ■ Malaise ■ Rapid, shallow respirations	Bacterial pneumonia

| Severe acute respiratory syndrome (SARS) | Productive cough (please note that this is a separate entry from above as the above info refers to pneumonia and this entry to SARS) | 38.6 (rectal) Celsius (≥101.3 Fahrenheit) | Affects children less severely than adults | ■ Coryza (younger than 12 years)
■ Headache (more common in children older than 12 years)
■ Sore throat
■ Myalgia
■ Nausea/vomiting
■ Diarrhea
■ No crackles or wheezing |

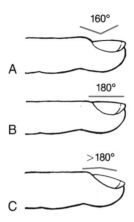

Figure 15-1

Clubbing of nails. **A,** Normal nail. Angle between nail and nail base is approximately 160 degrees. **B,** Early clubbing. Angle between nail and nail base is almost 180 degrees, caused by tissue proliferation on terminal phalanx. **C,** Late clubbing. Angle between nail and nail base is less than 180 degrees. Nail base is visibly swollen.

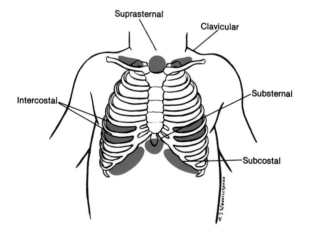

Figure 15-2

Areas where retractions are found.

(From Wong DL et al: *Whaley & Wong's nursing care of infants and children,* ed 6, St Louis, 1999, Mosby.)

Table 15-2 Breath Sounds

Sound	Relationship of Inspiration to Expiration	Diagram of Sound	Location Normal	Location Abnormal
Vesicular	Inspiration > Expiration		Throughout lung field	None
Bronchovesicular	Inspiration = Expiration		First or second intercostal space, at level of bifurcation of trachea and between scapulae	Peripheral lung
Bronchial	Inspiration < Expiration		Over trachea	Lung area

Table 15-3 Adventitious Sounds

Sound	Characteristics	Cause
Crackles (rales)		
Fine	Intermittent, high-pitched, soft popping sounds. Discontinuous. Heard late in inspiration. Do not clear with coughing. Indicative of fluid in small airways. Can be normal in newborns and older infants.	Pneumonia, congestive heart failure, tuberculosis
Coarse	Loud, bubbling, crackling, low pitched. Discontinuous. Heard predominantly on expiration. Can clear with coughing. Indicative of fluid in bronchioles and bronchi.	Resolving pneumonia, bronchitis, pulmonary edema, atelectasis
Wheezes		
Sonorous wheeze (rhonchi)	Continuous, low pitched, snoring. Heard predominantly on expiration. Clear with coughing. Indicative of narrowing of large airway or obstruction of bronchus.	Bronchitis

Sibilant wheeze (wheeze)	Continuous, musical, high pitched. Heard predominantly on expiration. Indicative of edema and obstruction in smaller airways. Can be audible without a stethoscope.	Asthma, foreign body obstruction, bronchitis
Stridor	Crowing sound, predominantly on inspiration. Continuous. Does not clear with cough.	Laryngotracheobronchitis
Pleural friction rub	Grating, rubbing, loud, high pitched. Can be heard during inspiration and expiration. Indicative of inflamed parietal and visceral pleura.	Inflamed pleural surfaces, pneumonia, tuberculosis
Crepitation	Coarse, cracking sensation as hand passes over affected area.	Injury, surgical intervention

Related Nursing Diagnoses

Altered tissue perfusion, cardiopulmonary: related to altered respiratory rate, use of accessory muscles, abnormal arterial blood gases, bronchospasm, dyspnea, nasal flaring, chest retraction.

Ineffective management of therapeutic regimen, families: related to complexity of therapeutic regimen.

Ineffective family coping, compromised: related to prolonged disease.

Altered parenting: related to illness.

Activity intolerance: related to imbalance between oxygen supply and demand.

Ineffective airway clearance: related to retained secretions, limited expansion of the chest wall, excessive mucus, presence of artificial airway, foreign body in airway, secretions in bronchi, exudates in alveoli, neuromuscular dysfunction, infection, asthma, allergic airways.

Ineffective breathing pattern: related to hyperventilation, pain, chest wall deformity, decreased energy, fatigue, neurologic immaturity, respiratory muscle fatigue.

Anxiety: related to change in health status.

Impaired gas exchange: related to alveolar-capillary membrane changes.

Risk for altered growth and development: related to infection, chronic illness.

Risk for altered development: related to chronic illness, technology dependence.

Risk for infection: related to exposure to pathogens, immunosuppression, inadequate acquired immunity, inadequate primary defenses, inadequate secondary defenses.

Sleep deprivation: related to stasis of secretions, fever.

Cardiovascular System

16

The heart is the primary focus of cardiovascular assessment in the infant and child. Assessment of peripheral circulation might be necessary under conditions such as application of casts. Auscultation provides the most significant data on cardiac status and receives the most emphasis, yet the importance of other assessments cannot be overlooked.

Rationale

Approximately 50% of all children have innocent heart murmurs. Screening and referral of children with murmurs assists in distinguishing between innocent and organic murmurs. Assessment of cardiac and vascular function is an essential component of many hospitalizations, particularly when surgery is performed and when drugs are administered. When cardiac problems have been identified, knowledgeable assessment aids in monitoring the effectiveness of treatment regimens and in early detection of complications.

Anatomy and Physiology

The heart is a muscular four-chambered organ located in the mediastinum. The upper chambers of the heart are the atria; the lower chambers are the ventricles. Septa divide the two ventricles and the two atria. Four valves prevent the backflow of blood into the chambers. The tricuspid valve, located between the right atrium and ventricle, and the bicuspid, or mitral valve, located between the left atrium and ventricle, are the atrioventricular valves. The pulmonic valve, located in the pulmonary artery, and the aortic valve, in the aorta, are the semilunar valves. Closure of the four valves produces vibrations that are thought to be responsible for heart sounds. S_1 refers to the "lubb" sound produced by closure of the atrioventricular valves, and S_2 to the "dubb" sound produced by closure of the semilunar valves. Table 16-1 summarizes the various sounds and their characteristics.

In its initial stage of development the heart is a straight tube. Between the second and tenth weeks of gestation it undergoes a series of changes to become a four-chambered organ. The heart begins beating during the third week of gestation. During fetal life it primarily distributes the oxygen and nutrients that have been supplied through the placenta. The fetal lungs are largely bypassed by shunts that exist during fetal life. At birth these shunts begin to close as pulmonary vascular resistance drops. Pulmonary vascular resistance approximates adult levels by 6 weeks. Pulmonary vascular resistance is still relatively high in the first month of life, and cardiac defects such as ventricular septal defect might not be detected.

The heart is large in relation to body size in the infant. It lies somewhat horizontally and occupies a large portion of the thoracic cavity. Growth of the lungs causes the heart to assume a lower position, and by 7 years of age the heart has assumed an adult position that is more oblique and lower. Heart size increases in adolescence in conjunction with rapid growth.

At birth ventricular walls are similar in thickness, but with circulatory demands the left ventricle increases in thickness. The thinness of the ventricle produces a low systolic pressure in the newborn. The systolic pressure rises after birth until it approximates adult levels by puberty. Blood vessels lengthen and thicken in response to increased pressures.

Equipment for Assessment of Cardiovascular System

■ Stethoscope (preferably with a small diaphragm)

Preparation

The child can sit or lie. Allow the child to handle the stethoscope. Listening to the parent's or nurse's heart or to their own hearts is often effective in dispelling anxieties in young patients. Ask the parent or child about heart disease in family members. Inquire whether the child has had difficulty in feeding (infant), undue fatigue, intolerance for exercise, poor weight gain, weakness, cyanosis, edema, dizziness, epistaxis, squatting, frequent respiratory tract infections, or delayed development. Ask the parent whether the

Table 16-1 **Heart Sounds**

Sound	Cause	Location	Characteristics
S_1 (lubb)	Mitral and tricuspid valves are forced closed at the beginning of systole (heart contraction).	Apex of heart	S_1 is longer and lower pitched than S_2. Synchronous with carotid pulse. Closure of valves usually heard as one sound, but slight asynchrony can produce audible splitting, best heard in the fourth left interspace.
S_2 (dubb)	Aortic and pulmonic valves are forced closed at the beginning of diastole (heart relaxation).	Base of heart	Short, high-pitched S_2 can be split during inspiration. Splitting is best heard in the aortic area. If the breath is held on inspiration, "physiologic split" is accentuated.
S_3	Vibrations are produced by rapid ventricular filling.	Apex of heart	Heard early in diastole. Dull, low pitched. Normal in children and young adults.
S_4	Resistance to ventricular filling after contraction of atria.	Apex of heart	Low pitched. Considered abnormal. Best heard when child is supine.

mother had any infection or took medications during pregnancy, age of mother at infant's birth, and presence of maternal diabetes or alcohol use. Inquire whether the child had problems at birth, such as low birth weight, prematurity, congenital infection, or respiratory difficulty. Inquire about temperament of the child and family responses to illness.

Assessment of Heart

Assessment	Findings
Inspection	
Observe the child's body posture.	**Clinical Alert**
	Squatting is seen in tetralogy of Fallot.
	Persistent slight hyperextension of the neck in infants can indicate hypoxia.
	Restlessness accompanied by abdominal pain, pallor, vomiting, unconsolable crying, and shock can indicate acute myocardial infarction in susceptible children.
Observe the child for cyanosis, mottling, and edema.	**Clinical Alert**
	Cyanosis, pallor, and mottling can indicate heart disease. Edema can indicate congestive heart failure. Edema of sacral and periorbital areas is more common in younger children.
	Edema of the extremities is more common in older children but in the younger child can more likely indicate renal failure.
	Cyanosis increases with crying in children with an atrioventricular canal defect and with some other cardiac defects.

Assessment	Findings
Inspection—cont'd	
Observe the child for signs of respiratory difficulty (grunting, costal retractions, flaring of the nares, adventitious chest sounds) and hacking cough.	**Clinical Alert** Respiratory difficulties and congested cough can indicate congestive heart failure or respiratory infection.
Inspect the child's nailbeds for clubbing, lengthening, widening, and splinter hemorrhages (thin, black lines).	**Clinical Alert** Clubbing indicates hypoxia. Splinter hemorrhages indicate emboli and might indicate bacterial endocarditis. Symmetric chest expansion is normal. In thin children the apical pulse, or point of maximal impulse (PMI), can be seen as a pulsation.
Examine the anterior chest from an angle. Observe for the symmetry of chest movement, visible pulsations, and diffuse lifts or heaves.	**Clinical Alert** A sternal lift or heave can signal congestive heart failure. A systolic heave can indicate right ventricular enlargement.
Palpation	
Using the fingerpads, palpate the anterior chest for the apical pulse or PMI. The location of the PMI is usually felt at the apex of the heart and is found in the fourth intercostal space in children 7 years of age or younger and in the fifth intercostal space in children older than 7 years.	The apical pulse normally is palpable in infants and young children. **Clinical Alert** A lower, more lateral PMI can indicate cardiac enlargement. An amplified PMI can indicate anemia, fever, or anxiety.

Assessment	Findings

Palpation—cont'd

The PMI is left of the midclavicular line until 4 years, midclavicular between 4 and 6 years, and to the right of the line by 7 years.

Fingertips are more useful for detecting pulsations, and the ball of the hand (palmar surface at the base of the fingers) is useful for detecting vibratory thrills or pre-cordial friction rubs. Thrills feel much like the belly of a purring cat.

Clinical Alert

Rubs and thrills are abnormal and should be reported.

Percussion

Percussion is used to estimate heart size by outlining cardiac borders. It is a difficult technique and has limited use-fulness in assessing the heart in infants and young children. The location of PMI is a more useful indicator of heart size.

Auscultation

Using both the bell (for low frequency; S_3, S_4 sounds) and the diaphragm (for high frequency; S_1, S_2 sounds), auscultate for heart sounds.

Assessment	Findings
Auscultation—cont'd	
Beginning in the second right intercostal space (aortic area), systematically move the stethoscope from the aortic to the pulmonic area (Figure 16-1). S_2 is best heard at the base of the heart (aortic and pulmonic areas). Move down to Erb's point, and then to the tricuspid and mitral areas. S_1 is heard at the beginning of the apical pulse, which facilitates differentiation of S_1 and S_2. Evaluate the sounds for: *Quality* (normally S_1 and S_2 are clear and distinct)	S_2 normally loudest in the aortic and pulmonic areas, near the base of the heart. S_2 normally splits on inspiration in children and becomes single on expiration. S_1 and S_2 are equal in intensity at Erb's point. S_1 is loudest in the mitral and tricuspid areas. Sinus arrhythmia is a normal variant in which the rate increases with inspiration and decreases with expiration. If unsure whether auscultation suggests sinus arrhythmia or a serious arrhythmia, ask the child to hold the breath.

Assessment	Findings
Auscultation—cont'd	
	With sinus arrhythmia, holding the breath results in a steady heart rate.
	Pulse rate may be lower in athletic children and adolescents.
	Clinical Alert
	Heart sounds will be auscultated primarily on the right side of the chest if the child has dextrocardia.
	S_1 is intensified during fever, exercise, and anemia.
	Accentuation of S_1 can also indicate mitral stenosis.
	A split S_2 that is fixed with the act of respiration can indicate an atrial septal defect.
	Pulse rate usually increases 8 to 10 beats for every degree of Fahrenheit increase.
Rate (synchronous with radial pulse)	S_1 that varies in intensity can indicate serious arrhythmia and must be reported.
Intensity (consistent with what would normally be found at each auscultatory point)	
Rhythm (normally regular)	
The child should be helped to assume at least two different positions during auscultation. If adventitious sounds are suspected, have the child assume sitting, standing, leaning forward, and left sidelying positions.	

Assessment	Findings

Auscultation—cont'd

Auscultate for additional sounds, such as S_3 and and S_4, which are best assessed with the infant or child lying on the left side. Assess for abnormal sounds such as clicks, murmurs, and precordial friction rubs. Murmurs should be evaluated and documented as to:

Location, or auscultatory area in which found.

Timing in the S_1-S_2 cycle

Intensity and whether intensity varies with the child's position. Intensity is usually graded on a 6-point scale, with grade I being very faint and grade VI being audible even with the stethoscope off the chest. Grade III is considered moderately loud.

PitchQuality (whether murmur is musical, blowing, or swishing)

S_3 is a normal finding.

Clinical Alert

Innocent or nonpathologic murmurs do not increase over time and do not affect the child's growth (Table 16-2). Innocent murmurs are usually systolic (Figure 16-2), medium-pitched, and best heard at the second and third left interspaces. Innocent murmurs can disappear with changes in position and can be accentuated during fever, stress, or exercise.

Organic murmurs are caused by congenital or acquired heart disease. Murmurs occurring before 3 years of age are usually related to congenital defects, and after 3 years to rheumatic heart disease. (Table 16-3) provides descriptions of murmurs associated with cardiac defects.

Murmurs associated with rheumatic heart disease include those of aortic and mitral stenosis and of aortic and mitral regurgitation. Additional sounds and murmurs must always be described and reported for further evaluation.

Assessment	Findings

Auscultation—cont'd

Precordial friction rubs are high-pitched grating or scratching sounds that are unaffected by breathing patterns. Pleural friction rubs stop when children hold their breath.

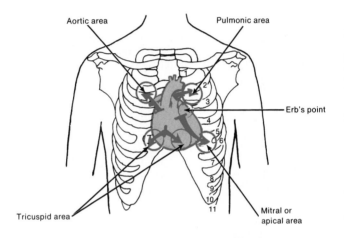

Figure 16-1
Cardiac auscultatory areas.
(From Hockenberry MJ et al: *Wong's nursing care of infants and children,* ed 7, St Louis, 2003, Mosby.)

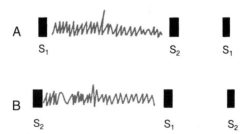

Figure 16-2
Timing of murmurs in S_1-S_2 cycle. **A,** Systolic murmur. **B,** Diastolic murmur.

Table 16-2 Innocent Murmurs

Type of Murmur	Age	Intensity	Quality	Other Characteristics
Pulmonary flow murmur (of the newborn)	Low–birth-weight newborn; disappears by 3 to 6 months of age	Grade I to IV (very faint to loud)	Rough	
Stills	>2 years	<Grade IV (loud)	Squeaking, twanging, musical	Best heard with child in supine position and with bell
Venous hum	3 to 6 years	<Grade IV (loud)	Continuous hum	Heard best with child in upright position; disappears when supine and if head is turned
Pulmonary ejection	8 to 14 years	<Grade IV (loud)	Slightly grating	

Adapted from Zator Estes ME: Health assessment & physical examination, ed 2, Clifton Park, 2002, Delmar Thomson Learning.

Assessment of Vascular System

Assessment of vascular integrity is necessitated by cast application and by other conditions that can impair blood flow. Femoral and dorsal pedal areas should be palpated if cardiac defects are suspected.

Assessment	Findings
Palpate the peripheral arteries for rhythm and for pulse rate, using the same finger. Use the same fingerpads to palpate the pulses simultaneously for equality.	Normally pulses are palpable, equal in intensity, and even in rhythm.
Palpate the radial pulse. The radial pulse is best felt in children older than 2 years of age and who do not evidence spasticity.	
Palpate the femoral pulse by applying deep palpation midway between the iliac crest and the symphysis pubis. The child must be in the supine position (Figure 16-3).	**Clinical Alert** Diminution or absence of the femoral, popliteal, dorsalis pedis, or posterior tibial pulses can indicate coarctation of the aorta. A brachial-femoral lag is abnormal, when the two pulses are palpated simultaneously.
Palpate the popliteal pulse by having the child flex the knee (Figure 16-4).	
Palpate the dorsalis pedis pulse along the upper medial aspect of the foot (Figure 16-5).	
Palpate the posterior tibial pulse posterior to the ankle on the medial aspect of the foot.	

Table 16-3 Murmurs Associated with Childhood Cardiac Defects

Defect	Location	Timing	Intensity	Pitch	Quality
Aortic stenosis	Right second interspace (aortic area)	Crescendo effect, occurring between S_1 and S_2	Variable	Medium	Harsh
Pulmonic stenosis	Pulmonic area, third left interspace	Crescendo effect, occurring between S_1 and S_2	Variable	Medium	Harsh
Mitral stenosis	Mitral area	Occurs between S_2 and S_1	Variable (Grade I to IV); can be accentuated by exercise	Low	Rumbling
Aortic regurgitation	Aortic area	Heard between S_2 and S_1; usually a short period follows S_2 before sound begins	Variable (Grade I to IV); most audible when child leans forward and exhales	High; best heard with diaphragm of stethoscope	Blowing Can be confused with breath sounds

Continued

Table 16-3   Murmurs Associated with Childhood Cardiac Defects—cont'd

Defect	Location	Timing	Intensity	Pitch	Quality
Mitral regurgitation	Mitral area	Occurs between S_1 and S_2	Variable; unaffected by respiratory cycle	High	Blowing
Ventricular septal defect	Left sternal border; third, fourth, and fifth interspaces	Heard between S_1 and S_2	Very loud	High	Blowing
Patent ductus arteriosus	Second left interspace	Continuous; louder in late systole (just before S_2); obscures S_2; softer in diastole	Loud	Medium	Harsh, machinery like
Tetralogy of Fallot	Second and third left interspaces	Heard between S_1 and S_2	Not well transmitted		

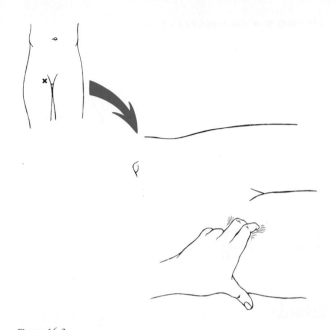

Figure 16-3
Femoral pulse.
(From Potter PA: *Pocket guide to health assessment,* ed 3, St Louis, 1994, Mosby.)

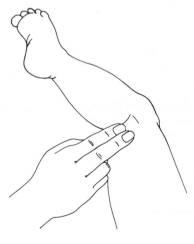

Figure 16-4
Popliteal pulse.

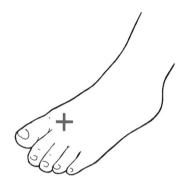

Figure 16-5
Dorsalis pedis pulse.

Related Nursing Diagnoses

Anxiety: related to change in health status.

Altered family processes: related to shift in health status of family member.

Fluid volume excess: related to compromised regulatory system.

Altered growth and development: related to chronic illness.

Knowledge deficit: related to diet, drug therapy, signs and symptoms of complications.

Risk for impaired skin integrity: related to fluid excess.

Impaired social interaction: related to fatigue, limited mobility.

Activity intolerance: related to imbalance between oxygen supply/demand.

Sleep pattern disturbance: related to shortness of breath.

Altered tissue perfusion, cardiopulmonary: related to edema, weak or absent pulses, blood pressure changes in extremities.

Decreased cardiac output: related to physical illnesses/anomalies.

Fatigue: related to poor physical condition.

Impaired physical mobility: related to limited cardiovascular endurance.

Ineffective management of therapeutic regimen: related to complexity of therapeutic regimen.

Altered parenting: related to physical illness, presence of stress.

Social isolation: related to altered state of illness.

Risk for altered development: related to complexity of therapeutic regimen.

Abdomen

17

Encased within the abdominal cavity are the organs and structures of the genitourinary, gastrointestinal, and hemopoietic systems. Assessment of the abdomen is really a multiple system assessment and commonly follows assessment of the thorax and lungs.

Lower bowel sounds can be affected by manual manipulation; thus the order of assessment is inspection, auscultation, percussion, and palpation. Because it is sometimes performed as part of the abdominal assessment, assessment of the anus is included in this chapter.

Rationale

The upper gastrointestinal tract is largely inaccessible to the nurse; thus examination of the abdomen primarily involves assessment of lower gastrointestinal and genitourinary structures. Many common childhood disorders involve the gastrointestinal and genitourinary systems, and the function of these systems can also be altered by factors such as surgery, stress, medications, or the hygienic care that the child receives.

Anatomy and Physiology
Gastrointestinal System

The primary functions of the gastrointestinal tract are the digestion and absorption of nutrients and water, elimination of waste products, and secretion of various substances required for digestion.

The liver, located in the right upper quadrant of the abdomen, has several important functions, including biosynthesis of protein; production of blood clotting factors; metabolism of fat, protein, and carbohydrates; production of bile; metabolism of bilirubin; and detoxification.

A primitive gut develops from the endoderm by the third week of gestation. This developing midgut grows so rapidly that by the fourth week of gestation it is too large for the abdominal cavity. Failure of the midgut to rotate and reenter the abdominal cavity at 10 weeks of gestation can produce a variety of disorders, such as omphalocele, and susceptibility to intussusception and bowel obstruction.

The anus arises from a pit invagination of the skin during embryonic development and is the terminal segment of the anal canal. Normally the anal canal is closed by action of the voluntary external sphincter and involuntary internal sphincter muscles. The canal is well supplied by somatic sensory nerves and is sensitive to touch. Externally it is moist and hairless.

Despite the development of the digestive tract in utero, the exchange of nutrients and waste is the function of the placenta. At birth the gastrointestinal tract is still immature and does not fully mature for the first 2 years. Because of this immaturity, many differences exist between the digestive tract of the infant or child and that of the adult. For example, the muscle tone of the lower esophageal sphincter does not assume adult levels until 1 month of age. This lax sphincter muscle tone explains why young infants frequently regurgitate after feedings. Intestinal peristalsis in children is rapid, with emptying time being 2½ to 3 hours in the newborn infant and 3 to 6 hours in older infants and children. Stomach capacity is 10 to 20 ml (0.3 to 0.7 oz) in the neonate, compared with 10 to 200 ml (0.3 to 7 oz) in the 2-month-old infant, 1500 ml (50 oz) in the 16-year-old adolescent, and 2000 to 3000 ml (68 to 101 oz) in the adult. The stomach is round and lies somewhat horizontally until 2 years of age. The parietal cells of the stomach do not produce adult levels of hydrochloric acid until 6 months. The gastrocolic reflex, or movement of the contents toward the colon, is rapid in young infants, as evidenced by the frequency of stools. The intestine, which underwent rapid growth in utero, undergoes further growth spurts when the child is 1 to 3 years of age and again at 15 to 16 years. After birth the musculature of the anus develops as the infant becomes more upright. The child then becomes able to voluntarily control defecation.

Genitourinary System

The kidneys lie posteriorly within the upper quadrants of the abdomen. The kidneys regulate fluid and electrolyte levels in the body through filtration, reabsorption, and secretion of water and electrolytes. Water is excreted in the form of urine. The bladder, located below the symphysis pubis, collects the urine for elimination.

The development of the kidneys begins early in gestation but is not complete until near the end of the first year of life. Until the epithelial cells of the nephrons assume a mature flat shape, filtration and absorption are poor. The loop of Henle gradually elongates, which increases the infant's ability to concentrate urine, as seen by fewer wet diapers near the first year of life. Increasing bladder capacity also contributes to decreased frequency of voiding. The infant's bladder capacity is 15 to 20 ml (0.5 to 0.7 oz), compared with 600 to 800 ml (20 to 27 oz) in the adult. The size of the kidneys varies with size and age. The kidneys of infants and children are relatively large in comparison with those of adults and are more susceptible to trauma because of their size.

Equipment for Assessment of Abdomen

- Warm stethoscope
- Warm hands
- Short fingernails

Preparation

Ask the parent or child about a family history of gastrointestinal or genitourinary tract disorders and about the child's prenatal history (maternal hydramnios is associated with intestinal atresia), mother's lifestyle during pregnancy, and child's growth. Inquire about whether the child had imperforate anus, failure to pass meconium, cleft palate or lip, difficulty in feeding, prolonged jaundice, or abdominal wall disorders (e.g., omphalocele or hernia) as a neonate. Ask if the child has had problems with feeding, such as anorexia, vomiting, or regurgitation, or if the child has engaged in fasting or dieting (see Chapter 7 and Chapter 24 for more information about assessment of eating disorders). If the child has had emesis or regurgitation, determine the time of occurrence, frequency, type (Table 17-1), amount, and force (nonprojectile or projectile). (See Table 17-2 for types of vomiting and associated etiologies). Inquire about whether the child has had pain (frequency, intensity, type, location; Table 17-3), itching (location), sleeplessness, swelling, tendency to bruise, thirst, dry mouth, unexplained fever, food allergies, sensitivity to diapers,

Table 17-1   Types of Emesis and Related Findings

Type of Emesis	Related Findings
Undigested formula or food	Rapid expulsion of stomach contents before digestion has occurred.
Yellow; might smell acidic	Contents originated in stomach.
Dark green (bile-stained)	Contents originated below the ampulla of Vater.
Dark brown, foul odor	Emesis produced by intestinal obstruction.
Bright red/dark red	Bright red signifies fresh bleeding. Dark red signifies old blood or blood altered by gastric secretions.

or alterations in bowel movements or urinary elimination patterns. If there is a problem with bowel movements, inquire about the frequency, amount, consistency, quality, and color of stool (Table 17-4; Table 17-5); use of laxatives and enemas; recent camping trips; and presence of dogs, cats, or turtles. If there are alterations in the pattern of urinary elimination, determine what they are and when they began. If problems with urination or bowel movements occur in toddlers, explore what these problems mean to parents. In the school-age child who experiences recurrent abdominal pain, explore possible stressors and responses to stressors. Inquire about body piercings, tatoos, and environmental factors such as daycare, crowded living conditions, and sharing of utensils and other personal items. When making inquiries of parents regarding bowel habits and vomiting, it is important to avoid asking "Does your child vomit?" or "Does your child have constipation or diarrhea?" because studies suggest that understanding of these terms varies. There is a tendency, for example, with bowel movements, to define diarrhea and constipation by frequency, rather than by consistency of the stool.

It is important that the child be relaxed during abdominal examination, particularly during palpation. Having the child void, if possible, before the examination assists with comfort during the assessment. Flexing the child's head or hips helps relax abdominal muscles. Asking the child to "suck in" or "puff out" the abdomen helps assess

Text continued on p. 264

Table 17-2   Characteristics and Common Etiologies of Vomiting in Children

Description of Vomiting	Associated Symptoms	Possible Etiology
Acute vomiting	Diarrhea Fever Abdominal pain or cramping (except with cholera infections) Nausea Meningeal symptoms (*Shigella* and *Salmonella* groups) Upper respiratory symptoms (found with Rotavirus)	Infections (e.g., Rotavirus, Norwalk virus, *Salmonella*, *Shigella, Escherichia coli, Giardia lamblia, Vibrio cholerae*—cholera)
Acute vomiting	Fever Irritability Poor feeding (infants and young children) and anorexia Pulling at the ear Complaint of earache Red, bulging eardrum	Acute otitis media
Acute vomiting	Fever Headache Irritability Photophobia	Bacterial meningitis

	Nuchal rigidity	
	Positive Kernig's sign	
	Positive Brudzinski's sign	
	Lethargy	
	Failure to feed (infants)	
	High-pitched cry (infants)	
	Tense or bulging fontanel (infants)	
	Macular or petechial rash	
Acute Vomiting	Periumbilical pain that moves to the right iliac fossa	Appendicitis
	Fever	
	Rebound tenderness	
Acute Vomiting	Disorientation	Alcohol poisoning
	Ataxia	
	Nystagmus	
	Drowsiness	
	Hypotension	
	Dysarthria	
Vomiting	Episodic colicky pain	Intussusception
	Pallor	
	Infant/child draws up legs	
	Red currant-jelly stools	

Continued

Table 17-2   Characteristics and Common Etiologies of Vomiting in Children—cont'd

Description of Vomiting	Associated Symptoms	Possible Etiology
Persistent vomiting	Palpable mass in the line of the colon	Gastroesophageal reflux
	Peak incidence in infants between 5 and 7 months	
	Effortless regurgitation or emesis	
	Frequently found in infants younger than 6 months but also occurs in children	
	Weight loss or failure to gain adequately (if vomiting is severe)	
	Anemia	
	Irritability	
	Heartburn (older children)	
Episodic vomiting	Headache	Migraine
	Visual symptoms (blurring, flashing lights, stars, scotomata, photophobia)	
	Dizziness	
	Abdominal pain	
	Strong family history of migraine	

Recurrent vomiting, possibly hematemesis	Local weakness Sensory disturbances Stabbing, burning pain that radiates to the back Chronic abdominal pain Family history Use of alcohol or tobacco or ulcerogenic drugs Presence of stress Presence of bacterium *Helicobacter pylori*	Peptic ulcer disease
Vomiting (morning, with or without feeding, becomes increasingly projectile)	Headache on waking or with sneezing Clumsiness Spasticity Irritability Weakness Seizures Positive Babinski's sign Decreased appetite	Brain tumor

Continued

Table 17-2 Characteristics and Common Etiologies of Vomiting in Children—cont'd

Description of Vomiting	Associated Symptoms	Possible Etiology
Forceful vomiting (non bile-stained, progressive)	Dehydration Weight loss Infant hungry following vomiting Visible peristalsis in the left hypochondrium Palpable mass between the umbilicus and right costal margin Usually presents in infants 3 to 6 weeks	Pyloric stenosis

Table 17-3 Characteristics and Common Etiologies of Acute Abdominal Pain in Children

Location	Characteristics	Possible Age Group	Etiology	Related Factors	Associated Symptoms
Lower abdomen, flank	Severe, colicky	Adolescent	Urolithiasis	■ Hypercalciuria ■ Urinary tract infection	■ Restlessness ■ Dysuria
Lower abdomen, especially suprapubic	Constant	Any	Cystitis	■ Bubble baths ■ Tight jeans ■ Nylon panties ■ Sexual activity	■ Urinary frequency ■ Dysuria
Lower abdomen		Any	Obstruction	■ Adhesions related to surgery ■ Ingestion of hairballs or trichobezoars ■ Developmental or psychologic problems	■ Frequent tinkling sounds (early obstruction) or high-pitched rumbles ■ Diminished bowel sounds (late obstruction) ■ Absence of bowel sounds (total obstruction)

Continued

Table 17-3 Characteristics and Common Etiologies of Acute Abdominal Pain in Children—cont'd

Location	Characteristics	Possible Age Group	Etiology	Related Factors	Associated Symptoms
Lower abdomen	Acute or chronic, crampy	Older school-age or adolescent	Ulcerative colitis	■ Infection ■ Dietary habits ■ Familial tendency	■ Diarrhea ■ Blood in stools ■ Growth failure
Bilateral, lower abdomen	Constant	Adolescent	Pelvic inflammatory disease	■ Multiple sex partners ■ Alcohol/drug use ■ Begins during or within week of menses	■ Guarding upon palpation ■ Fever ■ Pain with movement ■ Walks slightly bent over and tends to hold abdomen
	Constant	Adolescent	Endometriosis	■ Menses	
	Constant, crampy	Adolescent	Ectopic pregnancy	■ Amenorrhea	■ Morning vomiting

	Constant, crampy	Any	Constipation	■ Spinal injury ■ Meningomyelocele ■ Use of anticholinergics, laxatives ■ Eating disorders	■ Lack of stooling ■ Bloating ■ Presence of a mass
Nonspecific	Chronic	School-age adolescent	Psychogenic	■ Abuse ■ Depression ■ Eating disorders ■ Minor adjustment problems	■ Pain might interfere with stressful activities but not with pleasurable ones ■ Can be associated with specific situations ■ Eyes remain closed during palpation
Generalized		Any	Streptococcal pharyngitis	■ Infection	■ Erythematous pharynx ■ Fever ■ Pain

Continued

Table 17-3   Characteristics and Common Etiologies of Acute Abdominal Pain in Children—cont'd

Location	Characteristics	Possible Age Group	Etiology	Related Factors	Associated Symptoms
Periumbilical	Crampy	Older school-age or adolescent	Crohn's disease	■ Infection ■ Dietary habits ■ Familial tendency	■ Weight loss ■ Anorexia ■ Poor growth
	Colicky	Any	Lactose intolerance	■ Symptoms occur after milk ingestion ■ Cultural and hereditary factors	■ Borborygmi ■ Abdominal distention ■ Watery stools
	Crampy	Any	Gastroenteritis	■ Infection	■ Vomiting ■ Diarrhea ■ Dehydration ■ Fever
	Constant, upon deep inspiration	Any	Pneumonia	■ Infection ■ Aspiration	■ Cough ■ Fever ■ Malaise ■ Rales

	Colicky	Any	Diabetic ketoacidosis	■ Absent or inadequate supply of insulin	■ Polydipsia ■ Polyuria ■ Headache ■ Kussmaul's respirations
Periumbilical (nontender) in early stages followed by generalized and then right lower quadrant pain (tender)	Constant, increasing	Preschool, school-age, adolescent	Appendicitis	■ Hardened fecal material ■ Parasites ■ Foreign bodies	■ Anorexia ■ Vomiting ■ Fever ■ Leukocytosis ■ Rebound tenderness ■ Flex hip on affected side
Epigastric	Dull ache	Adolescent	Esophagitis	■ Self-induced vomiting	■ Vomiting
			Hepatitis	■ Exchange of blood or any bodily fluid or secretion ■ Fecal-oral transmission	■ Nausea and vomiting ■ Fever ■ Anorexia ■ Pruritus ■ Jaundice

Continued

Table 17-3 Characteristics and Common Etiologies of Acute Abdominal Pain in Children—cont'd

Location	Characteristics	Possible Age Group	Etiology	Related Factors	Associated Symptoms
	Sharp, constant, sudden	Adolescent	Pancreatitis	■ Alcohol ingestion ■ Lying supine can aggravate	
	Stabbing, burning, radiates to back	Adolescent	Duodenal ulcer	■ Blood group (O) ■ Familial tendency ■ Ulcerogenic drugs ■ Alcohol ■ Smoking ■ *Helicobacter pylori* ■ Stress	■ Hematemesis ■ Melena ■ Anemia ■ Poor eating habits
Epigastric area, right upper quadrant, shoulder, right scapula	Can be dull, crampy, acute, or gradual	Adolescent more common than children	Cholecystitis	■ Oral contraceptive use ■ Ingestion of fatty or acidic foods	■ Nausea ■ Bloating ■ Guarding upon palpation

Table 17-4 Variants in Stool Consistency and Related Findings

Type of Stool	Related Findings
Soft or liquid	Indicative of breastfeeding.
Light yellow, pasty; soft or pasty green	Common in formula-fed babies. Stool has been exposed to air for some time, and oxidation has occurred.
Black	Can indicate that the child is receiving iron or bismuth preparations or has gastric or duodenal bleeding.
Gray or clay colored	Biliary atresia might be present.
Undigested food in stool	Common in infants who are unable to completely digest foods, such as corn and carrots.
Currant-jelly stool (blood and mucus)	Indicative of intussusception, Meckel's diverticulum. Found with Henoch-Schönlein purpura (HSP).
Ribbonlike	Indicative of Hirschsprung's disease.
Frothy, foul smelling, bulky	Steatorrhea. Can indicate cystic fibrosis.
Firm, hard stool	Associated with diet, inadequate fluid or fiber intake, encopresis, obstructive disorders, irritable bowel syndrome, chemotherapy, medications, overly rigid toilet training.
Diarrhea (watery, bloody)	Can be related to infection (bacterial, viral, parasitic), dietary causes (overfeeding, excessive ingestion of sugar, or ingestion of heavy metals), irritable bowel syndrome.

Table 17-5 Characteristics of Selected Etiologies of Diarrhea in Children

Type of Diarrhea	Pattern of Diarrhea	Common Age Group Affected	Associated Symptoms	Possible Etiologies
Diarrhea Related to Infectious Causes				
Watery, profuse	Abrupt onset; can persist for more than a week. Can involve significant diarrhea; major cause of dehydration and hospitalization in children. Incubation period 1 to 3 days. Peak incidence in winter in temperate climates.	6 months to 24 months most affected Most common cause of severe diarrheal disease and dehydration in infants	Upper respiratory infection Fever ≥38° C (100° F) Nausea Vomiting Abdominal pain Dehydration (see Table 17-6 for description of degrees of dehydration)	Rotavirus
Watery	Incubation period of 1 to 3 days. Self-limiting; symptoms last 1 to 2 days, but reinfection can occur.	All ages	Low-grade fever Loss of appetite Abdominal pain Nausea Vomiting	Norwalk virus

Green, watery diarrhea with blood and mucus	Diarrhea follows sudden onset of nausea and abdominal cramps. Can be gradual or abrupt in onset.	All ages Common cause of acute gastroenteritis in children in developing countries	Malaise Headache Myalgia Fever Vomiting Abdominal distention Appears toxic Hemolytic uremic syndrome occurs with 10% of infections with enterohemorrhagic *E. coli*	Diarrheagenic *E. coli*
Watery diarrhea	Onset variable. Diarrhea contains pus and mucus after approximately first 12 hours. Incubation period 1 to 7 days.	Majority of cases in children younger than 9 years	High fever Convulsions can accompany fever Appears toxic Headache Nuchal rigidity Abdominal cramps precede stools	*Shigella* groups

Continued

Table 17-5 Characteristics of Selected Etiologies of Diarrhea in Children—cont'd

Type of Diarrhea	Pattern of Diarrhea	Common Age Group Affected	Associated Symptoms	Possible Etiologies
Diarrhea Related to Infectious Causes—cont'd				
Watery, profuse, foul-smelling diarrhea with blood	Incubation period 1 to 7 days.		Severe abdominal pain (periumbilical) Abdominal cramping Vomiting Fever	Campylobacter jejuni
Watery, profuse diarrhea containing blood and mucus	Intermittent, then continuous diarrhea. Incubation period can be as long as 5 days.	Rare in infants younger than one year	Usually characterized by lack of cramping and anal irritation	Cholera
Occasionally bloody diarrhea with mucus	Rapid onset. Incubation period 6 to 72 hours for gastroenteritis.	Can occur with all ages, but majority of cases are younger than 20 years	Fever Nausea Vomiting Colicky abdominal pain Can have headache and meningeal symptoms	Salmonella groups

Bloody diarrhea	More common in winter. Can relapse for weeks.	Highest incidence in children younger than 5 years	History of eating poultry or eggs or of handling turtles and other domestic animals	
		Commonly occurs in infants and toddlers	Fever >38.7° Celsius (101.6° Fahrenheit) Abdominal pain in right lower quadrant Vomiting	*Yersinia enterocolitica*
Profuse diarrhea	Self-limiting (improves in 24 hours).	All ages	Severe abdominal cramping Nausea Vomiting	*Staphylococcus*
Diarrhea Related to Parasites				
Large, pale stools with mucus	Threat to immunocompromised children. Children can be asymptomatic with light infection.	Young children affected less often than adolescents and adults	Nausea Vomiting Distention Abdominal pain Respiratory symptoms	Strongyloidiasis

Continued

Table 17-5   Characteristics of Selected Etiologies of Diarrhea in Children—cont'd

Type of Diarrhea	Pattern of Diarrhea	Common Age Group Affected	Associated Symptoms	Possible Etiologies
Diarrhea Related to Parasites—cont'd				
Diarrhea	Can be asymptomatic.		Abdominal pain Distention	Trichuriasis
Mild diarrhea	Gradual onset. Steatorrhea can also occur. Incubation period of 1 to 2 weeks and symptoms last 2 to 4 weeks.	Found in areas where there is poor sanitation	Nausea Vomiting Weight loss (can be significant) Malaise Flatulence Cramping	*G. lamblia* (also known as "beaver fever" or "backpacker's diarrhea")
Bloody, profuse diarrhea	Symptoms appear 2 to 6 weeks after initial infection.	Second leading protozoan cause of death	Fever Malaise Weight loss Severe abdominal pain Liver abscess	*Entamoeba histolytica*

Diarrhea Related to Noninfectious Causes

Bright red or currant-jelly stools	Diarrhea is painless. Stools can also be tarry.	Most sympto-matic cases involve children 10 years and younger	Symptoms vary with whether process is obstructive or inflammatory or involves hemorrhage	Meckel's diverticulum
Ribbonlike, foul-smelling stool	Can have history of delayed passage of meconium stool.		Constipation Vomiting Failure to thrive Abdominal distention relieved by rectal stimulation or enemas	Hirschsprung's disease
Bloody diarrhea	Urgency with stooling; diarrhea can be severe. Bleeding can be occult.		Mild to moderate weight loss Mild to moderate anorexia Some growth retardation Abdominal cramps	Ulcerative colitis

Continued

Table 17-5   Characteristics of Selected Etiologies of Diarrhea in Children—cont'd

Type of Diarrhea	Pattern of Diarrhea	Common Age Group Affected	Associated Symptoms	Possible Etiologies
Diarrhea Related to Noninfectious Causes—cont'd				
Diarrhea (can be bloody)	Mild gastrointestinal symptoms can be present for years.		Abdominal pain Epigastric pain Anorexia (can be severe) Weight loss (can be severe) Growth retardation Anal and perianal lesions Large joint arthritis	Crohn's disease
Watery, offensive stool with mucus and undigested food	Short interval between ingestion of food and diarrhea.	Most common cause of chronic diarrhea in children 1 to 5 years	Child can look healthy No identifiable pathogen	Toddler diarrhea ("pea and carrot diarrhea")
Chronic diarrhea	Diarrhea can be severe and watery in infants with congenital deficiency	Usually manifests between 3 and 7 years of age	Pain Bloating Flatulence	Lactose intolerance

Chronic diarrhea with unformed stools	of lactase. Symptoms begin within 30 minutes to several hours of consuming lactose. Stools initially bulky; progress to large, loose stools or diarrhea by 6 months of age. Stools frothy and very foul smelling.	Symptoms can begin at birth	Dyspnea Chronic cough Clubbing Rhinitis Chronic sinusitis Nasal polyps Chronic bronchial pneumonia Obstructive emphysema Malabsorption syndrome Failure to thrive in young children Gastroesophageal reflux Rectal prolapse	Cystic fibrosis

Continued

Table 17-5 Characteristics of Selected Etiologies of Diarrhea in Children—cont'd

Type of Diarrhea	Pattern of Diarrhea	Common Age Group Affected	Associated Symptoms	Possible Etiologies
Diarrhea Related to Noninfectious Causes—cont'd				
Chronic diarrhea	Changes in stools follow introduction of gluten into the diet. Stools bulky, fatty, foul smelling.		Failure to thrive Weight loss Abdominal distention Anorexia Irritability Muscle wasting	Celiac disease

Table 17-6 Assessment of Degree of Dehyration in Infants and Children

	Mild Dehydration	Moderate Dehydration	Severe Dehydration
Weight loss (% of body weight)	3% to 5 %	6% to 9 %	10% to 15%
Skin color	Pale	Gray	Mottled
Mucous membranes	Dry	Very dry	Parched
Skin elasticity	Decreased	Poor	Very poor
Blood pressure	Normal or increased	Can be lower	Lowered
Pulse	Normal or increased	Increased	Rapid, thready

Adapted from Hockenberry MJ et al: *Wong's nursing care of infants and children,* ed 7, St Louis, 2003, Mosby.

the degree of discomfort present before deeper probing. Flexing the child's knees permits greater visibility of the anal area. If the toddler or preschooler is apprehensive, having the parent hold the child supine on the lap with legs flexed and dangling can be helpful in completing the assessment. Talking to and playing with the child also assists in examination. Most children are ticklish, so briefly place a hand flat on the abdomen before beginning the examination. A very ticklish child can be assisted by placing the child's hand over the nurse's during palpation. During palpation, observe for changes in vocalization (e.g., cry becomes high-pitched) or sudden protective movements that can indicate pain or tenderness.

Assessment of Abdomen

Assessment	Findings
Inspection	
Inspect the contour of the abdomen while the infant or child is standing and while he or she is lying supine.	A pot-bellied or prominent abdomen is normal until puberty, related to lordosis of the spine. The abdomen appears flat when the child is supine. **Clinical Alert** An especially protuberant abdomen can suggest fluid retention, tumor, organomegaly (enlarged organ), or ascites. A large abdomen, with thin limbs and wasted buttocks, suggests severe malnutrition and can be seen in children with celiac disease or cystic fibrosis. A depressed abdomen is indicative of dehydration or high abdominal obstruction. A midline protrusion from the xiphoid process to the umbilicus or the symphysis pubis indicates diastasis recti abdominis.

Assessment	Findings
Inspection—cont'd	
Inspect the color and condition of the skin of the abdomen. Note the presence of scars, ecchymoses, and stomas or pouches.	Veins are often visible on the abdomen of thin, light-skinned children. **Clinical Alert** Yellowish coloration can suggest jaundice. Jaundice is found with hepatitis, cirrhosis, and gallbladder disease. Silver lines (striae) indicate obesity or fluid retention. Scars can indicate previous surgery. Ecchymoses of soft tissue areas can indicate abuse. Distended veins indicate abdominal or vascular obstruction or distention.
Inspect the abdomen for movement by standing at eye level to the abdomen.	**Clinical Alert** Visible peristaltic waves nearly always indicate intestinal obstruction, and in the infant younger than 2 months indicate pyloric stenosis. If an infant younger than 2 months is fed, the peristaltic waves become larger and more frequent if stenosis is present. Failure of the abdomen and thorax to move synchronously can indicate peritonitis (if the abdomen does not move) or pulmonary disease (if the thorax does not move).
Inspect the umbilicus for hygiene, color, discharge, odor, inflammation, herniation, and fistulas.	**Clinical Alert** A bluish umbilicus indicates intraabdominal hemorrhage. A nodular umbilicus indicates tumor.

Assessment	Findings
Inspection—cont'd	
	Protrusion of the umbilicus indicates herniation. Umbilical hernias protrude more noticeably with crying and coughing. Palpate the umbilicus to estimate the size of the opening. Drainage from the umbilicus can indicate infection or a patent urachus.
Auscultation	
Auscultate for bowel sounds by pressing both the bell and the diaphragm of the stethoscope *firmly* against the abdomen. Listen in all four quadrants (Figure 17-1) and count the bowel sounds in each quadrant for 1 full minute.	Normal bowel sounds occur every 10 to 30 seconds and are heard as gurgles, clicks, and growls. **Clinical Alert** High-pitched tinkling sounds indicate diarrhea, gastroenteritis, or obstruction. Absence of bowel sounds can indicate peritonitis or paralytic ileus.
Before deciding that bowel sounds are absent, the nurse must listen for a minimum of 5 minutes in each area where sounds are not heard. Bowel sounds can be stimulated, if present, by stroking the abdomen with a fingernail.	
Percussion	
Using indirect percussion, systematically percuss all areas of the abdomen.	Dullness or flatness is normally found along the right costal margin (see Figure 17-1) and 1 to 3 cm (0.4 to 1.2 in) below the costal margin of the liver.

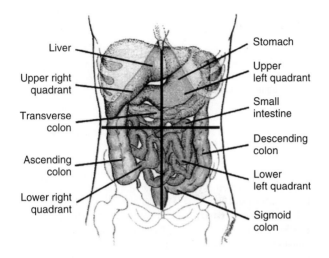

Figure 17-1
Anatomic landmarks of abdomen.
(From Potter PA, Perry AG: *Basic nursing theory and practice,* ed 4, St Louis, 1999, Mosby.)

Assessment	Findings
Percussion—cont'd	
	Dullness above the symphysis pubis can indicate a full bladder in a young child and is normal. Tympany is normally heard throughout the rest of the abdomen.
	Clinical Alert
	If liver dullness extends lower than expected, an enlarged liver might be suspected.
	Dullness in areas in which tympany would normally be expected can indicate tumor, ascites, pregnancy, or a full bowel.

Assessment	Findings

Palpation

If the child complains of pain in an abdominal area, palpate that area last.

Using superficial palpation, assess the abdomen for tenderness, superficial lesions, muscle tone, turgor (pinch the skin into a fold), and cutaneous hyperesthesia (pick up a fold of skin but do not pinch). Superficial palpation is performed by placing the hand on the abdomen and applying light pressure with the fingertips, using a circular motion. Note areas of tenderness.

Visceral pain, arising from organs such as the stomach and large intestine, is dull, poorly localized, and felt in the midline. Somatic pain, arising from the walls and the linings of the abdominal cavity (parietal peritoneum), is sharp, intense, focused, and well defined and will be at the same dermatomal level as the origin of the pain. Coughing and movement will aggravate pain arising from parietal

Clinical Alert

Sudden protective behaviors (e.g., grabbing the hand of the nurse), withdrawal, or a tense facial expression can indicate apprehension, pain, or nausea.

Pain on picking up a fold of abdominal skin indicates hyperthesia, which can be found with peritonitis.

Pain that is poorly localized, vague, and periumbilical can indicate appendicitis in the early stage. As the peritoneum becomes inflamed, the pain becomes localized and constant in the right iliac fossa.

Diffuse pain that mimics the pain associated with appendicitis, along with generalized lymphadenopathy, can indicate mesenteric lymphadenitis.

Assessment	Findings

Palpation—cont'd

origins. Do not ask,
"Does this hurt?" The
child, eager to please,
might say yes. A pain
measurement scale can
help children to rate
pain more specifically
and to differentiate
between pain and fear.
During palpation,
observe if the child's
eyes are closed; a child
with genuine pain will
tend to watch the
palpating hand closely.

Perform deep palpation,
either by placing one
hand on top of the other
or by supporting
posterior structures with
one hand while palpating
anterior structures with
the other. Palpate from
the lower quadrants
upward so that an
enlarged liver can be
detected.

Discomfort in the epigastrium on
deep palpation is related to
pressure over the aorta.

The spleen tip can be palpated 1 to
2 cm (0.4 to 0.8 in) below the
left costal margin during
inspiration in infants and young
children and is felt as a soft,
thumb-shaped object.

The liver can be palpated 1 to
2 cm (0.4 to 0.8 in) below the
right costal margin during
inspiration in infants
and young children. The
liver edge is firm and smooth.
It is often not palpable in
older children.

Kidneys are rarely palpable except
in neonates.

The sigmoid colon can be palpable
as a tender sausage-shaped mass
in the left lower quadrant. The
cecum can be palpated as a soft
mass in the right lower quadrant.

Assessment	Findings
Palpation—cont'd	

Clinical Alert

Tenderness in the lower quadrants can indicate feces, gastroenteritis, pelvic infection, or tumor.

Tenderness in the left upper quadrant can indicate splenic enlargement or intussusception.

Tenderness in the right upper quadrant can be related to hepatitis or an enlarged liver.

Pain in the costovertebral angle or abdominal pain can indicate upper urinary tract infection.

Tenderness in the right lower quadrant or around the umbilicus can indicate appendicitis.

Rebound tenderness can indicate appendicitis and might be elicited by applying pressure distal to where the child states there is pain.

Pain is experienced in the original area of tenderness when pressure is released.

An enlarged spleen indicates infection or a blood disease.

Palpation of an olive-sized mass in the epigastric area and to the upper right of the umbilicus can indicate pyloric stenosis in the young infant.

An enlarged liver is found with infection, blood dycrasias, sickle cell anemia, or congestive heart failure.

Enlarged kidneys can indicate tumor or hydronephrosis.

A distended bladder can be palpable above the symphysis pubis.

Assessment	Findings

Palpation—cont'd

Further assess for peri-
toneal irritation by
performing the psoas
muscle test. This test
can be performed in a
cooperative older child
if the nurse is assessing
for appendicitis. Have
the child flex the right
leg at the hip and knee
while you apply
downward pressure.
Normally, no pain is felt.

Clinical Alert
Pain suggests appendicitis.

Palpate for an inguinal
hernia by sliding the
little finger into the
external inguinal canal
at the base of the
scrotum (inguinal
hernia is more common
in boys) and ask the
child to cough.
If the child is young,
have child laugh or
blow up a balloon.

Clinical Alert
Report the presence of inguinal
hernia. An inguinal hernia is felt
as a bulge when the child laughs
or cries and can also be visible
as a mass in the scrotum.

Palpate for a femoral
hernia by locating the
femoral pulse. Place the
index finger on the pulse
and the middle or ring
finger medially against
the skin. The ring finger
is over the area where
the herniation occurs.

Clinical Alert
Report the presence of femoral
hernia. A femoral hernia is felt
or seen as a small anterior mass.
Femoral hernia is more
commonly found in girls.

Assessment of Anal Area

Assessment	Findings
With the child prone, inspect the buttocks and thighs. Examine the skin around the anal area for redness and rash.	**Clinical Alert** Asymmetry of the buttocks and thigh folds indicates congenital hip dysplasia. Redness and rash can indicate inadequate cleaning after bowel movements, infrequent changing of diapers, or irritation from diarrhea.
Examine the anus for marks, fissures (tears in the mucosa), hemorrhoids (dark protrusions), prolapse (moist tubelike protrusion), polyps (bright red protrusions), and skin tags.	The anus usually appears moist and hairless. **Clinical Alert** Scratch marks can indicate itching, which can indicate pinworm infestation. Fissures can indicate passage of hard stools. Defecation can be accompanied by bleeding if fissures are present. Bleeding can also accompany polyps, intussusception, gastric and peptic ulcers, esophageal varices, ulcerative colitis, infectious diseases, and Meckel's diverticulum. Rectal prolapse indicates difficult defecation and often accompanies untreated cystic fibrosis. Skin tags can indicate polyps and are usually benign. Lacerations and bruises of anus can indicate abuse.
Stroke the anal area to elicit the anal reflex.	The anus should contract quickly. **Clinical Alert** A slow reflex can indicate a disorder of the pyramidal tract.

Related Nursing Diagnoses

Anxiety: related to change in health status.

Pain: related to injury agents.

Constipation: related to insufficient physical activity, pharmacologic agents, megacolon, tumors, electrolyte imbalance, neurologic impairment, poor eating habits, insufficient fluid intake, dehydration, insufficient fluid intake.

Perceived constipation: related to faulty appraisal, cultural/family health beliefs.

Diarrhea: related to stress, anxiety, inflammation, infectious processes, malabsorption, irritation, parasites, contaminants, toxins.

Altered family processes: related to shift in health status of family member.

Fluid volume deficit: related to compromised regulatory mechanisms.

Fluid volume excess: secondary to liver disorders, renal disorders.

Knowledge deficit: related to disease process, dietary alterations, hygienic needs, dietary needs.

Altered parenting: related to physical illness.

Impaired skin integrity: related to nutritional deficit or excess, chemical factors, fluid deficit or excess.

Altered urinary elimination: related to urinary tract infection, anatomic obstruction, sensory motor impairment.

Ineffective therapeutic regimen: related to complexity of therapeutic regimen.

Lymphatic System

18

The lymphatic system includes the lymph nodes, spleen, thymus, and bone marrow. The superficial lymph nodes and the spleen are accessible for assessment and are discussed in this chapter. Assessment of the lymphatic system is often integrated with assessment of the neck, breast, and abdomen.

Rationale

The most common causes of visible lymphoid activity are infection and neoplasms. Infection is the most common cause of lumps in children's necks. An understanding of which areas are drained by the nodes is useful in further assessment of present or past infections. Detection of enlarged nodes and an enlarged spleen can be critical to the early diagnosis and treatment of serious disorders.

Anatomy and Physiology

The lymphoid system is a system of lymph fluid, collecting ducts, and tissues. Although the specific functions of lymphoid tissue are still not fully understood, the system is thought to play an important role in the production of lymphocytes and antibodies and in phagocytosis. The system also transports lymph fluids, microorganisms, and protein back to the cardiovascular system and absorbs fat and fat-soluble substances from the intestine.

Lymph enters open-ended ducts called *capillaries.* The capillaries form larger collecting ducts, which drain into tissue centers or nodes. Lymph from the nodes eventually drains into the venous system by way of even larger ducts.

Lymph nodes, the most numerous element in the lymphatic system, rarely occur singly, but usually in chains or clusters. The lymph nodes that are closer to the center of the body are usually smaller; thus cervical nodes are larger than axillary nodes.

The spleen is composed of lymphoid and reticuloendothelial cells. It is found under the ribs in the upper left quadrant of the abdomen. The amount of lymphoid tissue and the size of the lymph nodes vary with age. Infants have a small amount of palpable lymphatic tissue, which gradually increases until middle childhood, when the volume of lymphatic tissue reaches its peak. By middle adolescence the volume of lymphatic tissue begins to diminish, until it reaches the adult level of 2% to 3% of total body weight. Children are more likely to develop generalized adenopathy in response to disease, and even mild infections result in swollen nodes or "swollen glands."

Equipment for Assessment of Lymphatic System

■ Ruler

Preparation

Inquire about recent contact with persons with infectious diseases. Ask if the child has been experiencing weakness, easy fatigability, fever, bruising, bone pain, or chronic or recurrent infection. Ask if there is a family history of blood disorders or cancer.

Assessment of Lymph Nodes

Assessment	Findings
Using the distal portion of the fingers and gentle but firm circular motions, palpate the head, neck, axillae, and groin to detect enlarged lymph nodes (Figure 18-1). Note the color, size, location, mobility, temperature, consistency, and tenderness of enlarged nodes. Tender nodes should be assessed last. Measure enlarged nodes.	Small (less than 1 cm, or 0.5 in), movable, nontender nodes are normal in young children. **Clinical Alert** Nodes that are enlarged because of infection are firm, warm, fluctuant, and movable, and their borders are diffuse. Redness can overlie nodes that are enlarged because of infection. Enlargement of preauricular nodes commonly suggests eye infection. Enlargement of the preauricular, mastoid, and deep cervical nodes can indicate infection of the ear.
To palpate nodes in the areas anterior and	Enlargement of nodes in the jaw area can signify infections of the

Assessment	Findings
posterior to the sterno-cleidomastoid muscle, move the fingertips against the muscle. To palpate nodes in the head and neck, have the child flex the head forward or bend toward the side being examined. To palpate nodes in the axillae, roll the tissues against the chest wall and muscles of the axillae. Have the child hold the arms in a relaxed, slightly abducted position at the sides. To palpate nodes in the inguinal area, place the child in a supine position.	tongue or mouth. Enlargement of nodes in the supraclavicular region often indicates metastases from the lungs or abdominal structures. Bilateral lymph node enlargement can indicate infectious mononucleosis. Nodes enlarged as a result of cancer are usually nontender, fixed, hard, of variable size, and matted. No discoloration is present. Enlarged nodes can also indicate metabolic disorders, hypersensitivity reactions, and primary hematopoietic disorders.

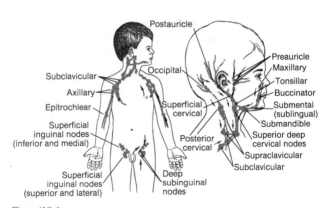

Figure 18-1

Location of lymph nodes and direction of lymph flow.

(From Hockenberry MJ et al: *Wong's nursing care of infants and children,* ed 7, St Louis, 2003, Mosby.)

Assessment of Spleen

Assessment	Findings
With the child supine, place one hand under the child's back and the other hand on the left upper quadrant of the child's abdomen. Ask the child to "Suck in your breath." The spleen tip can be felt during inspiration on deep palpation.	The spleen can be palpated 1 to 2 cm (0.4 to 0.8 in) below the left costal margin in infants and children. **Clinical Alert** A spleen that extends more than 2 cm (0.8 in) below the costal margin can indicate leukemia, thalassemia major, sickle cell anemia, or infectious mononucleosis.

Related Nursing Diagnoses

Activity tolerance: related to generalized weakness.

Compromised family coping: related to situational crisis, knowledge deficit.

Hyperthermia: related to illness.

Altered protection: related to abnormal blood profiles.

Risk for infection: related to immunosuppression, inadequate secondary defenses.

Altered parenting: related to physical illness.

Risk for altered body temperature: related to illness.

Reproductive System

19

Assessment of the reproductive system in infants and children includes inspection of the external genitalia. Examination of internal genitalia is performed by nurses specially prepared in this skill.

Rationale

Examination of the external genitalia enables screening for common disorders that arise from prenatal development and influences. Examination enables the nurse to detect infections that require further evaluation. Assessment of the reproductive system often provides a beginning point for teaching and discussion related to sexuality and hygiene.

Anatomy and Physiology
Female Genitalia

The female genitalia includes the external and internal sex organs. The external sex organs, or vulva, include the mons pubis, a fatty pad overlying the symphysis pubis (Figure 19-1); the labia majora, rounded folds of adipose tissue extending down and back from the mons pubis; the labia minora, two thinner folds of skin medial to the labia majora, which, following prominence in the newborn period, atrophy to become nearly invisible until adolescence; and the clitoris, an erectile body situated at the anterior end of the labia minora. The labia minora are homologous to the male scrotum, and the clitoris to the male penis. Underlying the labia minora is a boat-shaped area termed the *vestibule.* At the posterior end of the vestibule is the vaginal opening, or introitus, which can be partially obscured by the hymen, a vascular mucous membrane. The perineum is the area between the vaginal opening and the anus. The urethral opening, or urinary meatus, lies between the vaginal opening and the clitoris.

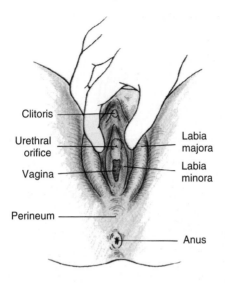

Figure 19-1
External female genitalia.
(From Potter PA, Perry AG: *Basic nursing: theory and practice,* ed 4, St Louis, 1999, Mosby.)

On either side of the urethral opening can be seen Skene's glands, or the paraurethral ducts. Bartholin's glands, which secrete lubricating fluid during intercourse, are situated on either side of the vaginal opening, but the openings to the glands usually cannot be seen.

The vagina is a hollow tube extending upward and backward between the urethra and the rectum. The cervix joins the vagina, which has a slitlike opening, termed the *external os,* that provides an opening between the uterus and the endocervical canal. The uterus is a muscular pear-shaped organ suspended above the bladder. In the prepubescent girl the uterus is 2.5 to 3.5 cm (1 to 1.4 in) long, compared with 6 to 8 cm (2.4 to 3.2 in) in the mature woman. The uterine, or fallopian, tubes extend from the uterus to the ovaries and produce a passageway in which ova and sperm meet.

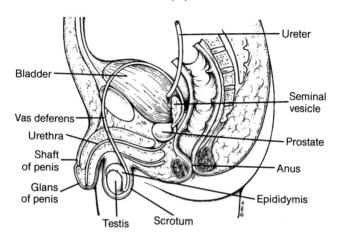

Figure 19-2
Male genitalia.
(From Whaley LF, Wong DL: *Nursing care of infants and children*, ed 4, St Louis, 1991, Mosby.)

Male Genitalia

The external male genitalia include the penis and scrotum. The penis consists of a shaft and a glans (Figure 19-2). The shaft is formed primarily of erectile tissue. The glans is a cone-shaped structure at the end of the penis and contains both erectile and sensory tissue. The corona is the crownlike area where the glans arises from the shaft. A loose fold of skin, termed the *prepuce* or foreskin, overlies the glans. This skin is removed during circumcision. The urethra is within the penile shaft, with the slitlike urethral meatus located slightly centrally at the tip of the glans.

The scrotum is a loose, wrinkled sac located at the base of the penis. The scrotum has two compartments, each of which contains a testis, epididymis, and parts of the vas deferens. The testes, epididymis, and vas deferens are considered internal male sex organs.

The testes are ovoid and somewhat rubbery. The testes in the infant are 1.5 cm (0.6 in) long. Testicular length remains virtually unchanged until puberty, when the testes gradually enlarge to the adult length of 4 to 5 cm (1.6 to 2 in). The left testis lies slightly lower than the right. Primary functions of the testis are sperm and hormone production. During ejaculation, sperm drains into the epididymis, and then into the vas deferens before passing into the urethra.

The genetic sex type of the embryo begins during cell division, when X and Y chromosomes are distributed. Initially, internal and external genitalia are not differentiated (Figure 19-3, *A*). External differentiation begins by about the seventh week of gestation. Under the influence of androgens, enlargement and fusion of primitive urogenital structures occurs and male genitalia are formed (Figure 19-3, *B*). The testes descend from the abdominal cavity at between 7 and 9 months of gestation. If the tube that precedes their descent fails to close, an indirect inguinal hernia is produced.

The male reproductive system remains unchanged until maturity. Testicular enlargement is a visible sign of sexual maturation, which can begin by 10 years of age. Accompanying the initial increase in testicular size are a coarsening, reddening, and wrinkling of the scrotal sacs and the growth of a few pubic hairs (the child has no pubic hair). Height and weight increase, and hair growth appears

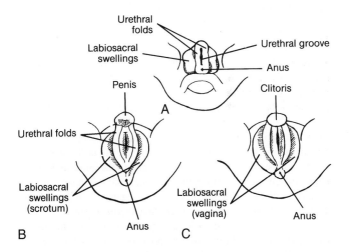

Figure 19-3
Initial stages in embryonic genital development. **A,** Undifferentiated stage. **B,** Initial differentiation of external genitalia in male embryo. **C,** Initial differentiation of external genitalia in female embryo.

on the face about 2 years after the appearance of pubic hair. During further development the penis enlarges, the voice changes, and body odor appears. The genital skin continues to pigment and the external sex organs continue to enlarge until full maturation is reached. At maturity pubic hair covers the symphysis pubis and medial aspects of the thighs. Reproductive capability accompanies sexual maturity, which is accomplished between 14 and 18 years of age.

In the embryo, development of female genitalia involves shrinkage and minimal fusion of primitive urogenital structures (Figure 19-3,C). Primordial follicles are formed during the sixth month of gestation, but must wait until puberty for further development. Breast development is usually the first sign of sexual maturation, although growth of pubic hair can precede breast enlargement. The initial pubic hair, located at the sides of the labia, is fine. Gradually the hair coarsens and covers the sides of the labia and the perianal area at full maturation. Internal and external sex organs enlarge. The onset of menstruation provides observable evidence of reproductive maturation (Figure 19-4).

Equipment for Assessment of Reproductive System

- Glove for pelvic examination
- Drape
- Speculum

Preparation

A casual, matter-of-fact approach facilitates examination of the reproductive system. Much of the examination can be accomplished during assessment of the abdomen and anus in the infant and young child. Inform parents (if appropriate) and child of results of the finding as the assessment progresses because this helps relieve anxiety. A child other than an infant should be adequately covered at all times with clothing, such as a top that opens in the front, or a drape. Alternative positions for examination, such as semisitting on the parent's lap, with the child's feet on the nurse's knees, might be more comfortable. An adolescent should be given the option of having a supportive person, such as a friend, present during examination. It is important to ensure privacy and confidentiality and if a parent is present, it must be made clear the adolescent is the patient by directing questions at him or her. It is important to recognize that children and parents from some cultures (e.g., Hispanic) are particularly modest and might require additional assistance to become comfortable.

The first pelvic examination is usually performed when the female child is 18 to 21 years old or as soon as she becomes sexually active, when there is a history of trauma or abuse, when there is vaginal discharge, menorrhagia, primary amenorrhea, secondary amenorrhea for more than 3 months, abdominal pain, or at the adolescent's request. Adolescents at high risk (sexual intercourse before 18 years, multiple partners, intercourse without a condom, partners with history of intercourse, smoking, sexually transmitted diseases, and absence of three consecutive, negative Pap smears) should be screened yearly.

Inquire whether the female child has had itching, pain on urination, abdominal pain, or vaginal discharge. If the girl is older, inquire whether menses have commenced, the date of the last menstrual period, length of cycle, amount of flow, if the adolescent knows how to or is practicing breast self-examination, dietary and exercise regimen, type of contraception used (if sexually active), number of sexual partners, and experiences with sexual abuse and rape. Inquire about family history of breast cancer and ovarian cancer. If the child has missed three consecutive menses, inquire about eating habits.

Inquire whether the male child has had decreased urination, forced urination, a strong urinary stream, pain on voiding, discharge or drip from the penis, and whether using a condom (if sexually active). Inquire if adolescent knows how or is practicing testicular self-examination.

Assessment of Female Breasts

Assessment is accomplished with the adolescent sitting with arms at her sides. Because the adolescent must disrobe to the waist or wear a front-opening gown, ensure that the room is warm. Privacy is essential. Tell the adolescent that you are going to examine her breasts. A gentle, matter-of-fact approach assists in putting her at ease. If the adolescent is unfamiliar with breast self-examination, this is a good opportunity to explain what is being done and to encourage her to imitate the examination maneuvers. Adolescents might be too embarrassed to touch their breasts, and the nurse's approach should vary with the patient's degree of psychologic comfort.

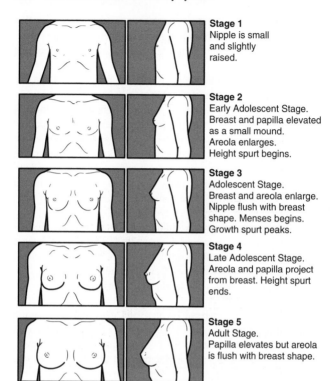

Stage 1
Nipple is small and slightly raised.

Stage 2
Early Adolescent Stage. Breast and papilla elevated as a small mound. Areola enlarges. Height spurt begins.

Stage 3
Adolescent Stage. Breast and areola enlarge. Nipple flush with breast shape. Menses begins. Growth spurt peaks.

Stage 4
Late Adolescent Stage. Areola and papilla project from breast. Height spurt ends.

Stage 5
Adult Stage. Papilla elevates but areola is flush with breast shape.

Figure 19-4
Tanner stages in development of secondary sexual characteristics in females.

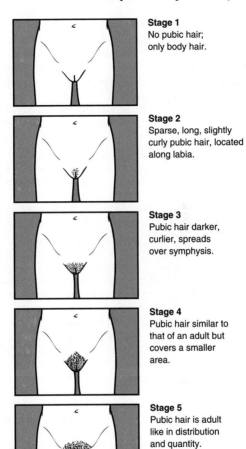

Stage 1
No pubic hair;
only body hair.

Stage 2
Sparse, long, slightly
curly pubic hair, located
along labia.

Stage 3
Pubic hair darker,
curlier, spreads
over symphysis.

Stage 4
Pubic hair similar to
that of an adult but
covers a smaller
area.

Stage 5
Pubic hair is adult
like in distribution
and quantity.

Figure 19-4—cont'd

Assessment	Findings
Inspect the breasts. Note their size, contour, symmetry, and color while the child or adolescent is sitting, trunk exposed, and arms at side.	Contour and size of the breasts and changes in the areola indicate sexual maturity. Some difference in size of the breasts is usually normal.
	One breast can develop before the other, and the adolescent might need reassurance that this is normal.
	Clinical Alert
	Breast development before 8 years of age can be normal but requires careful assessment.
	Delayed breast development (none by age 13 years) should be evaluated along with the development of secondary sexual characteristics.
	Dimpling and alterations in the contour of the breast can indicate cancer.
	Redness can signal infection.
	Striae can be related to obesity or pregnancy. (New striae in the fair-skinned adolescent are red and in the dark-skinned adolescent are ruddy and dark-brown. Old striae in the fair-skinned adolescent are silver and in dark-skinned adolescents are lighter than the skin color.)
Inspect the nipple and areola. Note the color, size, shape, and the presence and color of any discharge.	The color, size, and shape of the nipple and areola provide information about sexual maturity.
	Nipple inversion is a normal variation and can be present from puberty.
	Clinical Alert
	Recent inversion, flattening, or depression of the nipple in a more mature adolescent or edema of the nipple or areola can indicate the presence of cancer.

Assessment	Findings
	Discharge is an abnormal finding and can be related to a number of hormonal and pharmacologic causes. It should, however, be referred to a physician.
Have the adolescent place her arms above her head, and then on her hips. These maneuvers help accentuate dimpling or retraction that might be missed. Note axilla hair.	African American girls develop axillary hair sooner than Caucasian counterparts (Tanner stages are based on studies of white, English girls) and sometimes before pubic hair. Asian adolescents tend to have finer and sparser hair.
Palpate the breast tissue with the patient supine and with her hands behind her neck. If breasts are large, place a pillow under the patient's shoulder on the side that is to be examined. This distributes the breast tissue more evenly. Use the pads of the fingers flat on the breast to gently compress the tissue against the chest wall. Systematically palpate the entire breast, including the periphery, areola, nipple, and tail using a pattern such as parallel lines, concentric circles, or consecutive clock times, using a rotary motion. During palpation note consistency of tissues and areas of tenderness. If masses are present, note size, shape, consistency, number, mobility, definition, tenderness, erythema, and lymphadenopathy.	Normal young breast tissue has firm elasticity. The stimulation of examination can cause erection of the nipple and wrinkling of the areola. Coolness in the room can also elicit erection of the nipple.

Assessment	Findings
Palpate abnormal masses and note their location (by quadrant or clock), size (in centimeters or inches), shape (round, discoid, irregular, matted), consistency (soft, firm, hard, fluid, cystic), tenderness (whether palpation elicits pain), mobility (fixed or freely movable), definition (well-circumscribed or not), presence of erythema, and lymphadenopathy.	**Clinical Alert** Fixed or movable, hard, irregular, and poorly circumscribed nodules can suggest cancer. Mobile, nontender, round or dislike, well-delineated nodules can indicate fibroadenoma.

Assessment of Female Genitalia

Assessment is best accomplished with the child supine or semireclining. If a young child, the examination can be performed with child semireclining in the parent's lap; if an adolescent, she might prefer to assume a semisitting position and to have a mirror to see what is taking place. Encouraging the child to keep her heels together provides distraction. Before beginning a pelvic examination, have the adolescent empty her bladder.

Assessment	Findings
Inspect the mons pubis for hair. Note color, quality, quantity, and distribution of hair, if present.	Soft, downy hair along the labia majora signals early sexual maturation. In the mature female, pubic hair forms an inverted triangle.
Inspect the labia majora and labia minora for size, color, skin integrity, masses, and lesions.	Labia should appear pink and moist. **Clinical Alert** Rash over the mons pubis and labia can indicate contact dermatitis or infestations. Redness and swelling of labia can indicate infection, masturbation, or sexual abuse. Fusion of labia can indicate male scrotum. Labial adhesions can be seen in infants.

Assessment	Findings
	Painful, clear, raised vesicles that fuse together to form an ulcer on the genitals are indicative of Herpes simplex.
	Hard, nontender, red, sharply demarcated and indurated lesions (chancre) and yellow discharge are indicative of syphilis.
	Venereal disease in the young child is a sign of sexual abuse.
	Urogenital abnormalities are found in infants born to mothers who used cocaine prenatally.
Note the size of the clitoris.	**Clinical Alert**
	A clitoris larger than normal can indicate labioscrotal fusion.
	In some cultures, female circumcision is practiced, which can produce extensive scarring and adhesions.
Palpate for Skene's and Bartholin's glands.	Skene's and Bartholin's glands are normally not palpable.
	A small amount of clear, mucousy discharge is normal.
	Clinical Alert
	If Bartholin's or Skene's glands are palpable, infection or cysts might be present.
Inspect urethral and vaginal openings for edema, redness, and discharge.	**Clinical Alert**
	Redness of the urethra can indicate urethritis.
	Hymen tears, enlarged hymenal opening, irregular or thickened hymenal edges, and attenuation of hymenal tissue can indicate abuse.
	Redness and foul-smelling discharge from the vagina can indicate a foreign body, infection, sexual abuse, or pinworms.

Assessment	Findings
	A white, cheesy discharge from the vagina indicates a candidal infection.
	Pregnancy is the most common cause of abnormal bleeding, but bleeding can also be related to foreign bodies, STDs, bleeding disorders, or endocrine disorders.
	Dysfunctional uterine bleeding can occur in the absence of these conditions.
	Vaginal discharge and dysuria can indicate chlamydial infection.
	Refer the child for further examination if a vaginal opening cannot be seen.
Initiate the speculum examination in the adolescent after inspection of external structures. Use a plastic or metal speculum that has been lubricated and warmed with warm water. Usually the narrow Pederson speculum is used.	**Clinical Alert** Adnexal tenderness and cervical motion tenderness, as well as tenderness in the lower abdomen, can indicate pelvic inflammatory disease.
Initiate the bimanual examination following the speculum examination. Inability to feel ovaries is not unusual, especially if the adolescent is overweight.	

Assessment of Male Genitalia

Assessment	Findings
Inspect the penis for size, color, skin integrity, masses, and lesions.	An obese child might appear to have a small penis because of overlying skin folds.

Assessment	Findings
Note whether the child is circumcised. If uncircumcised and older than 3 years of age, attempt to gently retract the foreskin. Do not forcibly attempt to retract the foreskin; in infants, the prepuce is tight. Forcible retraction can damage the thin membrane and cause adhesions	The foreskin is normally adherent in children younger than 3 years.

Clinical Alert

A penis that is large in relation to the child's stage of development can suggest precocious puberty or testicular cancer. An abnormally small penis can indicate a clitoris.

Chancres are indicative of syphilis and need to be reported.

Condyloma acuminatum, or genital warts, is a venereal disease and can indicate sexual activity in an adolescent or sexual abuse in a young child. Warts appear as soft, skin-colored discrete growths that are whitish pink to reddish brown. Warts can be pedunculated or broad based and can enlarge to cauliflower-like masses. Warts on the anus or rectum are associated with anal intercourse.

Small, round or oval, dome-shaped papules with a central umbilicum, from which thick, creamy material can be expressed, are found with molluscum contagiosum.

A foreskin that cannot be easily retracted in a child older than 3 years can indicate phimosis.

Assessment	Findings
Inspect the urinary meatus for shape, placement, discharge, and ulceration. If possible, note the strength and steadiness of the urinary stream.	The urinary meatus is normally *slightly* ventral at the tip of the penis and slitlike. **Clinical Alert** A urinary meatus that is ventral is called *hypospadias*. A meatus that is dorsal is called *epispadias*. A round meatus can indicate meatal stenosis related to repeated infections.
Inspect the quality, quantity, and distribution of pubic hair. Inspect the base of the penis for scratches and inflammation. Inspect the scrotum for color, size, symmetry, edema, masses, and lesions. Palpate the testes by holding a finger over the inguinal canal while palpating the scrotal sac. Cold, touch, exercise, and stimulation cause the testes to ascend higher into the pelvic cavity. A retractile testicle can be pushed back into the scrotum by placing firm pressure on the inguinal canal before palpating the abdomen or genitalia or by having the child sit tailor fashion or blow on a windmill. A retractile testicle can be distinguished from a lymph node by its mobility; it can be massaged down	A prepubertal boy normally does not have pubic hair (Figure 19-5). The left testis is lower than the right. A testis should be present in each sac, freely movable, smooth, equal in size, and about 1.5 cm (0.6 in) until puberty. A retractile testis is usually bilateral. **Clinical Alert** The absence of a testis in the scrotal sac can indicate temporary ascent of the testis into the pelvic cavity or an undescended testicle. If the one testis is undescended, the affected hemiscrotum will appear small in contrast to the other hemiscrotum. Reassess. If testes still cannot be felt, refer the child if older than 1 year. Before 1 year the testicle might descend without intervention. If both testes are undescended, this can indicate pseudohermaphroditism, especially if hypospadias or a small penis is also present. Delayed pubertal

Assessment	Findings
the canal although it will spring back.	changes can indicate chronic illness or abnormalities in the anterior pituitary gland, hypothalamus, or testes. Scratches and inflammation at the base of the penis can indicate lice. Check for nits on the pubic hair.

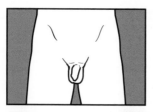

Stage 1

Prepubescent. No pubic hair; only fine body hair. Penis and scrotum childhood size and proportion.

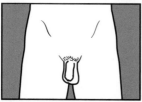

Stage 2

Sparse growth of long, slightly dark hair at base of penis. Scrotum and testes enlarge. Scrotal skin reddens.

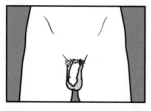

Stage 3

Hair becomes darker, curlier, coarser. Hair spreads over symphysis. Penis, scrotum, and testes enlarge.

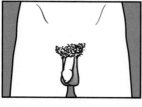

Stage 4

Hair similar to that of an adult but has not spread to thighs. Penis increases in diameter and length; glans developed. Scrotum enlarges and darkens.

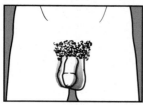

Stage 5

Hair spreads to medial surface of thighs. Genitals are adultlike.

Figure 19-5
Tanner stages in development of secondary sexual characteristics in males.

Related Nursing Diagnoses

Pain: related to injury agents.

Altered family processes: related to shift in health status of family member.

Infection: related to trauma, inadequate primary defense, insufficient knowledge to avoid pathogens.

Knowledge deficit: related to normal development, safe sexual practices, breast or testicular self-examination, home contraceptive practices.

Self-esteem disturbance: related to disturbances in body image, role performance, guilt/shame.

Impaired skin integrity: related to excretions, moisture, discharge, abuse.

Impaired tissue integrity: related to mechanical factors.

Sexual dysfunction: related to misinformation or lack of knowledge, vulnerability, psychosocial abuse, physical abuse, altered body structure/function.

Altered sexuality: related to conflicts with sexual orientation or variant preferences.

Fear: related to physical/social conditions, fear of others, separation from support system in potentially stressful situations, knowledge deficit.

Altered parenting: related to physical illness.

Musculoskeletal System 20

The nurse can obtain a great deal of data about the musculoskeletal system by watching the child walk, sit, and carry on various activities during other portions of the health assessment. Specific assessments aid in screening for childhood disorders such as clubfoot, developmental dysplasia of the hip, and scoliosis.

Rationale

Movement is so much a part of a child's activities that it is important to screen for disorders that can affect a child's socialization, exercise patterns, participation in sports, and ability to engage in self-care. Early diagnosis and intervention in disorders such as developmental dysplasia of the hip can possibly prevent more exhaustive treatment as the child grows.

Anatomy and Physiology

The musculoskeletal system provides support for the body and enables movement. The musculoskeletal system is composed of bones, muscles, tendons, ligaments, cartilage, and joints.

The skeleton arises from mesoderm. At birth the epiphyses of most bones are made of hyaline cartilage. Shortly after birth, secondary ossification centers appear in the epiphyses. The epiphyses ossify, except for the epiphyseal plate, which separates the epiphyses and the diaphyses. The epiphyseal plate is replaced by bone until only the epiphyseal line remains. When the epiphyses are completely ossified, no further bone lengthening occurs.

Muscle fibers are developed by the fourth or fifth month of gestation. The number of muscle fibers remains constant throughout life. Muscle growth is accomplished by increase in the size of the fibers. Muscle mass decreases from one fourth of total body weight at birth to one sixth of total body weight at adolescence. Transient increases in nonlean mass (subcutaneous fat) occur just before the growth spurt, especially in boys, accompanied by decreases 1 to 2 years later. Lean body mass increases, chiefly muscle, occur after the growth spurt, with the increase greater in males than in females.

Preparation

Inquire whether the infant sustained trauma or injury at birth. Inquire whether there is a family history of bone or joint disorders and whether the child has experienced delays in gross or fine motor development, trauma, joint stiffness and swelling, fever, or pain. If the child has or has had pain, it is important to determine the location, type, intensity, and time of occurrence of the pain. Sharp pain that lessens during rest can indicate injury. Constant dull pain that awakens the child might indicate tumor or infection. Inquire about participation in sports activities (type of sport, level of training involved, amount of contact, previous injuries) and diet. Minimal clothing assists with assessment of the spine.

Assessment of Musculoskeletal System

Assessment	Findings
If the child is able to walk, observe the gait. Note the presence of casts and braces.	Infants and toddlers tend to walk bowlegged. A wide-based gait is normal in the infant and toddler.
	Clinical Alert
	Limping can indicate developmental dysplasia of one hip (especially in toddlers). If both hips are involved, the child has a waddling gait. (Table 20-1 lists further indications of developmental dysplasia of the hip.)
	Limping also indicates scoliosis, Legg-Calvé-Perthes disease, infection of the joints of the lower extremities, a slipped capital femoral epiphysis, or stress fractures of the metatarsals.

Assessment	Findings
	Weight bearing on the toes *(pes equines)* and short heel cords indicate muscular disease or cerebral palsy.
Observe the curve of the infant's or child's spine and note the symmetry of the hips and shoulders while the child is standing erect. Test for scoliosis by having the child bend forward at the waist and observing the child from side; note asymmetry or prominence of rib cage.	The spine is normally rounded in the infant younger than 3 months. A lumbar curve forms at 12 to 18 months. Lumbar lordosis is normal in young children. **Clinical Alert** Rigidity of the spine while sitting up can indicate infection of the central nervous system or tension. Kyphosis (hunchback) can indicate wedge-shaped or collapsed vertebrae secondary to myelomeningocele, spinal tumors, Scheuermann's disease, tuberculosis of the spine, or sickle cell anemia. Kyphosis can also indicate habitual slouching. The persistence of lateral curvature of the spine indicates scoliosis. If the child can voluntarily correct the curve or if it disappears when the child is recumbent, the curve might be functional. A persistent curve, accompanied by unequal height of the shoulders and iliac crests when the child is standing erect and asymmetric elevation of the scapula when the child is leaning forward (Figure 20-1), indicates structural scoliosis.
Observe the lumbosacral area for abnormalities of the overlying skin (pigmented skin, hairy patches, or dimpling).	Pigmented skin, hairy patches, or dimpling in the lumbosacral area can indicate spina bifida occulta.

Assessment	Findings
Note the mobility of the spine, especially the cervical spine.	No resistance or pain should be felt when the child bends or when the neck is flexed or moved from side to side.
	Clinical Alert
	Pain, crying, or resistance when the neck is flexed indicates meningeal irritation and is known as Brudzinski's sign. Lateral inclination of the head can indicate congenital torticollis.
	Limitations in movement of the cervical spine can indicate cervical fusion, which is found in some children with fetal alcohol syndrome.
	Limitations in shoulder movement and pain across the upper back can be related to packing heavy book bags.
Inspect and palpate the upper extremities. Note the size, color, temperature, range of motion, and mobility of the joints and abnormalities in the upper extremities. Inspect the palmar creases (Figure 20-2).	**Clinical Alert**
	Short, broad extremities, hyperextensible joints, and simian creases can indicate the presence of Down syndrome.
	The Sydney line is found in children with rubella syndrome.
	Abnormal palmar creases can indicate fetal alcohol syndrome.
	Abnormally long and tapering fingers, tall and thin build, and hypermobility of joints can indicate Marfan syndrome.
	Short, bowed, and fragile bones and hyperextensible joints are found with osteogenesis imperfecta.
	Polydactyly (external digits) and syndactyly (webbing) are abnormal findings and may or may not indicate more serious underlying conditions.
	Warmth and tenderness of the joints can indicate rheumatoid arthritis. Tenderness also indicates Lyme disease or Henoch-Schönlein purpura (HSP).

Assessment	Findings
	Widening of the wrist joints can indicate rickets.
	Limitation of elbow extension and pain can indicate subluxation of the head of the radius.
	Limitation of movement in elbows, knees, and ankles, as well as complaints of tingling or aching, warmth, redness, and swelling can indicate hemarthrosis, which accompanies hemophilia.
	A solid palpable mass along a bone can indicate a tumor.
	Pain in the elbow that is aggravated by use can indicate tennis elbow or Little League elbow.
	Pain in the shoulder, loss of internal rotation, and increased external rotation can indicate Little League shoulder.
	Pain in the shoulder can indicate swimmer's shoulder.
Assess the strength of the upper extremities by asking the child to squeeze your crossed fingers.	The strength of the upper extremities should be equal. **Clinical Alert** Unilateral weakness can indicate hemiparesis or pain. The feet of infants and toddlers are flat, and the legs are bowed until walking has been firmly established.
Inspect and palpate the lower extremities. Assess for abnormalities of mobility, length, shape, and pulses.	**Clinical Alert** Fibrosis and contracture of the gluteal and quadriceps muscles occur as complications of intramuscular injections. Observe for limited knee flexion (quadriceps involvement) or hip flexion (gluteal involvement).

Assessment	Findings
Assess for *genu varum* (bowleg or lateral bowing of the tibia) or *genu valgum* (knock-knee) by instructing the child to stand with ankles together.	Knock-knee is present until the child is past 7 years of age. **Clinical Alert** A space greater than 5 cm (2 in) between the knees indicates *genu varum.* Toddlers are generally bowlegged until leg and back muscles develop fully; unilateral bowleggedness after 2 or 3 years of age can be pathologic. A space greater than 7.5 cm (3 in) between the malleoli in the child older than 7 years indicates *genu valgum.*
Assess for the presence of clubfoot by lightly scratching the inner and outer soles of the feet. Observe whether the foot assumes a normal angle (i.e., right angle) to the leg when stimulated.	**Clinical Alert** Return of the foot, after stimulation, to a right angle in relation to the leg can indicate metatarsus varus in an infant with adduction and inversion of the forefoot. Inability of the foot to right itself after stimulation can indicate talipes equinovarus (inversion of the forefoot, plantar flexion, and heel inversion) or talipes calcaneovalgus (eversion of the forefoot and dorsal flexion).
Assess the child for meningeal irritation by flexing the child's hips and then straightening each of the knees (Kernig's sign). Assess for developmental dysplasia of the hip (see Table 20-1).	**Clinical Alert** Pain and resistance to straightening of the knees indicate meningeal irritation.

Assessment	Findings
Assess for strength in the lower limbs by asking the child to push against your hands with the soles of the forefeet.	Strength should be symmetric in the lower limbs. **Clinical Alert** Unequal strength can indicate hemiparesis or pain. Pain with plantar flexion against resistance can indicate Achilles tendonitis. Pain in the arch or heel is related to repetitive stretching of the plantar fascia. Pain along the anterior or medial aspect of the midshaft or distal third of the tibia is indicative of shin splints.
Palpate knees for tenderness, warmth, and consistency.	**Clinical Alert** Tenderness, warmth, and boggy consistency can indicate synovitis. Pain, diffuse swelling, and limitation of movement can indicate sprain. Bone and joint pain, pallor, fatigue, hemorrhage, and anorexia can indicate leukemia.
If large amounts of fluid are suspected in the knee, instruct the child or adolescent to lie down. Grasp the patella firmly on each side with the left thumb and index finger. With right fingers, push down on the patella. Feel for a click or fluid wave (ballottement test).	Normal finding is absence of movement of patella. **Clinical Alert** Click or fluid wave indicates large amount of knee joint effusion. Absence of pain and clicking are normal findings.
If child or adolescent states knee "locks" or "gives way," perform McMurray's test. With the child supine, ask the child to flex the affected knee and hip.	**Clinical Alert** Clicking or pain can indicate a torn meniscus of the knee joint. Overprominence of the tibial tubercle, pain, and tenderness can indicate Osgood-Schlatter disease or Sinding-Larsen syndrome (pain is

Assessment	Findings
Place the thumb and index finger of one hand on either side of the knee; with the other hand, rotate the lower leg and foot laterally, holding the heel. Slowly extend the knee, noting pain or clicking. Rotate the lower leg and foot medially, observing for pain and clicking.	slightly lower). Chronic knee pain, especially after forced extension or overuse of the leg, can indicate patellofemoral syndrome. Knee joint laxity is the most valid indication of the severity of a sprain; athlete will complain of joint being loose or unstable.

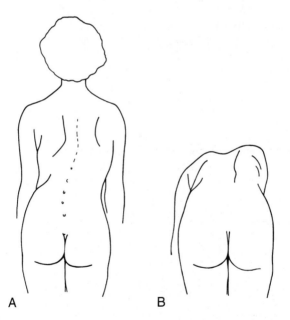

Figure 20-1
Scoliosis. **A,** When child stands, spine assumes lateral curvature and thoracic convexity is present. **B,** When child bends, chest wall on side of convexity is prominent and scapula on side of convexity is elevated.

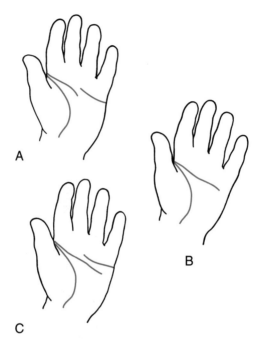

Figure 20-2
Palmar creases. **A,** Normal creases. **B,** Simian crease. **C,** Sydney line.

Table 20-1 Assessment for Presence of Developmental Dysplasia of the Hip

Test/Sign	Assessment	Abnormal Findings
Galeazzi or Allis' sign	Place the infant supine with the hips and knees flexed so that heels are as close to the buttocks as possible.	The knees are unequal in height. (Finding might not be apparent in the infant younger than 6 weeks.)
Unequal thigh folds	Place the infant or child prone. Observe symmetry of the thigh folds.	Unequal thigh folds.
Ortolani's test	Place the infant supine. With your thumbs on the inside of both thighs and your fingertips resting over the trochanter muscles, flex (do not force) both hips and knees. Slowly abduct each knee until the lateral aspect of each knee touches the examining table. This test is the most reliable in the infant from birth to 3 months.	A click or clunk is heard on abduction. Affected hip will not fully abduct.
Barlow's test	Place the infant supine. Flex and slightly adduct both hips while lifting the femur and applying downward pressure to the trochanter. This test is reliable from birth to 2 or 3 months of age.	Instability of hip joints.

Continued

Table 20-1 Assessment for Presence of Developmental Dysplasia of the Hip—cont'd

Test/Sign	Assessment	Abnormal Findings
Trendelenburg gait	Observe the gait of the child.	When the child bears weight on the affected side, the unaffected side of the pelvis drops (Figure 20-3).
Asymmetric inguinal folds and limited hip abduction.	Place the child supine and flex the hips. Gently abduct the hips while hips are in flexion (hip abduction is the most sensitive indicator of developmental dysplasia past 2 or 3 months).	Asymmetry of folds. Limited abduction on the affected side.

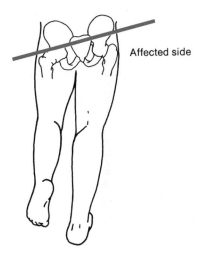

Affected side

Figure 20-3
Trendelenburg gait.

Related Nursing Diagnoses

Risk for infection: related to invasive procedures, trauma.

Altered tissue perfusion: related to mechanical reduction of arterial flow.

Impaired tissue integrity: related to impaired physical mobility, mechanical factors.

Impaired skin integrity: related to mechanical factors, physical immobilization.

Risk for impaired skin integrity: related to physical immobilization, mechanical factors, skeletal prominence.

Impaired role performance: related to health alterations, pain, fatigue.

Altered parenting: related to lack of knowledge about child health maintenance, physical illness.

Altered family processes: related to shift in health status of a family member, situation crisis.

Impaired physical mobility: related to musculoskeletal impairment; decreased muscle strength, control, or mass; reluctance to initiate movement; loss of integrity of bone structures; joint stiffness; pain.

Impaired walking: related to illness, use of mobility aids.

Risk for impaired neuromuscular dysfunction: related to trauma, orthopedic surgery, fractures, mechanical compression.

Dressing/grooming/toileting/hygiene self-care deficit: related to musculoskeletal impairment.

Altered growth and development: related to effects of physical disability.

Knowledge deficit: related to information misinterpretation, unfamiliarity with information resources.

Pain: related to injury agents.

Chronic pain: related to physical disability.

Nervous System

21

Assessment of the nervous system involves observation and testing of mental status, motor functioning, sensory functioning, cranial nerve functioning, reflexes, and infant automatisms. The thoroughness of assessment depends on the presenting complaint, contributing data from the health assessment, the reason for the assessment, the condition, and the child's age.

Much of the neurologic assessment can be integrated with other areas of the assessment. Parents can be valuable aides in performing the neurologic assessment of a child because they are more aware of the child's usual functioning. Parental concerns are important in alerting health professionals to delays, impairments, behavioral changes, and need for anticipatory guidance.

In performing the neurologic assessment, the nurse must be aware of age-appropriate levels of functioning.

Rationale

A thorough neurologic assessment is necessary whenever a child has sustained a fall, has suffered an injury to the head or spine, complains of headaches, or has a temperature of unknown origin. Children who have an apparent developmental delay or impairment and those with identified neurologic disorders should also undergo neurologic assessment. Neurologic impairment can delay a child's development and functioning and must be identified early to minimize long-term disability.

Anatomy and Physiology

The nervous system is a complex integrated system, and its scope is beyond that of this text. Essentially the nervous system is composed of the brain, spinal cord, and peripheral nervous system. The brain is divided into the brainstem, cerebrum, and cerebellum.

Except for the first cranial nerve, the cranial nerves emerge from the brainstem. The brainstem and the spinal cord are continuous. Consciousness arises from interaction between the cerebrum and brainstem. The cerebellum is primarily responsible for coordination. The full number of adult nerve cells is established midway through the prenatal period. Neurons, responsible for memory, consciousness, sensory and motor responses, and thought control, increase in size but not number after birth. Glial cells increase in both size and number until the age of 4 years. Dendrites, responsible for the transmission of impulses across synapses, increase in number and branchings. Axons increase in length. The size of the brain increases from 325 gm (11 oz) at birth to 1000 gm (2.2 lb) by 1 year of age (the adult brain weighs 1400 gm, or approximately 3 lb). Myelinization, begun in the fourth month of gestation, progresses throughout early infancy and childhood, until the child is able to move voluntarily and to engage in higher cortical functions. The order in which myelinization occurs corresponds to the normal sequence of development.

Equipment for Assessment of Nervous System

- Two safety pins
- Closed jars containing solutions with distinctive odors
- Cotton balls
- Reflex hammer

Preparation

Ask whether there is a family history of genetic disorders, learning disorders, or birth defects. Inquire whether the mother had difficulties during pregnancy or delivery. Ask the parent about prenatal history, consumption of drugs (such as alcohol, cocaine, heroin, and marijuana) during pregnancy, type of delivery, birth weight of the infant or child, and whether the infant or child had problems after birth. Ask whether the child has or has had recurrent headaches, neck stiffness, seizures, irritability, or hyperactivity. If the child has sustained an injury, determine the time of occurrence, the events surrounding the injury, the area of impact, whether consciousness was lost, and memory loss for events just before or after the injury. If concussion has been sustained, inquire about symptoms of postconcussion syndrome (PCS) (see box on p. 311).

Symptoms Associated with Concussion (PCS)

Somatic

Headaches
Dizziness
Blurred vision
Nausea
Vomiting
Balance problems
Photophobia
Sensitivity to noise
Numbness or tingling

Cognitive

Difficulty concentrating
Difficulty remembering
Feeling slow
Feeling as if in a fog

Affective

Irritability
Lability
Sleep disturbances
Sadness
Nervousness

Assessment of Mental Status

Mental status can be assessed formally and informally throughout the examination and includes intellectual or cognitive functioning, thought and perceptions, mood, appearance, and behavior (see Chapter 24 for a more detailed discussion of assessment of mental health). Intellectual functioning can be formally assessed through the use of the Denver Developmental Screening Test II (Denver II) (see Chapter 22), which is administered at specified intervals in some agencies but can be administered anytime a problem is suspected. Illness, injury, a strange environment, cultural and language differences, and the examiner's approach can all influence intellectual functioning, mood, and understanding, so the nurse should compare findings against the parent's observations of the child's behavior.

Assessment	Findings
Level of Consciousness (LOC)	
Level of consciousness remains the most reliable and earliest indicator of changes in neurologic status and is a less variable indicator than vital signs, reflexes, and motor activity. LOC can be assessed using a pediatric version of the Glasgow Coma Scale (Figure 21-1).	Normal children will score 15 on the Glasgow Coma Scale. **Clinical Alert** A score of 8 or less on the Glasgow Coma Scale indicates coma.
Responses in each category are rated on a scale from 1 to 5. Whenever possible, have a parent present because a child might not respond actively to an unfamiliar person in an unfamiliar environment. It is also important to ask the parent about the child's normal level of responsiveness.	A variety of drugs affect pupil size and reaction to light. Pupils are pinpointed and fixed with narcotic ingestion; they are dilated and reactive to light with central nervous system stimulants and hallucinogens. Photophobia occurs with bacterial meningitis, PCS, and some infectious diseases.
Posttraumatic Amnesia (PTA)	
If traumatic brain injury has occurred, recall of events before and after the event can be useful in assessing the extent of the injury. In concussion, this information is included in a variety of grading systems (Table 21-1). Inquire about the child's memory of the event (e.g., "Tell me what happened. What were you doing just before that? After that?").	

Assessment	Findings

Memory and Orientation

Assess memory and orientation by asking the child for his or her name; city or town of residence; grade or birth date; and day, time, and year (older children). With athletes, studies suggest it might be more useful to ask questions that assess short-term memory, such as "What period were we in?" "What rink are we at?" and "Which side scored the last goal?"

Clinical Alert

Cognitive function remains relatively intact in sports-related concussions; assessment of general orientation is therefore less sensitive than for other head injuries. Questions of short-term memory are more sensitive with sports-related injuries.

Headache and confusion may be the presenting symptoms in athletic related head injuries.

Athletes may not recognize that they have had a head injury or may be reluctant to report symptoms for fear of not being able to participate in sport.

Posture and Motor Behavior

Assess the child's level of activity, control of impulses, appropriateness of behavior to situation and developmental stage, repetitive movements, presence of culturally appropriate eye contact and interaction, withdrawal, cooperativeness, and argumentativeness.

Motor behavior will vary with the age of the child and stage of development, what is acceptable within the family, and cultural norms.

Clinical Alert

Soft signs represent more primitive responses than might be expected for age and can indicate minimum brain dysfunction. Signs normally disappear with maturation. These include unusual body movement (e.g., mirroring), short attention span, easy distractibility, impulsivity, lability, hyperactivity, poor coordination, perceptual defects, learning difficulties, and language or articulation difficulties.

Assessment	Findings
Posture and Motor Behavior—cont'd	
	Hyperactivity, irritability, and diminished impulse control can indicate attention deficit disorder (ADD) or fetal alcohol syndrome.
	Aggressiveness, irritability, disobedience, and emotional lability can indicate PCS when injury has occurred.
	Hyperactivity, hypoactivity, and other behavioral changes can accompany the use of commonly abused drugs.
	Withdrawal, diminished eye contact (unless culturally appropriate), slumped shoulders, and slowed movements can indicate depression.
	Opisthotonus or hyperextension of the neck and spine, accompanied by pain on flexion of the neck, can indicate meningeal irritation or inflammation and should be immediately referred.
Hygiene and Grooming	
Observe hygiene and grooming in older children and adolescents. Inquire if there have been changes in grooming habits lately that are of concern.	**Clinical Alert** Neglect of personal hygiene can indicate family stress, depression, PCS, fatigue related to sleep disturbances or injury, or substance abuse.
Mood	
Observe mood and intensity of mood (see Chapter 24 for detailed assessment).	

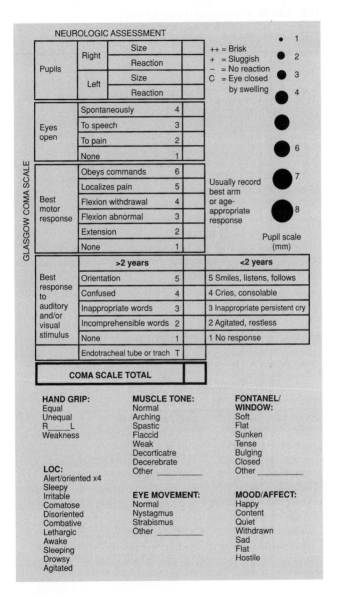

Figure 21-1
Pediatric adaptation of Glasgow Coma Scale.
(From Hockenberry MJ et al: *Wong's nursing care of infants and children,* ed 7, St Louis, 2003, Mosby.)

Table 21-1   McGill Concussion Grading System

Grade	Assessments
Grade 1	No loss of consciousness, no PTA
Grade 1A	No PCS seconds of confusion
Grade 1B	PCS and/or confusion (disorientation, inability to maintain coherent stream of thought or goal-directed movements, heightened distractibility) that resolves within 15 minutes
Grade 1C	PCS and/or confusion that lasts longer than 15 minutes
Grade 2	PTA that lasts less than 30 minutes and/or loss of consciousness that lasts less than 5 minutes
Grade 3	PTA that lasts longer than 30 minutes and/or loss of consciousness that lasts longer than 5 minutes

Adapted from LeClare S et al: Recommendations for grading of concussion in athletes, *Sports Med* 31:629-636, 2001.

Assessment of Motor Function

Motor function can be assessed during assessment of the musculoskeletal system.

Assessment	Findings
Observe the infant or child for obvious abnormalities that can influence motor functioning. Specifically, observe the size and shape of the head and inspect the spine for sacs and tufts of hair.	**Clinical Alert** A large head, enlarged frontal area, and tense fontanels (if open) can indicate hydrocephalus. A dimple with a tuft of hair or a sac protruding from the spinal column can indicate spina bifida occulta. A small head or microcephaly is associated with chromosomal abnormalities, prenatal exposure to toxic agents, maternal infections, and trauma during the perinatal period or infancy.

Assessment	Findings
Observe for handedness.	Infants and toddlers do not display *marked* preference for one hand, although they might show some preference.
	Clinical Alert
	Singular use of one hand by a very young child can indicate paresis of the opposite side.
	Failure to develop handedness in a school-age child can indicate failure of the brain to develop dominance.
Test muscle strength and symmetry by asking the child to squeeze your fingers, press soles of feet against your hands, and push away pressure exerted on arms and legs.	**Clinical Alert** Report any asymmetry.
Place all joints through range of motion. Note flaccidity or spasticity.	Infants normally have the most flexible range of motion.
	All school-age children should be able to perform these activities.
	Clinical Alert
	Retroflexion of the head, stiffness of the neck, and extension of the extremities accompanies the meningeal irritation of meningitis and intracranial hemorrhage.
	Head lag after 4 months is an early sign of neurologic damage.
	Hypotonia is associated with Down syndrome.

Assessment	Findings
Cerebellar function can be tested by asking the child to hop, skip, or walk heel-to-toe. A Romberg's test can be performed by asking the child to stand still, eyes closed and arms at side. Stand near the child to catch the child if leaning occurs.	**Clinical Alert** Leaning to one side during a Romberg's test indicates cerebellar dysfunction.

Assessment of Sensory Function

Sensory function is assessed during testing of cranial nerve function.

Assessment of Cranial Nerve Function

The function of most of the cranial nerves can be evaluated during other areas of the health assessment (Table 21-2). Particular attention is paid to function of the cranial nerves when neurologic impairment is possible, suspected, or actually present, and should be a routine part of assessment in a child with a head injury.

Assessment of the cranial nerves varies with the child's developmental and cognitive levels. Testing of several functions depends on the child's ability to understand and cooperate; therefore, such functions cannot be tested in the infant or young child.

Assessment of Deep Tendon Reflexes

Assessment of deep tendon reflexes (Figure 21-2) provides information about the intactness of the reflex area. Compare the symmetry and strength of reflexes. Superficial reflexes such as the abdominal reflex, anal reflex, and cremasteric reflex can also be evaluated (Table 21-3) but are usually assessed during other areas of the health assessment. Findings from assessment of deep tendon and superficial reflexes are variable in infancy. Their absence or intensity is not diagnostically significant unless asymmetry is present.

Text continued on p. 324

Table 21-2 Testing of Cranial Nerve Function

Cranial Nerve	Assessment of Function	Area of Health Assessment into Which Testing Can Be Integrated
I Olfactory	Have the child close eyes and, blocking one nostril at a time, correctly identify distinctive odors (e.g., coffee, oranges).	Head and neck
II Optic*	Check the child's visual acuity, perception of light and color, and peripheral vision. Examine the optic disk.	Eye
III Oculomotor*	Check pupil size and reactivity. Inspect the eyelid for position when open. Have the child follow light or a bright toy through the six cardinal positions of gaze.	Eye
IV Trochlear†	Have the child move eyes downward and inward.	Eye
V Trigeminal*	Palpate the temple and jaw as the child bites down. Assess for symmetry and strength. Determine whether the child can detect light touch over the cheeks (a young infant roots when the cheek areas near the mouth are touched). Approaching from the side, touch the colored portion of the eye lightly with a wisp of cotton to test the blink and corneal reflexes.	Eye
VI Abducens†	Ask the child to look sideways. Assess the ability to move eyes laterally.	Eye
VII Facial*	Test the child's ability to identify sweet (sugar), sour (lemon juice), or bitter (quinine) solutions with the anterior tongue. Assess motor function by asking the older child to smile, puff out the cheeks, or show the teeth. (Observe the infant while smiling and crying.)	Head and neck

*Some portions of function can be assessed in infants and younger children.
†Only older children can participate in testing.

Continued

Table 21-2 Testing of Cranial Nerve Function—cont'd

Cranial Nerve	Assessment of Function	Area of Health Assessment into Which Testing Can Be Integrated
VIII Acoustic	Test the child's hearing (see Chapter 12).	Ear
IX Glossopharyngeal[†]	Test the child's ability to identify the taste of solutions on the posterior tongue.	Head and neck
X Vagus	Assess the child for hoarseness and ability to swallow. Touch a tongue blade to the posterior pharynx to determine if the gag reflex is present (cranial nerves IX and X both participate in this response). *Do not stimulate the gag reflex if there is any suspicion of epiglottitis.* Check that the uvula is in the midline.	Head and neck
XI Accessory[†]	Have the child attempt to turn the head to the side against resistance. Ask the child to shrug shoulders while downward pressure is applied.	Head and neck
XII Hypoglossal[†]	Ask the child to stick out the tongue. Inspect the tongue for midline deviation. (Observe the infant's tongue for lateral deviation when crying and laughing.) Listen for the child's ability to pronounce "r" (rabbit, run, Robert). Place a tongue blade against the side of child's tongue and ask the child to move it away. Assess for strength.	Head and neck

[*]Some portions of function can be assessed in infants and younger children.
[†]Only older children can participate in testing.

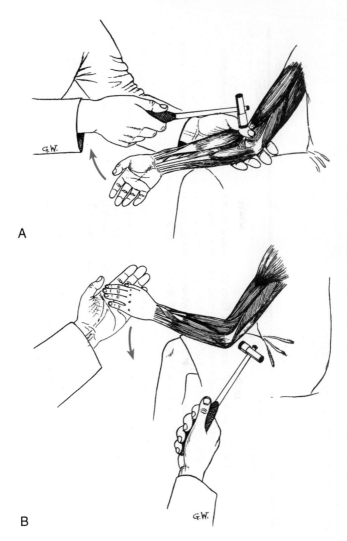

Figure 21-2
Assessment of deep tendon reflexes. **A,** Biceps. **B,** Triceps.
(From Whaley LF, Wong DL: *Nursing care of infants and children,* ed 4, St Louis, 1991, Mosby.)

Table 21-3 Assessment of Deep and Superficial Reflexes

Reflex	Method of Assessment	Usual Finding
Deep Tendon Reflexes		
Biceps	Partially flex the child's forearm. Place your thumb over the antecubital space and strike with the reflex hammer (Figure 21-2, A).	Forearm flexes slightly
Triceps	Bend the child's arm at the elbow while supporting the forearm. Strike the triceps tendon above the elbow (Figure 21-2, B).	Forearm extends slightly
Brachioradialis	Place the child's arm and hand in a relaxed position with the palm down. Strike the radius 2.5 cm (1 in) above the wrist.	Forearm flexes and palm turns upward
Knee jerk or patellar	Have the child sit on a table or on the parent's lap with legs flexed and dangling. Strike the patellar tendon just below the kneecap.	Lower leg extends

Achilles	Have the child sit on a table or on the parent's lap with legs flexed, and support the foot lightly. Strike the Achilles tendon.	Foot plantar flexes (points downward); rapid, rhythmic plantar flexion of the foot can occur in newborn infants (as many as 10 flexions might be noted)
Superficial Reflexes		
Abdominal	Stroke the skin toward the umbilicus. Assess the reflex in all four quadrants. The abdominal reflex might not be present for the first 6 months. (Can be incorporated into assessment of the abdomen.)	Umbilicus moves toward the stimulus
Cremasteric	Stroke the upper inner thigh. (Can be integrated into assessment of the abdominal or genital area.)	Testes retract into the inguinal canal
Anal	Stimulate the skin in the perianal area. (Can be incorporated into assessment of the rectal area.)	Brisk contraction of the anal sphincter occurs

Assessment of Infant Reflexes

Infant reflexes or automatisms (Table 21-4) are particularly useful in assessing the function of the central nervous system. Reflexes should be formally assessed if there is any suggestion of a central nervous system disorder. Many reflexes can be assessed during other parts of the health assessment. Knowledge of the reflex aids in education of the parents.

Assessment of Pain

The response of children to pain follows developmental patterns (Table 21-5) and is influenced by temperament, coping abilities, and previous exposure to pain and painful procedures. When assessing pain, the use of various assessment strategies aids in obtaining a more accurate assessment of the pain. These strategies include questioning the child (in words that are appropriate to developmental level and language) and the parents, observing behavioral and physiologic responses, and using pain scales (Table 21-6). The Preverbal, Early Verbal Pediatric Pain Scale (PEPPS) (see the box on pp. 332-333) is a pain-measurement tool that is useful with toddlers and for taking and evaluating action. Headache is a common symptom in children and can indicate several disorders (Table 21-7).

Table 21-4 Infant Reflexes (Automatisms)

Reflex	Description	Method of Assessment	Significance of Findings
Blinking (corneal or dazzle)	Closes eyelids in response to bright light. Present during first year of life.	Shine light into infant's eyes.	Absence of reflex suggests blindness.
Babinski's sign	Toes fan and big toe dorsiflexes. Disappears after 1 year.	Stroke sole of foot along outer edge, beginning from heel.	Fanning of toes and dorsiflexion of great toe after 2 years of age suggests lesion in extrapyramidal tract.
Crawling	Infant makes crawling movements with arms and legs when placed on abdomen. Disappears at about 6 weeks.	Place infant prone on flat surface.	Asymmetry of movements suggests neurologic disorder.
Dance or stepping	Infant's feet move up and down when feet lightly touch firm surface. Present for approximately first 4 weeks.	Hold infant so that feet lightly touch firm surface.	Persistence of reflex beyond 4 to 8 weeks is abnormal.
Extrusion	Tongue extends outward when touched. Present until 4 months of age.	Touch tongue with tip of tongue blade.	Persistent extension of tongue can indicate Down syndrome.

Continued

Table 21-4 Infant Reflexes (Automatisms)—cont'd

Reflex	Description	Method of Assessment	Significance of Findings
Galant's (trunk incurvation)	Back moves toward side that is stimulated. Present for first 4 to 8 weeks.	Stroke infant's back along side of spine from shoulder to buttocks.	Absence of reflex can indicate transverse spinal cord lesions.
Moro's	Arms extend, fingers fan, head is thrown back, and legs might flex weakly. Arms return to center with hands clasped. Spine and lower extremities extend. Strongest during first 2 months. Disappears at 3 to 4 months.	Change infant's position abruptly or jar table.	Persistence of reflex beyond 4 months suggests brain damage. Persistence beyond 6 months highly indicates brain damage. Asymmetry of responses indicates hemiparesis, fracture of clavicle, or injury to brachial plexus. Absence of response in lower extremities indicates congenital hip dislocation or low spinal cord injury.

Continued

Neck righting	When infant is supine, shoulder and trunk and then pelvis turn toward direction in which infant is turned. Appears at 3 months and persists until 24 to 36 months.	Place infant supine. Attempt to attract infant's attention to one side.	Absence or persistence beyond 10 months suggests central nervous system disorders.
Body righting	When infant is supine, all body parts follow when hips and shoulders are turned to one side.	Place infant supine. Turn hips and shoulders to side.	
Labyrinth righting	Infant able to raise head when prone or supine. Appears at 2 months and disappears by 10 months.	Place infant prone or supine.	
Parachute reflex	When infant is suspended horizontally and suddenly dipped downward, hands and fingers extend forward. Appears at 6 to 8 months and persists indefinitely.	Suspend infant and drop head and trunk.	

Table 21-4   Infant Reflexes (Automatisms)—cont'd

Reflex	Description	Method of Assessment	Significance of Findings
Palmar grasp	Infant's fingers curve around finger placed in infant's palm from ulnar side. Palmar grasp disappears by 3 to 4 months.	Place finger into infant's palm from ulnar side. If reflex is weak or absent, offer infant bottle or soother because sucking enhances reflex.	Asymmetric flexion indicates paralysis. Persistence of grasp reflex indicates cerebral disorder.
Placing	Infant lifts leg off table as if stepping on to table. Time of disappearance variable.	Hold infant upright, under arms. Place dorsal side of foot briskly against table or other hard surface.	
Rooting	Infant turns in direction that cheek is stroked. Reflex disappears at 3 to 4 months but can persist until 12 months, especially during sleep.	Stroke corners of infant's mouth or midline of lips.	Absence of reflex indicates severe neurologic disorder. Exaggerated rooting reflex together with ineffective sucking is associated with cocaine-dependent mothers.

Startle	Infant extends and flexes arms in response to loud noise. Hands remain clenched. Reflex disappears after 4 months of age unless there are neurologic impairments. Infants with neurologic impairments can evidence increased sensitivity to sound.	Claps hands loudly.	Absence of reflex indicates hearing impairment.
Sucking	Infant sucks strongly in response to stimulation. Reflex persists during infancy and can occur during sleep without stimulation.	Offer infant bottle or soother.	Weak or absent reflex suggests developmental delay or neurologic abnormality.
Tonic neck	Infant assumes fencing position when head is turned to one side. Arm and leg extend on side to which head is turned and flex on opposite side. Normally reflex should not occur each time head is turned. Disappears at 3 to 4 months.	Turn head quickly to one side.	It is considered abnormal if response occurs each time head is turned. Persistence indicates major cerebral damage.

Table 21-5   Developmental Responses to Pain

Age	Motor Response	Expressive Response	Ability to Anticipate Pain
Young infants	Generalized. Includes thrashing, rigidity, exaggerated reflex withdrawal, lack of sucking, disorganized sucking, starts to eat or drink and discontinues.	Cries loudly, closes eyes tightly, opens mouth in squarish manner, grimaces.	No link between approaching stimulus and pain.
Older infants	Localized. Withdrawal of affected area. Sucking and feeding behaviors as for young infants.	As for young infant except eyes can be open.	Physical resistance after painful stimulus occurs.
Young children	Thrashes arms, legs. Uncooperative, reluctant to move, lies rigid, guards area, restless.	Cries, screams loudly, moans, verbalizes pain, clings to support person, asks for support, irritable.	Anticipates pain.
School-age children	Includes behaviors found in young child, as well as muscular rigidity (clenched fists, body stiffness, closed eyes, frowning), muscle tension, and withdrawal.	Includes responses found in young child, as well as stalling or bargaining behavior.	Behaviors seen less before procedure; more pronounced during pain experience.
Adolescents	Less motor activity than for younger children. Demonstrates muscle tension, body control.	Uses more sophisticated language to verbalize pain. Less verbal protest.	Uses anticipation to prepare self.

Table 21-6 Pain Assessment Tools for Children and Adolescents

Tool	Instructions
Adolescent pediatric pain tool (APPT)	Ask adolescent to color in areas of pain on anterior and posterior body outlines. Ask adolescent to make marks as big or as small as pain.
Wong-Baker FACES Pain Rating Scale	

0	1	2	3	4	5
No Hurt	Hurts little bit	Hurts little more	Hurts even more	Hurts whole lot	Hurts worst

Explain to the child that each face is for a person who feels happy because he has no pain (hurt) or sad because he has some or a lot of pain. Face 0 is very happy because he doesn't hurt at all. Face 1 hurts just a little bit. Face 2 hurts a little more. Face 3 hurts even more. Face 4 hurts a whole lot. Face 5 hurts as much as you can imagine, although you don't have to be crying to feel this bad. Ask the child to choose the face that best describes how he or she is feeling. Recommended for children age 3 and older.

Numeric scale	Ask the child to rate pain on a line from 0 to 10, with 0 being no pain and 10 being the worst possible pain. Useful for children who know how to count and who understand the concepts of more and less.

FACES Pain Rating Scale from Hockenberry MJ et al: *Wong's nursing care of infants and children*, ed 7, St Louis, 2003, Mosby.

Preverbal, Early Verbal Pediatric Pain Scale

Heart Rate

4—>40 beats/min above baseline
3—31-40 beats above baseline
2—21-30 beats above baseline
1—10-20 beats above baseline
0—baseline range

Facial

4—Severe grimace; brows lowered and tightly drawn together, eyes tightly closed
2—Grimace; brows drawn together, eyes partially closed, squinting
0—Relaxed facial expression

Cry (Audible/Visible)

4—Screaming
3—Sustained crying
2—Intermittent crying
1—Whimpering, groaning, fussiness
0—No cry

Consolability/State of Restfulness

4—Unable to console, restlessness, sustained movement
2—Able to console, distract with difficulty, intermittent restlessness, irritability
1—Distractable, easy to console, intermittent fussiness
0—Pleasant, well integrated

Preverbal, Early Verbal Pediatric Pain Scale—cont'd

Body Posture

4—Sustained arching, flailing, thrashing, and/or kicking

3—Intermittent or sustained movement with or without periods of rigidity

2—Localization with extension or flexion or stiff and nonmoving

1—Clenched fists, curled toes, and/or reaching for or touching wound or area

0—Body at rest, relaxed positioning

Sociability

4—Absent eye contact, response to voice and/or touch

2—With effort, responds to voice and/or touch, makes eye contact, difficult to obtain and maintain

0—Responds to voice and/or touch, makes eye contact and/or smiles, easy to obtain and maintain; sleeping

Sucking/Feeding

2—Lack of sucking, refusing food or fluids

1—Disorganized sucking, attempting to eat or drink but discontinues

0—Sucking, drinking, and/or eating well

0—N/A; NPO and/or does not use oral stimuli

Total score:

Modified from Murphy E et al: Development of a pain assessment scale for the preverbal, early verbal child, Abstract No 160, Presented at the Third International Symposium on Pediatric Pain, Children and Pain: Integrating Science and Care, Philadelphia, June 1994, copyright WB Saunders.

Table 21-7 Characteristics and Etiologies of Headaches in Childhood and Adolescence

Characteristics of Pain	Location	Factors that Aggravate or Provoke	Associated Symptoms	Possible Etiology
Aching, mild, diffuse, tightness and pressure; gradual onset	Usually bilateral; can be generalized; can involve back of head and neck	■ School and relationship stressors ■ Long periods in one position (e.g., working at a computer, playing video games)	■ Depression ■ Anxiety	Tension headache
Aching, progressive, recurrent; worse on arising	Occipital or frontal areas	■ Lowering head ■ Bowel movements, coughing, sneezing	■ Vomiting, with or without feeding ■ Decreased appetite ■ Increasingly projectile vomiting ■ Clumsiness ■ Changes in reflexia ■ Spasticity ■ Irritability ■ Seizures ■ Weakness ■ Positive Babinski's sign	Brain tumor

Aching, throbbing; variable severity; can be recurrent	Above eye (frontal sinus), in cheekbones, over gums (maxillary sinus)	▪ Bending ▪ Coughing ▪ Sneezing ▪ Jarring the head	▪ Fever ▪ Nasal discharge ▪ Nasal congestion ▪ Halitosis	Sinusitis
Aching, steady, dull, in and around eyes	Around and over eyes	▪ Activities requiring use of eyes such as reading, schoolwork, video games, television	▪ Child might say eyes are tired ▪ Redness of conjunctiva ▪ Frequent rubbing of eyes ▪ Squinting ▪ Clumsiness ▪ Nausea following close work ▪ Closes one eye	Errors of refraction; strabismus
Steady, severe; abrupt onset, often after falling asleep; clustered over days or a week, with relief for weeks or months	One sided; high along the nose; over and behind the eye	▪ Can be provoked by alcohol use	▪ Coryza ▪ Reddening and tearing of the eye	Cluster headaches

Continued

Table 21-7 Characteristics and Etiologies of Headaches in Childhood and Adolescence—cont'd

Characteristics of Pain	Location	Factors that Aggravate or Provoke	Associated Symptoms	Possible Etiology
Steady, aching; gradual onset following injury to head; more common in infancy than in older children	Variable location	■ Injury, sometimes forgotten because of passage of time	■ Alterations in levels of consciousness ■ Irritability ■ Difficulty feeding ■ Excessive crying ■ Weakness along one side	Subdural hematoma
Severe, worsening; interferes with sleep	Variable	■ Injury to the head, often to the parietotemporal region	■ Possible loss of consciousness at time of injury ■ Drowsiness; difficult to arouse ■ Confusion ■ Difficulty with speaking ■ Irritability, crying ■ Unsteady gait (older child) ■ Refusal of feeding ■ Nausea	Epidural hemorrhage

				Meningitis
Steady, throbbing, severe	Generalized	▪ Movement of the neck	▪ Swelling in front of or above earlobe that increases in size ▪ Increased head circumference (infant) ▪ Pupil changes ▪ Papilledema (older child) ▪ Hemiparesis ▪ Accompanies fever, chills, vomiting ▪ Irritability ▪ Agitation ▪ Vomiting ▪ Seizures ▪ Photophobia ▪ Poor feeding ▪ Resists flexion of neck ▪ Positive Kernig's and Brudzinski's signs	

Continued

Table 21-7   Characteristics and Etiologies of Headaches in Childhood and Adolescence—cont'd

Characteristics of Pain	Location	Factors that Aggravate or Provoke	Associated Symptoms	Possible Etiology
Throbbing, aching; variable severity; rapid onset	Usually frontal or temporal, but can be occipital; can start behind eye and radiate outward; can be one or both sides	■ Alcohol ■ Some foods (chocolate milk, cheese, soft drinks, food additives) ■ Tension ■ Premenstrual ■ Noise, bright lights	■ Nausea, vomiting ■ Abdominal pain ■ Visual disturbances ■ Local weakness ■ Sensory disturbances	Migraine
Variable quality and severity; following head injury	Can be localized	■ Mental and physical activity ■ Excitement ■ Bending ■ Alcohol ■ Noise, lights	■ Can occur following injury to the head ■ Poor concentration ■ Irritability ■ Restlessness ■ Fatigue	Concussion

Related Nursing Diagnoses

Constipation: related to neurologic impairment, abdominal muscle weakness.

Impaired verbal communication: related to decrease in circulation in brain.

Diversional activity deficit: related to frequent lengthy treatment.

Self-care deficit: related to cognitive or neuromuscular impairment.

Altered role performance: related to physical illness.

Altered growth and development: related to physical disability.

Impaired physical mobility: related to sensoriperceptual impairments, neuromuscular impairments.

Altered family processes: related to transition, crisis.

Ineffective family coping, compromised: related to role disorganization, prolonged disease, situational crisis.

Impaired skin integrity: related to mechanical or chemical factors, impaired physical mobility.

Pain: related to injury agents.

Impaired social interaction: related to limited physical mobility.

Social isolation: related to alterations in mental status, altered state of wellness.

Altered thought processes: related to neurologic disturbance.

Impaired memory: related to neurologic disturbance, acute hypoxia.

Risk for disuse syndrome: related to paralysis.

Dysreflexia: related to bladder or bowel dysfunction, lack of caregiver knowledge, skin irritation.

Bowel incontinence: related to lower motor nerve damage.

Ineffective airway clearance: related to neuromuscular dysfunction.

Risk for injury: related to balancing difficulties, cognitive difficulties, reduced coordination, seizures.

GENERAL ASSESSMENT

IV

Development

22

Development is multifactorial and is the interplay among temperament, environment, and biophysical factors. Many observations about development can be made informally during the health interview and during the neurologic and musculoskeletal assessments; however, some observations need to be made more formally using tools such as the Denver Developmental Screening Test II (Denver II) and other objective tests.

The nurse needs to be aware that *"normal" encompasses a wide range of behavior at any given stage* and that delays in development can only rarely be attributed to one factor. Knowledge of behaviors that can be expected at various stages is essential to assessment of development.

Rationale

Complete periodic, systematic assessment of development enables early detection of problems, identification of parental and child concerns, anticipatory guidance, and teaching about age-appropriate expected behaviors. Judgments about an infant's or child's development must *never* rest solely on one assessment of development. Illness, stress, the examiner's approach, and a strange environment can alter a child's usual performance.

Preparation

Ask the parent to describe the infant's or child's development. Inquire whether the parent has specific concerns about the infant's or child's development (e.g., indistinct speech or language delays). Ask about the mother's prenatal history, including miscarriages stillbirths, exposure to medications or radiation, drug or alcohol use, maternal endocrine disorders, toxemia, hydramnios, infection, or abnormal bleeding. Inquire about the birth history of the infant or child, including type of delivery, fetal distress, birth weight, prematurity, respiratory problems, jaundice, hypoglycemia, seizures, irritability, poor muscle tone, or feeding problems. Inquire about family history of health concerns.

Assessment of Development Using the Denver II

Developmental screening tests are used as part of the developmental assessment. Developmental screening involves comprehensive health assessment and partnerships, including partnership with the parents. Several developmental screening tests are available (e.g., Ages and Stages Questionnaire, Revised Prescreening Developmental Questionnaire, Batelle Developmental Inventory), but the Denver developmental tests (DDST, DDST-R, Denver II) remain among the most widely used. The Denver II is not an IQ test but a series of standard developmental tasks that are used for children from birth to 6 years to determine how a child compares developmentally with other children of the same age. The test assesses personal, social, fine motor, adaptive, language, and gross motor skills and is useful for monitoring children who are at risk for developmental delays. The tests do not tell *why* developmental delays have occurred and should not be used for diagnosis.

Equipment for Assessment with Denver Screening Tests

■ *Approved* Denver II manuals, test kit, and forms

Method of Assessment

Before beginning the screening, tell the parents that the results will be discussed with them after all the items have been finished. Explain that the test involves activities that are familiar to infants and children and that there is nothing painful about the screening. In screening infants and children, approach the testing like a game. Take a toy out of the kit when needed for a particular item and replace the toy before moving on to the next item.

It is important to note that stress, illness, fear, shyness, and separation from the parent can affect the outcome of screening. In addition, the nurse must adjust the age of the child for prematurity. For children 24 months and younger, adjust for prematurity by subtracting the number of weeks of missed gestation from the child's current age; test at that age.

After the child's age is determined, draw a line through from top to bottom to connect the age intervals at the top and bottom of the sheet. The items that intersect the line indicate what is to be tested for the child's age. Begin by testing items to the left of the age line. Score each item that is tested as

- Fail (F)
- Pass (P)
- Refused (R)
- No opportunity (NO)

A *caution* is failure of the child to perform an item passed by 25% to 90% of children of that age. A *delay* is failure to pass an item to the left of the age line. A *normal* test is one with no delays and a maximum of one caution. A *suspect* test is one or more delays and/or two or more cautions. If a child cannot be tested or in the case of a suspect test, retest in 1 to 2 weeks.

When the screening is complete, ask the parents whether the child's performance is what they would expect at other times. If they respond that it is, then explain the results.

Before administering the screening, it is important to consult the instruction manual for the Denver II for complete details about administering the Denver II.

Significance of Findings

All children are not expected to pass all items. If a child fails one or more items that fall completely to the left of the age line, consider the child's developmental and health histories before deciding whether to retest at a later date.

Assessment of Growth and Development

Assessment of development requires knowledge of what can be expected at various stages in development. Table 22-1 gives a general summary of normal growth and development that can be used during observation of an infant or child.

Text continued on p. 365

Table 22-1 Normal Growth and Development in Children

Age	Physical/Motor	Language	Cognition	Socialization
1 month	Average weekly weight gain 140-200 gm (5-7 oz) until 6 months of age Average monthly gain in length 2.5 cm (1 in) until 6 months of age Obligate nose breather Head sags when not supported Back rounded in sitting position Hands held in fists Can turn head to side when prone Makes crawling movements when prone	Cries when uncomfortable Makes low throaty sounds	**Sensorimotor Stage (birth to 18 months)** Egocentric No intentionality; no expectations	Regards faces intently
2 months	Posterior fontanel closes Can lift head 45 degrees	Crying differentiated Coos	Responds differently to different objects	Might smile socially

	when prone When supported in sitting position, head is held up but bobs forward Visually pursues objects and sounds Hands held open more Grasp reflex fading	Vocalizes Voluntarily repeats activities, thereby demonstrating beginning connection between action and result Anticipates feeding Begins to separate self from others	Recognizes familiar face and unfamiliar situations Stops crying when parent approaches
3 months	Holds hands in front and stares at them Holds rattle but does not reach for it Raises chest, supported on forearms Little head lag Visually pursues sound by turning head	Squeals Laughs Vocalizes in response to other voices	As for 2 months

Continued

Table 22-1   Normal Growth and Development in Children—cont'd

Age	Physical/Motor	Language	Cognition	Socialization
	Able to bear some weight on legs when held in standing position Palmar grasp reflex weakening			
4 months	Holds head steady in sitting position Almost no head lag when pulled to sitting position Sits erect if propped Lifts head and shoulders 90 degrees when prone Turns from back to side Plays with hands Reaches for objects but overshoots Grasps objects with both hands	Makes consonant sounds (b, g, k, n, p) interspersed with vowel-like sounds Vocalization varies with mood	As for 2 months	Sociable Bored if left alone Demands attention by fussing

Visually pursues objects that
have been dropped

Begins drooling

Moro's, tonic neck, extrusion,
and rooting reflexes
disappear

Sleeps 10-12 hours at night

Naps two to three times a day

5 months

No head lag

Back straight when pulled to
sitting

Bears most of weight on legs
when standing

Sits for longer periods if
back supported

Plays with feet

Takes objects to mouth at will

Teeth might begin to erupt

Birth weight doubled

As for 4 months

Searches for objects
at point of
disappearance

Recognizes partially
hidden objects

Repeats interesting
actions

Wide repertoire of
activities (kicking,
batting, pulling,
patting) that produce
novel results

Imitates others

Recognizes
strangers

Can have rapid
mood swings

Vocalizes
displeasure if
preferred
object is taken

Continued

Table 22-1 Normal Growth and Development in Children—cont'd

Age	Physical/Motor	Language	Cognition	Socialization
6 months	Average weekly weight gain 90-150 gm (3-5 oz) for next 6 months Chews and bites Can hold own bottle but prefers it to be held Lifts chest and abdomen off flat surface, bearing weight on hands Sits in highchair with back straight Can turn completely from stomach to back to stomach Picks up objects that have been dropped Manipulates small objects Pulls feet to mouth Adjusts posture to visually pursue an object	Vocalizes to mirror Makes one-syllable sounds (ma, da, uh) Begins to mimic sounds (e.g., coughing)	As for 5 months	Shows fear of strangers Holds out arms when wants to be picked up Becomes excited when familiar persons approach Laughs when head is covered with towel

Age	Motor	Language	Cognitive	Social
7 months	Exhibits Landau reflex (when held prone, head raises and spine and legs extend) Sits in tripod position Lifts head off table if supine Bounces if held in standing position Transfers cube from hand to hand Holds cube in each hand Bangs cube on table Rakes at small objects Can approach toy and grasp it with one hand Responds to own name Evidences taste preferences	Chains syllables (mama, dada) but does not attach meaning Is able to produce four distinct vowel sounds	As for 5 months	Increasing fear of strangers Imitative Coughs, snorts to attract attention Closes lips in response to dislike of food Bites and mouths Plays peek-a-boo
8 months	Sits alone steadily Can stand holding on to something Beginning pincer (thumb-finger) grasp Regards a third cube while holding a cube in each hand	Makes d, t, w sounds Responds to simple commands	As for 5 months Coordination of secondary schemes Object permanence	Increased stranger anxiety and fear of separation from parent Begins to respond to "no-no" Searches for hidden objects

Continued

Table 22-1 Normal Growth and Development in Children—cont'd

Age	Physical/Motor	Language	Cognition	Socialization
	Releases objects voluntarily Rings bell purposely Reaches for toys out of reach Might have night awakenings Patterns emerge in bowel and bladder elimination			Shows interest in pleasing parent
9 months	Pulls self to standing position Crawls, perhaps backward at first Recovers sitting position if leaning forward, but cannot do so if leaning sideways		Beginning of intelligence Assigns symbols to events Goal-directed activities	Might show fear of going to bed or of being alone
10 months	Crawls, pulling self forward by hands Stands holding on to furniture Might cruise (step sideways holding on to furniture) Recovers balance readily if sitting	Comprehends dada, mama Might say one word	As for 9 months	Waves bye-bye Extends toys to others but does not release toy Repeats activities that attract attention Plays pat-a-cake Cries when scolded

11 months	Creeps with abdomen off floor Pivots when sitting (reaches backward to pick up an object) Intentionally drops objects for them to be picked up Places objects inside each other Holds crayon to make mark on paper	Imitates speech sounds	As for 9 months	Expresses frustration when restricted Plays so-big, up-down, peek-a-boo
12 months	Birth weight tripled Head and chest circumference equal Cruises well Walks with help Can sit from standing without help Drinks from cup and eats from spoon but requires help Cooperates in dressing Neat pincer grasp	Says two or more words in addition to mama and dada Recognizes objects by name Imitates sounds of animals	As for 9 months	Responds to simple commands Explores actively Clings to mother in unfamiliar situations Might take security objects Shows emotions

Continued

Table 22-1   Normal Growth and Development in Children—cont'd

Age	Physical/Motor	Language	Cognition	Socialization
	Turns several pages of book at a time Lumbar nerve develops, with resulting lordosis when walking			
13-18 months	Anterior fontanel closes Abdomen protrudes Walks with wide-based gait Walks up stairs with help; creeps down stairs Throws ball overhand Seats self on small chair Climbs Pulls toys behind and pushes light furniture Imitates housework Puts shaped objects into holes Scribbles vigorously Imitates vertical and circular strokes	Can say 4-6 words by 15 months and 10 words or more by 18 months Points to desired object Points to two or three body parts (18 months)	Trial and error learning Active experimentation Solicits help of adults to bring about results Understands relationship between object and use	Drinks well from cup but might drop it when finished Holds cup well in both hands Uses spoon but turns bowl of spoon downward before it reaches mouth Might discard bottle Less fearful of strangers Hugs and kisses significant others and pictures in books

Age	Physical	Language	Cognitive	Socialization
	Builds tower of two or three cubes Sleeps 10-12 hours; has one afternoon nap Might uncover self during sleep			Temper tantrums begin Beginning sense of ownership Takes off simple clothes
24 months	Average yearly weight gain 1.8-2.7 kg (4-6 lb) Chest circumference larger than head circumference Physiologic systems stable except for reproductive and endocrine systems Gait steadier, more adult Jumps crudely	Approximately 300 words in vocabulary Short sentences of two or three words Uses pronouns Gives first name Verbalizes need for food, drink, and toilet	**Preoperational Stage (2 to 7 years)** *Preconceptual thinking (about 2 to 4 years)* Inventions of new means through mental combinations Beginning of mental problem solving and play	Dawdles Negativistic Temper tantrums decrease Treats other children as objects Wants to make friends but doesn't know how

Continued

Table 22-1   Normal Growth and Development in Children—cont'd

Age	Physical/Motor	Language	Cognition	Socialization
	Might pedal tricycle			Cannot share possessions
	Walks up and down stairs with two feet on each step; holds on to rail			Engages in parallel play
	Picks up objects without falling		Has insight and forethought	Shows increased independence from mother
	Kicks ball forward without overbalancing		Able to delay imitation for several days	Chews with mouth closed
	Turns doorknob and unscrews lids			Uses straw
	Builds tower of six or seven cubes			Puts on simple clothing
	Turns pages of book one at a time			
	Might be daytime toilet trained			
30 months	Birth weight quadrupled	Gives first and last names		Separates more easily from parent
	Primary dentition complete			

Age	Motor	Language	Adaptive	Personal-Social
36 months	Builds tower of eight cubes Copies circle from model Throws large ball 1.2-1.5 m (4-5 ft) Takes a few steps on tiptoe Average yearly weight gain 1.8-2.7 kg (4-6 lb) Balances on one foot for 5 seconds Jumps from a low step Walks upstairs, alternating feet Might attempt to dance but balance still insecure Pours fluid well from a pitcher Begins to use scissors Strings large beads Builds tower of 9 or 10 cubes Copies cross (X) from model Washes hands	Enjoys rhymes and singing Vocabulary of about 900 words Talks in sentences of about six words Uses telegraphic speech Asks many questions	Repeats three numbers Remainder as for 30 months	Notices sex difference Independent in toileting except for wiping Less negativistic Friendly Begins to understand taking turns Able to share but uses "mine" often Begins to learn meaning of simple rules, but rules subject to own interpretation Names appropriate sex of others Boys tend to identify more strongly with father

Continued

Table 22-1   Normal Growth and Development in Children—cont'd

Age	Physical/Motor	Language	Cognition	Socialization
	Might be nighttime toilet trained Sleeps 10-15 hours; takes fewer naps			Can dress with minimal assistance Feeds self completely Begins to use fork but holds it in fist Uses adult form of chewing Might have fears, especially of dark or animals
48 months	Length at birth doubled Balances on one foot for 10 seconds Hops on one foot Catches bounced ball Laces shoes Imitates bridge with cubes Uses scissors to cut out picture	Vocabulary of 1500 words Knows simple songs Exaggerates, boasts, might be mildly profane Understands concepts of under, on top of, beside, in front of	*Intuitive thought (4 to 7 years)* Time linked with daily events Counts but does not clearly understand what numbers mean Believes thoughts cause events Cannot conserve	Tattles Might have imaginary playmate Independent Aggressive; takes out aggression on family members Exhibits mood swings

Age				
	Immunoglobulin G reaches adult levels Draws man in three parts	Understands simple analogies	matter Egocentricism decreases Repeats four numbers Names one or more coins	Engages in cooperative group play without rigid rules (associative play) Enjoys entertaining Do's and dont's important Identifies with parent of opposite sex
5 years	Permanent dentition begins Handedness established Jumps rope Walks backward heel-to-toe Might be able to tie shoelaces Can form some letters correctly Might print first name Draws man in six or seven parts	Vocabulary of about 2100 words Talks constantly Asks meanings of words	Uses time words with more comprehension Interested in facts associated with environment Names four or more colors Names coins Names days of week	Comfortable Trustworthy Fewer fears Eager to do things the right way Might seek out mother more often because of more outside activities such as school

Continued

Table 22-1 Normal Growth and Development in Children—cont'd

Age	Physical/Motor	Language	Cognition	Socialization
6 years	Uses scissors or pencil well Copies triangle and diamond Dexterity increasing Jumps rope Skates, rides bicycle Can sew crudely	Describes objects in pictures	Knows right from left Recognizes many shapes Reads from memory Obeys three commands in succession	Identifies strongly with parent of same sex Enjoys bossing others Might be defiant and rude Jealousy of younger siblings more apparent Might have temper tantrums Cheats to win Enjoys table games
7 years		Mechanical in reading Might skip words	**Concrete Operations Stage (7-11 years)** Repeats three numbers	Enjoys teasing Girls play with girls,

Age	Motor	Language	Cognitive	Social/Emotional
8-9 years	Increased speed and smoothness in motor activities Uses common tools such as hammer and household utensils More individual variation in skills	such as he, it	backward Reads time to quarter hour Age of relational thinking; able to classify, seriate, arrange in hierarchies Learns principle of conservation Knows date Gives days of week and months in order	and boys with boys Modest about sexual matters Anxious over failures Occasional periods of shyness or sadness Increasing interest in spiritual matters Expansive; wants to become involved in everything Actively seeks company of others Likes clubs and fads Hero worship begins Likes to help Might reject Santa Claus, Easter Bunny

Continued

Table 22-1   Normal Growth and Development in Children—cont'd

Age	Physical/Motor	Language	Cognition	Socialization
			Counts backward from 20 to 1 Makes change correctly from a quarter	Might show lack of interest in God
10 years	Slow increase in height Rapid increases in weight Body changes associated with puberty may begin to appear Remainder of teeth erupt Cooks, sews, paints, draws Washes and dries own hair	Likes writing letters Reads for enjoyment or practical purposes	Performs complex operations on problems as long as problems are concrete	
			Formal Operational Stage (about 11 years and beyond)	
11-14 years	Maximum increase in height, weight (in North America, girls have peak weight spurt	Spends long periods on telephone	Logical thinking and ability to use abstract thought	Differences intolerable Conforms to group standards

at an average of 12.7 years, and adult stature is reached at an average of 13 years; boys have their peak height and weight spurt at an average of 14 years)	develops	Tries on various roles
	Clumsy and inconsistent in abstract thinking	Ambivalent
Girls might commence menses		Mood swings
Girls might look more obese	Thinking is reflective, futuristic, multidimensional	Boys gravitate toward sports; girls discuss clothes, makeup
Secondary sex characteristics appear		
Might be clumsy and have poor posture	Low point in creativity	Daydreams a great deal
Might have fatigue		
Immunoglobulins A and M reach adult levels		
14-17 years	Able to maintain an argument	Introspective
Girls reach physical maturity	Increased capacity for abstract reasoning	Self-centered
Secondary sex characteristics well advanced	Enjoys intellectual powers	Emotions still labile
	Concerned with philosophic and social problems	Parent-child relationship might reach low point; major conflicts over independence

Continued

Table 22-1   Normal Growth and Development in Children—cont'd

Age	Physical/Motor	Language	Cognition	Socialization
			Creative period	and control
				Disengagement from dependent parent-child relationship occurs
				Fears rejection by peers
				Adheres to group norms
				Sexual preference becoming established
17-20 years	Physically mature		Complex thinking	Dating becomes important
			Creativity fading	Pursues career
				Sexual identity established
				More comfortable with self
				Fewer conflicts with family
				Peer group less important
				Emotions more controlled
				Forms stable relationships
				Might publicly identify as gay, lesbian, or bisexual

Assessment of Speech and Language

Early assessment and detection of speech and language disorders are important in planning interventions that will assist the child with interactions, learning, and later, employment and career. *Language* refers to the system of symbols used to convey meaning to others and can be expressive (speaking) or receptive (understanding). *Speech* refers to the production of language, including articulation of sounds, rhythm (e.g., stuttering), tone, and quality (e.g., hyper-nasality). Communication impairments often occur in conjunction with other developmental delays or severe disabilities (cerebral palsy, mental retardation, autism) and can also reflect hearing deficits. To assess children for speech and language difficulties, it is important to distinguish what is developmentally appropriate and what would be considered deviations (Table 22-2).

Table 22-2   Indications of Normal Development of Speech and Language and of Impairments in Childhood

Age	Normal Development	Intelligibility	Signs of Communication Impairment
1 year	Able to say two to three words with meaning Omits most final and some initial consonants Imitates animal sounds	Intelligible about 25% of time if listener not familiar with child	Lack of response to noise Failure to localize sounds Failure to follow directions Absence of babble or inflection
2 years	Two- to three-word phrases Articulation lags behind vocabulary Uses pronouns ("I," "you")	50% intelligible in context	Failure to speak any meaningful words spontaneously Failure to respond to sound consistently Failure to follow directions Uses gestures rather than words
3 years	Four- to five-word sentences About 900 words in vocabulary Rhythm shows hesitations and repetitions	75% intelligible	Omission of initial or final consonants on frequent basis Use of vowels instead of consonants

Age			
4-5 years	Uses "what," "who," "where," plurals, prepositions, pronouns Uses complete sentences Able to use most grammatical forms correctly Vocabulary of about 1500-2100 words	100% intelligible although some sounds still imperfect	Failure to use sentences of at least three words Stutters Many sound substitutions Omits word endings Noticeable impairment of sentence structures By age 7, sound substitutions, omissions, or distortions are indicative of communication impairment Unusual confusions or reversals, inappropriate vocal pitch, and poor voice quality might be indicative of impairment
5-6 years	Vocabulary of 3000 words Might still distort s, z, sh, ch, j sounds Comprehends "because," "if," "why"		

Related Nursing Diagnoses

Impaired verbal communication: related to decrease in circulation in brain, psychologic barriers, physical barriers, anatomic defects, brain tumor, differences related to developmental age, absence of significant others, physiologic conditions, alteration of central nervous system, emotional conditions.

Altered growth and development: related to separation from significant others, environmental and stimulation deficiencies, effects of physical disability, inconsistent responsiveness.

Risk for altered development, prenatal: related to maternal age, substance abuse, genetic or endocrine disorders, poor prenatal care, inadequate nutrition, poverty, illiteracy, (individual) prematurity, seizures, brain damage, hearing impairment, vision impairment, chronic illness, dependence on technology, failure to thrive, lead poisoning, chemotherapy, radiation therapy, natural disaster, behavior disorder, substance abuse, (environmental) poverty, violence, abuse, mental retardation, severe learning disability.

Impaired social interaction: related to limited physical mobility, communication barriers.

Social isolation: related to inability to engage in satisfying personal relationships, unaccepted social behavior, inadequate personal resources, immature interests, alterations in physical appearance, altered state of wellness.

Altered parenting: related to lack of access to resources, lack of resources, social isolation, poor home environment, lack of knowledge about child health maintenance, inability to recognize and act on infant cues, physical illness, premature birth, handicapping condition or developmental delay.

Risk for altered parent/infant/child attachment: related to ill infant.

Altered family processes: related to situation transition or crisis.

Assessment of Child Abuse

23

Rationale

Although the exact number of cases of child abuse and neglect is difficult to determine because of problems in identification and reporting, estimates place the incidence of child abuse and neglect in the United States at approximately 900,000 cases annually or 12 out of every 1000 children. Neglect constitutes about 40% to 50% of all cases, emotional abuse about 10% to 20%, and sexual abuse approximately 10%. By far, parents are the most frequent abusers of their children. The preeminence of abuse and neglect necessitates that nurses be alert to specific maltreatment indicators when assessing children.

Development of Abuse

Child abuse, defined as intentional physical, psychologic, sexual, or social injury or damage, maltreatment, or corruption of a child, can be traced to parents, siblings, relatives, friends, professionals, and others who encounter the child. *Neglect* usually refers to intentional or unintentional failure to supply a child with the basic necessities of life.

Familial violence/abuse is generally considered to be the way in which a family system expresses its dysfunction. These families, which demonstrate several common characteristics (Table 23-1), might be geographically and emotionally isolated and tend to discount, deny, or be unaware of the seriousness of their problems. Several factors (see the box on p. 371) can place a family at risk for violence and abuse; awareness of these factors can assist the nurse in assessing families at all stages in family development.

Assessment of Abuse and Neglect in Children

Assessment of abuse and neglect should be ongoing and an integral part of a total health assessment. Findings that indicate abuse

Table 23-1   Characteristics of Abusive and Violent Families

Characteristic	Manifestations
Boundary	Rigid, inflexible. Little contact with outside social support systems. Within the family, there might be blurring of generational boundaries so that a daughter, for example, takes on the role of adult female sexual partner. Parent might seek gratification from child.
Affective tone	Helplessness, crisis, anger, powerlessness, depression. Competition for caring. Little empathy or evidence of nurturance, caring.
Control	Caring confused with conflict and abuse. Imbalance in power, often male or adult dominated. Members facilitate victim roles.
Instrumental functioning	Confusion about roles. Adult and child roles might be reversed. Intense attention to tasks or ineffective performance of tasks. Inappropriate age-related expectations of children.
Communication	Poor; double messages, mixed messages. Threats, sarcasm, blaming, demeaning communication. Incongruence in communication. Lack of meaningful communication. Family secrets common.
Role stereotyping	Traditionalist. Rigid. Role confusion, blurring, reversal. Parental coalition limited or absent.

(see the box on p. 372) must be clearly documented and reported. Sexual abuse is more likely to be seen with girls and severe physical abuse with boys. Firstborns are more likely to be abused than those born later, and children with disabilities are at risk for abuse. Care must be taken to describe, not interpret, behaviors and communications. In assessing for abuse, it is important to accurately describe findings and to be alert to whether reports of injury are congruent

Factors That Place Families at Risk for Child Abuse and Neglect

History of childhood abuse, neglect, deprivation in parent(s)

Decreased knowledge of parenting skills and normal child development

Parental age at time of child's birth younger than 18 years

Low level of educational attainment (parent education less than 12 years)

Marital discord

Interspousal violence

Parental separation

Parent living alone or in unstable relationship

Unstable socioeconomic conditions, including homelessness, low income, poverty, lack of steady employment, and frequent moves

History of parental substance abuse/chemical dependency within past 6 months

Depression or emotional illness of mother (during pregnancy) or of parents

Poor or delayed parent/child attachment

Violent older siblings

Chronically ill parent(s)

Diminished self-esteem in parent(s)

Blended family

Prematurity of infant(s)

Developmental delays in child(ren)

Social isolation

Illegitimacy

Approval of physical force and/or violence within family or culture as way to solve problems

---

with the child's age and the events (e.g., a newborn cannot roll across a bed). If a child indicates that abuse has occurred, the child's report must be accepted and the child must be shown acceptance, unconditional positive regard, and active listening. Further exploration of abuse in the young child can be facilitated by trained professionals through play, particularly through drawings and dramatic activities.

Indicators of Abuse and Neglect in Children

Emotional Abuse, Deprivation, and Neglect

Self-reports of abuse

Failure to thrive (feeding difficulties, abnormally low height and weight, hypotonia, delayed dentition, developmental delays, passivity)

Feeding disorders (rumination, anorexia)

Speech disorders

Wetting/soiling

Sleep disorders

Psychosomatic complaints (headaches, nausea, abdominal pain)

Self-stimulation behaviors (rocking, head-banging, sucking)

Lack of stranger anxiety (infancy)

Withdrawal, indifference

Anxiety, fear, low self-confidence

Inhibition of play

Antisocial behavior (stealing, cruelty, destructiveness)

Substance abuse

Running away

Poor school progress or changes in school performance, school truancy, or school phobia

Suicide attempts

Excessive criticism, name calling, and/ or embarrassment of child by parent

Unresponsiveness or diminished responses to child's needs and interactions by parent

Physical Abuse and Neglect

Self-reports of abuse

Bruises and welts (on soft tissue areas such as buttocks, mouth, thighs, or torso; can be in various stages of healing; shape of bruises can approximate fingers, blunt objects); differentiate bruises from mongolian spots (areas of deep blue pigmentation in sacral and gluteal areas; found in infants of Native American, African, Asian, or Hispanic descent), café-au-lait spots (pale tan macules), and bruises related to bleeding disorders (occur with minimal trauma over bony points)

Indicators of Abuse and Neglect in Children—cont'd

Burns (can be friction, immersion, or pattern burns; located on soles of feet, hands, buttocks, back; cigarette burns are round; immersion burns have lines of demarcation)

Fractures (multiple; various stages of healing; spiral fractures; fractures of skull, face, nose, ribs, and long bones more common)

Lacerations and abrasions (especially found on backs of arms, legs, torso, external genitalia, face, mouth, lips, or gums; human bite marks can be evident)

Whiplash

Chemical injuries (unexplained poisoning or illness)

Failure to thrive, graphed weight/height below 5th percentile with no biologic cause

Signs of malnutrition (thinness, abdominal distention)

Unattended needs (glasses, dental work, physical injuries, immunization)

Poor physical hygiene (severe diaper rash, dirty hair, persistent body odor)

Unclean or inappropriate dress

Frequent accidents because of neglect

Unusual wariness or fear of adults

Withdrawal and/or lack of reaction

Inappropriate displays of friendliness and affection

Acting out (hitting, punching, biting, vandalism, shoplifting)

Absenteeism from school

Arriving early at school and staying late

Dullness, lethargy, inactivity

Begging and stealing food

Consistent lack of supervision

Sexual Abuse

Self-reports of abuse

Bruises; bleeding; fissures; lacerations of external genitalia, vagina, or anus

Abnormalities of hymen

Labial fusion

Anal laxity, anal gaping

Swelling of scrotum/penis (sucking injury)

Continued

Indicators of Abuse and Neglect in Children—cont'd

Bloody or stained underwear
Difficulty walking and/or sitting
Venereal disease in young child
Vaginal or penile discharge
Chronic pelvic pain
Recurrent vaginal infections
Pain on urination
Repeated incidences of chlamydial urethritis (males)
Persistent sore throats of unknown origin
Hickeys on the body
Pregnancy in adolescent females
Withdrawal
Preoccupation with fantasies
Unusual or precocious sexual behavior and knowledge with
    younger children, peers, or adults (provocative exhibition
    of genitalia, fondling, mutual masturbation)
Sudden changes in behavior (nightmares, fears, phobias,
    regression, acute anxiety)
Unexplainable rage when exposed to perpetrator
Noticeable personality changes
Anger at mother (in incestuous relationships)
Poor peer relationships
Infantile behaviors
Self-mutilation
Suicidal thoughts or attempts
Abuse of drugs or alcohol

Related Nursing Diagnoses

Fatigue: related to malnutrition, anemia, poor physical condition.

Posttrauma syndrome: related to abuse, serious threats or injury to
self or others, witnessing trauma.

Rape-trauma syndrome: related to rape by family member or
friend.

Altered parent/infant/child attachment: related to sexual abuse,
multiple stressors, maturity of parents, childhood abuse or neglect
of parents, violence in parental relationship.

Altered parenting: related to compromised family coping, history of being abused, poor problem-solving skills, social isolation, lack of access to resources, change in family unit or circumstances, poor communication skills, preference for physical punishment, lack of knowledge, physical illness, developmental delay, lack of readiness for parenthood, multiple births, difficult delivery, mental illness.

Impaired social interaction: related to absence of available significant others or caregivers, self-concept disturbance, fear, guilt.

Risk for altered development: related to inadequate nutrition, poverty, violence, abuse, brain damage.

Risk for altered growth: related to malnutrition, deprivation, violence, abuse, caregiver maladaptive feeding behaviors.

Knowledge deficit: related to cognitive limitation, information misinterpretation, lack of exposure, lack of interest in learning, unfamiliarity with information resources.

Infection: related to trauma, broken skin, tissue destruction, inadequate secondary defenses.

Impaired physical mobility, secondary to musculoskeletal impairment, loss of integrity of bone structure: related to developmental delay, pain.

Self-esteem disturbance: related to disturbances in body image, role performance, personal identity related to dysfunctional family relationships, physical or sexual abuse.

Sexual dysfunction: related to abuse.

Risk for self-mutilation: related to guilt, abuse, dysfunctional family.

Risk for violence, self-directed: related to social isolation, poor rapport with family, suicidal ideation, despair, lack of social resources.

Risk for violence, directed at others: related to abuse, history of witnessing family violence, suicidal ideation, impulsivity.

Assessment of Mental Health

24

The alert practitioner will detect concerns during the complete health assessment of children and adolescents that might lead to determination of the need for a more focused assessment of mental health. The cognitive and emotional development of children and adolescents produce greater variability in assessment of mental health and can make interpretation challenging; because of this, multiple approaches are recommended to increase reliability in findings. There are many standardized tests available that can be utilized with the techniques of observation and interviewing, which remain acceptable approaches in mental health assessment.

Assessment of mental health requires understanding of normal development, which will guide conclusions about what is normal for the age of the child or adolescent and what should be explored further. Additionally, knowledge of what is expected in development assists in adapting the assessment to the age of the child or adolescent, eliciting cooperation , and determining the emotional state of the child. Finally, in assessing mental health status, it is important to consider that childhood disorders with an organic basis might first present with abnormal behavior and that disorders with a psychosocial basis can have physical effects.

Rationale

It was once thought that young children, in particular, lacked the cognitive and emotional development to experience disorders such as depression. Statistics, however, related to major depressive disorder and suicide in children and adolescents suggest that mental health problems are of considerable concern worldwide. In the United States, the prevalence of major depressive disorder is as high as 1% among preschool children, 1% to 9% among school-age children, and 4% to 8% among adolescents. Suicide in young children is relatively rare and is thought to be more common in adolescents because of the ability to plan ahead. The incidence in older children and adolescents increases with the co-morbidity of other disorders and is second only to injuries as the leading cause of death in adolescents. Studies suggest that children who present with depression frequently have a history of attention deficit hyperactivity disorder (ADHD), oppositional defiant disorder, or conduct disorder. Subsequent to the onset of depression, adolescents are at increased risk for alcohol abuse, suicide, nicotine dependence, and anxiety disorders.

Extended mental health assessment should be considered whenever there is a central nervous system disorder (whether developmental or acquired); history of even mild untreated head trauma or major life or traumatic events; sudden changes in school performance, behavior, everyday cognitive functioning, or behavior patterns; changes in sensory function; neglect or abuse; and reports of symptoms suggesting mental health disorders.

Preparation

Assessment should begin with simpler aspects of mental health functioning and then progress to more complex or distressing elements later in the interview, when trust and rapport are established and if the need is determined. Standardized tests and behavior scales, such as the Beck Depression Inventory or the Children's Depression Inventory, can be used to assist in the assessment.

Much of the assessment related to mental health can be readily obtained in other areas of the health assessment. Good observational skills and the ability to establish rapport are essential to performing reliable mental health assessments in children and adolescents. Rapport is established through attentive and nonjudgmental listening. A play area with toys can be helpful when working with young children.

Typically, the parent or caregiver will present the history, but older children and adolescents benefit from privacy and assurance that conversation with them is confidential, unless their safety is at risk. When young children express a desire to share a secret, it might signal the need to disclose important information. Although this information might be important to diagnosis, treatment, or protection of the child, it is important to discuss with the child how secrets that involve harm to the child have to be told to someone and to invite the child to participate in deciding who should be told.

Inquire as to when the problem began; how current behavior is similar to or different from what is usually expected in the child or adolescent; severity, duration, and impact of problem; and significant events occurring before or concurrently with the problem. Inquire about family history of disorders, especially related to history of mental or emotional disorders, substance abuse, self-harm, epilepsy, delayed development, and learning problems. Ask about prenatal influences (drug or alcohol use during pregnancy, smoking, hospitalizations, surgeries), birth and perinatal events (type of delivery, use of anesthetics during birth, bruising, special medical treatments, number of weeks at birth, birth weight), traumatic events, developmental milestones, abuse, changes in the family, school performance, and substance use.

Assessment of Mental Health

Assessment	Findings
Appearance	
Observe for hygiene: age-appropriate dressing, evidence of self-harm (e.g., cuts on arms or wrists), needle tracks, hair pulling, picking, weight, distinct facies.	**Clinical Alert** Poor hygiene can indicate depression, suicide risk, abuse, neglect, or homelessness.
	Short palpebral fissure, flat midface, short nose, indistinct philtrum, and thin upper lip are distinguishing features in fetal alcohol syndrome.
Behavior	
Observe the child for age-appropriate attention to play or questions; ease in completing tasks or following instructions; distractibility; fidgeting or squirming;	**Clinical Alert** Easy distractibility, lack of attention when spoken to, and difficulty following through on directions can indicate attention deficit

Assessment	Findings

Behavior—cont'd

tendency to climb on things or handle things even when asked not to do so; ease or discomfort with quiet play; level of shyness; withdrawal; excessive talk-ativeness; blurting out answers, not waiting for turns; lack of interest in surroundings or caregiver; avoidance of eye contact; over-sensitivity to sounds; repetition of sounds; inappropriate laughing or crying; eye blinking; lip licking; twitching; head jerking; staring at nothing; motor retardation; discomfort with contact with caregiver.

disorder (ADD), anxiety, or childhood schizophrenia.

Excessive talkativeness, blurting out, inability to sit still, excessive climbing, disregard for instructions, and difficulty organizing activities can indicate ADD or ADHD, fetal alcohol syndrome, anxiety, or schizophrenia (children older than 5 years).

Discomfort with normal touch, lack of eye contact, oversensitivity to sounds, and lack of response to voice, especially in the presence of early feeding difficulties and developmental delays, can indicate autism spectrum disorder in young children.

Hyperactivity, hypoactivity, and other behavioral changes can accompany commonly used drugs (Table 24-1).

Observe mood (angry, tense, sad, worried, happy, irritable, labile, suspicious, impulsive).

Tension or expressions of worry can represent a healthy response to stressful events, including hospitalization or assessment.

Clinical Alert

Suspiciousness can indicate presence of delusions and hallucinations.

Anger, in the presence of defiance, blaming, and argumentativeness, can indicate oppositional defiance disorder or extreme stress.

Irritability, anxiety, hypoalertness, or diminished affect or

Assessment	Findings
Behavior—cont'd	
	responsiveness can indicate posttraumatic stress disorder when a traumatic event or situation has occurred, especially if there are also disturbing recollections or nightmares, sleep disturbances, memory impairment, difficulty concentrating, and headaches.
	Irritability, emotional lability, aggressiveness, and disobedience can indicate posttraumatic concussion syndrome when injury to the head has occurred.
	Irritability, anxiety, mood swings, disorientation, and hypervigilance can be indicative of drug or alcohol abuse.
	Changes in sleeping and eating patterns can indicate increased risk for suicide in the depressed child and adolescent.
Observe verbalizations for expressions of worthlessness or guilt ("I mess up everything I do," "I'm not good at anything," "All I do is cause problems"), expressions of aggression ("I am going to kill you"), and appropriateness to situation.	**Clinical Alert**
	Expressions of worthlessness and guilt are more common in adolescents than in younger children with depression (Table 24-2).
	Talking to self or responding to voices not heard can indicate hallucinations.
Inquire about changes to eating, sleeping, and elimination.	
Eating	
Has there been a change in weight or appetite recently?	**Clinical Alert**
	Over concern with weight, attempts to control weight,

Assessment	Findings

Behavior—cont'd

What kinds of foods are preferred? Has there been a change in preferences recently?

Have there been attempts to control weight? (If there is a positive response to this inquiry, inquire whether there have been variations in weight, whether there are times when child eats so much it hurts, whether the child eats when upset or nervous or bored, whether vomiting has been tried after eating, amount of exercise child or adolescent engages in per day, and whether laxatives or diet pills are being used. Ask, "How much would you like to weigh?")

excessive exercising, purging techniques, and ritualism around eating can indicate anorexia nervosa, especially in adolescent girls.

History of early feeding difficulties are found with autism spectrum disorder, including refusal of foods, requirement for specific presentation of foods and utensils, narrowly restricted food choices, and persistent choice of low-texture foods.

Hunger accompanies withdrawal from amphetamines; decreased appetite occurs with withdrawal from marijuana.

Changes in sleeping and eating patterns can indicate increased risk for suicide in the depressed child and adolescent.

Sleeping

Inquire about sleep patterns, changes in sleep patterns, nightmares.

Excessive sleepiness, especially daytime sleepiness, can indicate sleep disorder; substance abuse; or depression.

Insomnia can indicate use of amphetamines and accompanies withdrawal from alcohol, marijuana, and sedatives/hypnotics.

Fear of going to sleep unless near parents; nightmares about separation, especially in the presence of school avoidance; and excessive concern with separation from parent can indicate separation anxiety disorder or generalized anxiety.

Assessment	Findings
Behavior—cont'd	

Elimination

Ask about nighttime wetting and daytime wetting or soiling, regression in toilet training.	Regression to nighttime wetting can indicate stress in the preschool-age child.
	Fecal incontinence by the age of 4 years can indicate neglect, lax training methods, or developmental delays. Fecal incontinence in the child older than 4 years who has previously achieved fecal continence can indicate stress, changes in the child's life, or depression.
Inquire about interests, friends, school, community.	**Clinical Alert**
Ask, "What kinds of things (hobbies, pets) do you enjoy?" or "What kinds of things did you enjoy until recently?" If the child is younger than 3, inquire about playfulness and changes in playfulness.	In the child younger than 3, lack of playfulness and expression can indicate depression, autism spectrum disorder, or sensory disorders.
	Withdrawal from activities previously enjoyed, transient enjoyment in activities, or preoccupation with morbid activities can indicate depression.
Ask, "What worries or scares you?"	Excessive preoccupation with fantasy friends or responses to voices not heard by others can indicate hallucinations.
	Excessive fears or worries can indicate generalized anxiety or depression.
	Lack of interest in making friends, difficulty pretending at play, lack of awareness of feelings of others, significant difficulty with language, and difficulty relating to others can indicate Asperger's syndrome.
Ask the child about his or her friends. "Who is your	Withdrawal from friends can indicate depression.

Assessment	Findings
Behavior—cont'd	
best friend? How about other friends?"	Sudden changes in friends, dropping grades, and social isolation can indicate drug or alcohol abuse.
"What kinds of things do you do with your friends?"	
"Whom do you talk to when you need help with school work?"	
"Have your friends changed lately?"	Fighting, bullying, threatening, destruction of property, and stealing can indicate a conduct disorder or physical abuse.
"Do people sometimes annoy you? What do you do when they annoy you?"	
Ask the child about school. "What grade are you in school?"	Loss of interest in school and dropping grades can indicate depression, substance abuse, or child abuse.
"What do you like about school?"	
"Has schoolwork changed for you? If so, how has it changed?"	
"What are your teachers like?"	
"How many days of school have you missed recently?"	
Inquire about coping strategies. "What do you do when you get scared? What about when you get mad or frustrated?"	
"Whom do you talk to?"	
Inquire about alcohol and drug use. "Do you use drugs or alcohol?" If affirmative, ask about frequency and amount ("How many joints do you smoke a week?"), age at which use began, and situations in which drugs and alcohol are used.	
Inquire about suicide ideation and attempts.	**Clinical Alert**
"Are there things that you do	Depression and well-described plans, including

Assessment	Findings

Behavior—cont'd

that you know are risky?" "Have you thought about harming yourself or others?" "If so, how would you do it?" "Have you attempted suicide before?" "Did you get help afterward?"

the method and time, who will be at the funeral, and other funeral plans, indicate significant risk for suicide, especially in adolescents (see the box below for other indications of suicide risk).

Sudden involvement in high-risk behaviors, such as drug use, promiscuity, or reckless driving, or noncompliance with treatment (e.g., refusal to take insulin) can indicate suicide risk in the depressed child or adolescent.

Suicide ideation can accompany early crash with cocaine.

Warning Signs for Child and Adolescent Suicide Risk

Putting personal affairs in order (e.g., giving away treasured possessions, making up with friends)

Verbal cues such as "When I am not here anymore," "I wish I were dead," or saying goodbye to family members and friends

Withdrawal from family and friends

No desire to socialize

Fatigue; lack of energy or sudden burst of energy (especially if previously low in energy)

Feelings of sadness, not caring

Easily frustrated

Emotional outbursts or sudden decline in outbursts

Decline in school performance, frequent absences

Neglect of appearance

Changes in sleeping and eating patterns

Table 24-1 Behaviors and Terms Associated with Drug and Alcohol Abuse

Substance	Terms Associated with Substance	Behaviors and Physical Responses Associated with Intoxication	Developmental Effects of Prenatal Exposure
Alcohol	Mountain dew, alley juice, moonshine, sauce, booze, hootch	Decreased alertness, slurred speech, nausea, vertigo, staggering, emotional lability, stupor, unconsciousness. *Girls are more sensitive to alcohol effects and require less alcohol for impairment. Use of oral contraceptives also slows elimination of alcohol from the body.*	Fetal alcohol effects, fetal alcohol syndrome
Barbiturates	Downers, goofers, barbs, idiot pills, peanuts, sleepers	Drowsiness, relaxation, slurred speech, slow and shallow respirations, decreased pulse rate and blood pressure, cold and clammy skin, depression, poor judgment, motor impairment.	Unknown
Gamma-hydroxybutyrate (GHB) and Rohypnol	Easy lay, roofies	Relaxation, lightheadedness, dizziness, drowsiness, slurred speech, muscle incoordination, euphoria. *Drugs are easily disguised and slipped into drinks; this should be suspected if unexpected drowsiness, lightheadedness, and incoordination occur after drinking.*	

Continued

Table 24-1   Behaviors and Terms Associated with Drug and Alcohol Abuse—cont'd

Substance	Terms Associated with Substance	Behaviors and Physical Responses Associated with Intoxication	Developmental Effects of Prenatal Exposure
Narcotics	Dreamer, dust, hard stuff, morf, white stuff, big Harry, horse, joy powder, smack, stuff, white lady, China white	Euphoria, clouding of consciousness, impairment of intellectual functioning, dreamlike state, respiratory depression, pupillary constriction, cyanosis, watery eyes, needle marks on arms.	Increased rate of sudden infant death syndrome (SIDS), hyperactivity
Cocaine	C, candy, Cecil, coke, crack, nose, nose candy, rock, snow, stardust, white horse	Euphoria, disinhibition, irritability, anxiety, insomnia, lack of energy and motivation, psychomotor retardation, dilated pupils, increased blood pressure, hyperactivity, impulsivity, hypervigilance, hypersexuality. During early and middle crash, there may be depression. Suicidal ideation can be present during early crash, as well as agitation.	Developmental delay, increased risk of SIDS, hyperactivity, hypertonia (children younger than 2 years), head circumference smaller (younger than 2 years)

Amphetamines	Beans, berries, black beauties, browns, co-pilots, dice, drives, eye openers, lead rollers, pep pills, speed, white crossed, zip	Sweating, dilated pupils, agitation, irritability, insomnia, hyperactivity, paranoia, confusion, aggressiveness, restlessness, anorexia, tachycardia, increased blood pressure, slurred speech, euphoria, seizures, flashbacks, panic, hallucinations. Withdrawal can be accompanied by fatigue, hunger, increased sleep, and severe depression.	
Methamphe-tamines	Ice, meth, crystal meth, crystal, glass, crank	Similar effects to amphetamines.	
Ecstasy	X, XTC	Alertness; increased energy; increased blood pressure, temperature, and thirst; euphoria; jitteriness; teeth clenching; pupil dilation; death.	Unknown
Hallucino-gens (LSD, PCP, DMT, STP)	Acid, cube, heavenly haze, sugar, angel dust, elephant, goon, magic mist, hog	Vomiting, tremors, panic, agitation, depression, aggression, nystagmus, sweating, paranoia, elevated blood pressure, hallucinations, dilated pupils.	

Continued

Table 24-1 Behaviors and Terms Associated with Drug and Alcohol Abuse—cont'd

Substance	Terms Associated with Substance	Behaviors and Physical Responses Associated with Intoxication	Developmental Effects of Prenatal Exposure
Cannabis	Bush, joint, reefer, pot, smoke, straw, weed, hemp, hooter, jive	Laughter, confusion, panic, drowsiness, reddened eyes, increased vital signs, increased appetite, blurred vision, depression, irritability, emotional swings, decreased motivation, impaired memory. Withdrawal can be accompanied by insomnia, hyperactivity, and increased appetite.	Infants can exhibit symptoms of withdrawal after delivery (irritability, disturbed sleep)
Inhalants		Giddiness, drowsiness, headache, nausea, fainting, loss of consciousness, respiratory arrest, muscular weakness, nystagmus, belligerence, tremor, emotional lability.	Unknown

		Poor school performance, increased risk of SIDS
Nicotine		Headache; nausea; increased pulse, blood pressure, and muscle tone. Withdrawal can be accompanied by increased appetite, nervousness, sleep disturbances, anxiety, and irritability.
Steroids	Steroids, roids, juice	Euphoria, energy, increased competitiveness, combativeness, muscle deposits, deeper voice, enlarged clitoris, heart damage with use of several weeks. Depression, irritability on withdrawal. *Can result in shorter height in adolescent males as steroids can prematurely end puberty and stop the rapid growth associated with puberty.*

Table 24-2   Common Manifestations of Major Depressive Disorder in Children and Adolescents

Age	Manifestations
Younger than 3 years	Temper tantrums, lack of playfulness, feeding problems.
3 to 5 years	Enuresis, encopresis, phobias, accident-proneness, over concern about minor infractions.
6 to 8 years	Complaints of headaches or abdominal pain, aggressiveness, resistance to new experiences or people.
9 to 12 years	Worry about homework, self-blame, fatigue and lethargy, changes in appetite, trouble with sleep, vague stomach ailments or complaints of headache, psychomotor agitation or retardation, excessive morbidity in thoughts, drop in grades, difficulties completing homework.
13 years and older	Feelings of worthlessness and guilt, risky behaviors (promiscuity, reckless driving, substance use and abuse), anger, irritability, uncommunicativeness, sleepiness, preoccupation with body image, delinquency, oversensitivity to criticism, avoidance of anything new or challenging, difficulty completing homework, drop in grades.

Related Nursing Diagnoses

Impaired verbal communication: related to developmental disorders, depression, ADD, schizophrenia, sensory disorders, situational stressors.

Interrupted family processes: related to situational crisis, child or adolescent illness.

Risk for injury: related to suicide ideation, self-neglect, disregard for personal safety, developmental disorders.

Impaired parenting: related to family stress, overprotectiveness, disengagement, frustration, anxiety.

Self-esteem: related to disturbances in body image, personal identity, feelings of worthlessness or guilt, physical or sexual abuse, loneliness, impaired social relationships, school performance.

Impaired skin integrity: related to self-harm, drug use.

Ineffective health maintenance: related to abuse, neglect, substance abuse, alcohol abuse, eating disorders.

Altered nutrition: related to disturbances in body image; vomiting, dieting, fasting, use of laxatives; depression; substance abuse; alcohol abuse.

Self-mutilation: related to poor self-esteem, developmental disorders, depression.

Risk for violence, self-directed: related to mental health, suicide plan, verbal cues.

Disturbed sleep pattern: related to anxiety, depression, nightmares.

Risk for violence, directed at others: related to impulsivity, compromised coping strategies, hallucinations, delusions, conduct disorder, substance abuse.

Social isolation: related to developmental disorder, depression, suicide ideation, disturbance in self-concept.

Altered thought processes: secondary to substance abuse, mental health issues.

Risk for constipation: related to stress, situational crisis, eating disorders.

Altered urinary elimination: related to stress, situational crisis.

CONCLUDING THE ASSESSMENT

V

Completing the Examination

25

- Signal to the child and the parent that the assessment is at an end.
- Provide an opportunity for the parent and child to ask questions or verbalize concerns.
- Assist the child to dress.
- Praise the child for cooperation during the examination. Offer reassurance and empathy to the child who has been frightened or upset.
- Express appreciation to the parent for assistance.
- Share assessment findings with the parent (and child, if appropriate). *If findings are abnormal, the beginning practitioner should confirm them with a more experienced nurse before sharing with the parents and child.*
- Findings that initiate concern for the *immediate welfare* of the child, such as respiratory difficulties and abnormal neurologic signs, should be *communicated directly and quickly* to the physician and appropriate health care providers.
- Findings should be organized and written down as soon as possible after assessment to avoid inaccurate or vague documentation of detail (see Appendix E).
- If unsure of the correct terminology, describe the findings.
- Avoid use of "good" and "normal." These terms are subjective and vary greatly from nurse to nurse. Use specific, descriptive terms. Measurements, when possible, should be included.
- Findings should be documented in a way that is organized, concise, specific, accurate, complete, confidential, and legible.

Appendixes

Developmental
Assessment

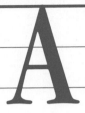

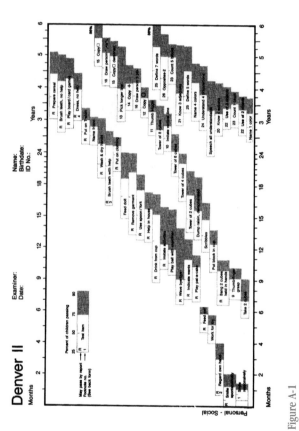

Figure A-1
Denver Developmental Screening Test II (Denver II).
(From Frankenburg WK, Dodds JB, University of Colorado Medical Center, 1990.)

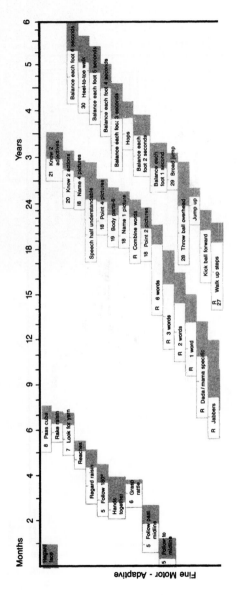

Figure A-1—cont'd

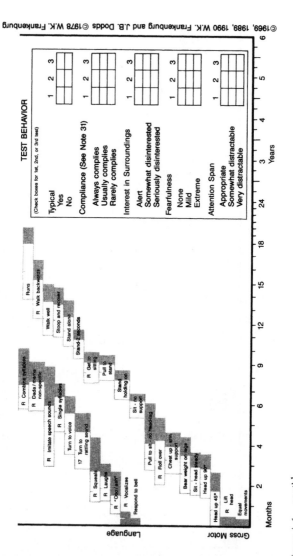

Figure A-1—cont'd

DIRECTIONS FOR ADMINISTRATION

1. Try to get child to smile by smiling, talking or waving. Do not touch him/her.
2. Child must stare at hand several seconds.
3. Parent may help guide toothbrush and put toothpaste on brush.
4. Child does not have to be able to tie shoes or button/zip in the back.
5. Move yarn slowly in an arc from one side to the other, about 8" above child's face.
6. Pass if child grasps rattle when it is touched to the backs or tips of fingers.
7. Pass if child tries to see where yarn went. Yarn should be dropped quickly from sight from tester's hand without arm movement.
8. Child must transfer cube from hand to hand without help of body, mouth, or table.
9. Pass if child picks up raisin with any part of thumb and finger.
10. Line can vary only 30 degrees or less from tester's line.
11. Make a fist with thumb pointing upward and wiggle only the thumb. Pass if child imitates and does not move any fingers other than the thumb.

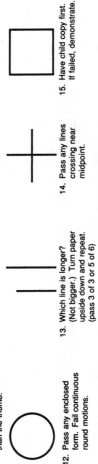

12. Pass any enclosed form. Fail continuous round motions.

13. Which line is longer? (Not bigger.) Turn paper upside down and repeat. (pass 3 of 3 or 5 of 6)

14. Pass any lines crossing near midpoint.

15. Have child copy first. If failed, demonstrate.

16. When scoring, each pair (2 arms, 2 legs, etc.) counts as one part.
17. Place one cube in cup and shake gently near child's ear, but out of sight. Repeat for other ear.

When giving items 12, 14, and 15, do not name the forms. Do not demonstrate 12 and 14.

Figure A-2

Directions for administration of numbered items on Denver II.
(From Frankenburg WK, Dodds JB, University of Colorado Medical Center, 1990.)

18. Point to picture and have child name it. (No credit is given for sounds only.)
    If less than 4 pictures are named correctly, have child point to picture as each is named by tester.

   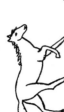 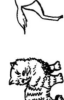

19. Using doll, tell child: Show me the nose, eyes, ears, mouth, hands, feet, tummy, hair. Pass 6 of 8.
20. Using pictures, ask child: Which one flies?... says meow?... talks?... barks?... gallops? Pass 2 of 5, 4 of 5.
21. Ask child: What do you do when you are cold?... tired?... hungry? Pass 2 of 3, 3 of 3.
22. Ask child: What do you do with a cup? What is a chair used for? What is a pencil used for?
    Action words must be included in answers.
23. Pass if child correctly places and says how many blocks are on paper. (1, 5).
24. Tell child: Put block on table; under table; in front of me, behind me. Pass 4 of 4.
    (Do not help child by pointing, moving head or eyes.)
25. Ask child: What is a ball?... lake?... desk?... house?... banana?... curtain?... fence?... ceiling? Pass if defined in terms
    of use, shape, what it is made of, or general category (such as banana is fruit, not just yellow). Pass 5 of 8, 7 of 8.
26. Ask child: If a horse is big, a mouse is ___? If fire is hot, ice is ___? If the sun shines during the day, the moon shines
    during the ___? Pass 2 of 3.
27. Child may use wall or rail only, not person. May not crawl.
28. Child must throw ball overhand 3 feet to within arm's reach of tester.
29. Child must perform standing broad jump over width of test sheet (8 1/2 inches).
30. Tell child to walk forward, ⟶ heel within 1 inch of toe. Tester may demonstrate.
    Child must walk 4 consecutive steps.
31. In the second year, half of normal children are non-compliant.

OBSERVATIONS:

Figure A-2—cont'd

Growth
Charts

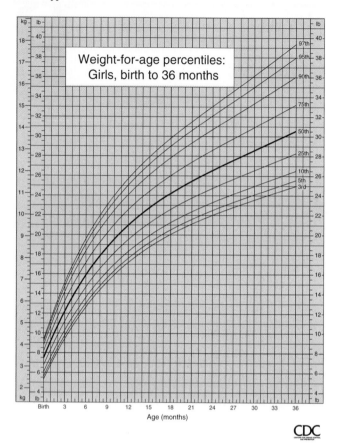

Figure B-1

Weight-for-age percentiles, girls, birth to 36 months, CDC growth charts: United States.

(Developed by the National Center for Health Statistics in collaboration with the National Center for Chronic Disease Prevention and Health Promotion, 2000.)

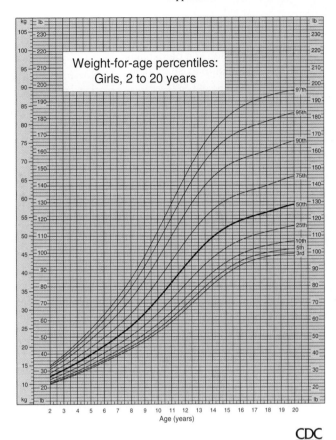

Figure B-2
Weight-for-age percentiles, girls, 2 to 20 years, CDC growth charts: United States.
(Developed by the National Center for Health Statistics in collaboration with the National Center for Chronic Disease Prevention and Health Promotion, 2000.)

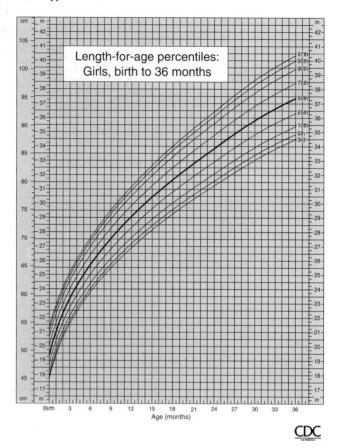

Figure B-3

Length-for-age percentiles, girls, birth to 36 months, CDC growth charts: United States.
(Developed by the National Center for Health Statistics in collaboration with the National Center for Chronic Disease Prevention and Health Promotion, 2000.)

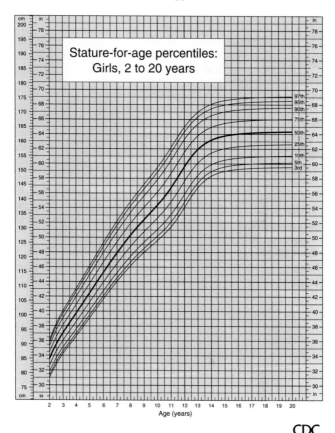

Figure B-4

Stature-for-age percentiles, girls, 2 to 20 years, CDC growth charts: United States.

(Developed by the National Center for Health Statistics in collaboration with the National Center for Chronic Disease Prevention and Health Promotion, 2000.)

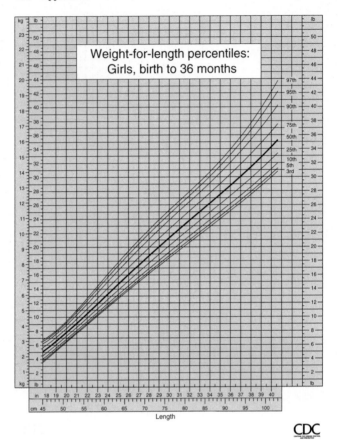

Figure B-5
Weight-for-length percentiles, girls, birth to 36 months, CDC growth charts: United States.
(Developed by the National Center for Health Statistics in collaboration with the National Center for Chronic Disease Prevention and Health Promotion, 2000.)

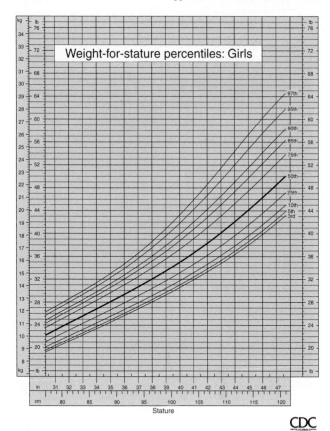

Figure B-6
Weight-for-stature percentiles, girls, 2 to 20 years, CDC growth charts: United States.
(Developed by the National Center for Health Statistics in collaboration with the National Center for Chronic Disease Prevention and Health Promotion, 2000.)

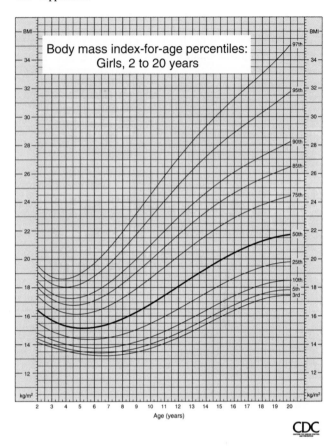

Figure B-7
Body mass index (BMI)-for-age percentiles, girls, 2 to 20 years,
CDC growth charts: United States.
(Developed by the National Center for Health Statistics in collaboration with the
National Center for Chronic Disease Prevention and Health Promotion, 2000.)

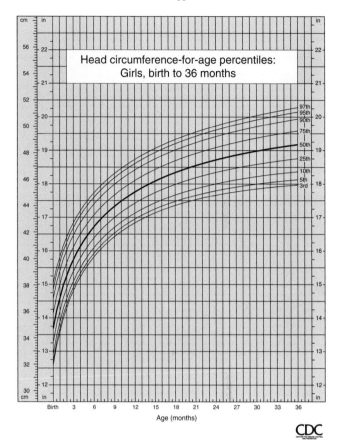

Figure B-8

Head circumference-for-age percentiles, girls, birth to 36 months, CDC growth charts: United States.

(Developed by the National Center for Health Statistics in collaboration with the National Center for Chronic Disease Prevention and Health Promotion, 2000.)

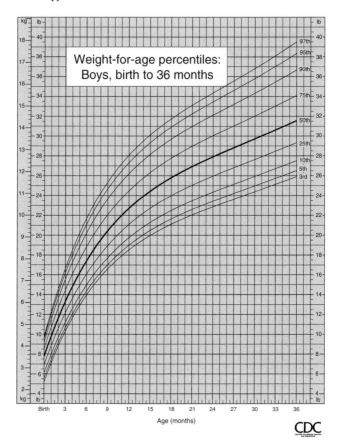

Figure B-9

Weight-for-age percentiles, boys, birth to 36 months, CDC growth charts: United States.

(Developed by the National Center for Health Statistics in collaboration with the National Center for Chronic Disease Prevention and Health Promotion, 2000.)

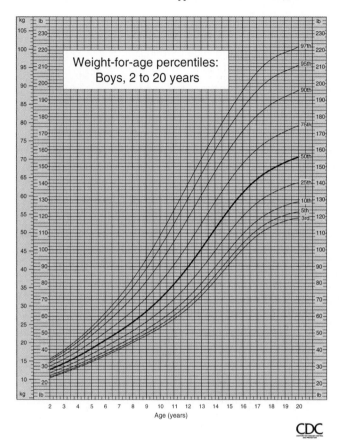

Figure B-10

Weight-for-age percentiles, boys, 2 to 20 years, CDC growth charts: United States.

(Developed by the National Center for Health Statistics in collaboration with the National Center for Chronic Disease Prevention and Health Promotion, 2000.)

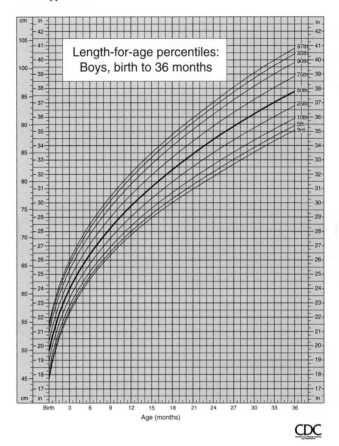

Figure B-11
Length-for-age percentiles, boys, birth to 36 months, CDC growth charts: United States.
(Developed by the National Center for Health Statistics in collaboration with the National Center for Chronic Disease Prevention and Health Promotion, 2000.)

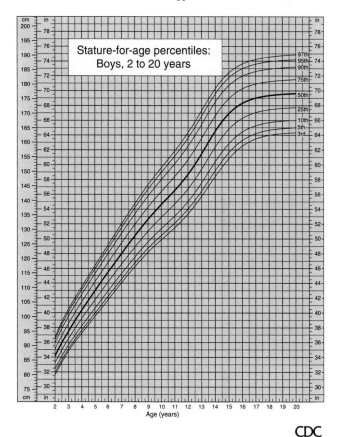

Figure B-12
Stature-for-age percentiles, boys, 2 to 20 years, CDC growth charts: United States.
(Developed by the National Center for Health Statistics in collaboration with the National Center for Chronic Disease Prevention and Health Promotion, 2000.)

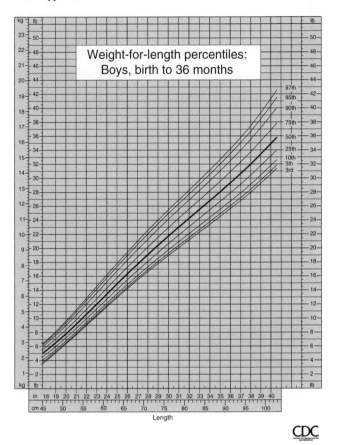

Figure B-13

Weight-for-length percentiles, boys, birth to 36 months, CDC growth charts: United States.

(Developed by the National Center for Health Statistics in collaboration with the National Center for Chronic Disease Prevention and Health Promotion, 2000.)

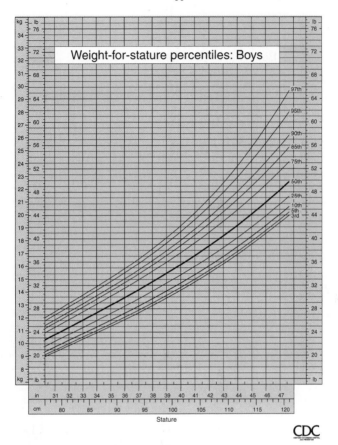

Figure B-14
Weight-for-stature percentiles, boys, 2 to 20 years, CDC growth charts: United States.
(Developed by the National Center for Health Statistics in collaboration with the National Center for Chronic Disease Prevention and Health Promotion, 2000.)

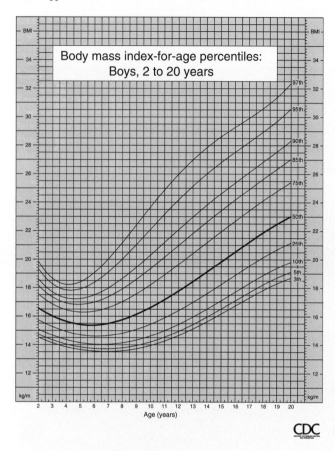

Figure B-15

Body mass index (BMI)-for-age percentiles, boys, 2 to 20 years, CDC growth charts: United States.

(Developed by the National Center for Health Statistics in collaboration with the National Center for Chronic Disease Prevention and Health Promotion, 2000.)

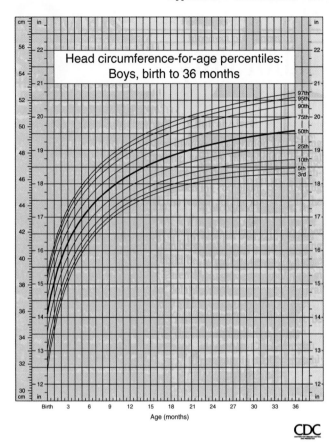

Figure B-16

Head circumference-for-age percentiles, boys, birth to 36 months, CDC growth charts: United States.

(Developed by the National Center for Health Statistics in collaboration with the National Center for Chronic Disease Prevention and Health Promotion, 2000.)

Normal
Laboratory
Values

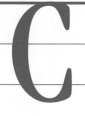

Table C-1 Hematology

Test	Age/Sex	Reference Range	
		Conventional Values	International Units
Hematocrit (Hct, HCT)		*% Packed Cells*	*Volume Fraction*
	Infant (2 mo)	28-42	0.28-0.42
	Child (6-12 yr)	35-45	0.35-0.45
	Adolescent: male	37-49	0.37-0.49
	Adolescent: female	36-46	0.36-0.46
	Critical values	<15 or >60	<0.15 or >0.60
Hemoglobin (Hb, Hgb)		*g/dl*	*mmol/L*
	Infant (2-6 mo)	10-15	6.1-9.0
	Child (1-12 yrs)	11-16	5.8-9.6
	Adolescent: male	14-16	7.4-9.3
	Adolescent: female	12-16	7.4-9.3
	Critical values	<5 or >20	<3.10 or >11.2

Continued

Table C-1 Hematology—cont'd

Test	Age/Sex	Reference Range	
		Conventional Values	International Units
Red blood cell (RBC) count (erythrocyte count)		*Million Cells/mm³ (μL)*	*×10¹² Cells/L*
	Infant	3.8-5.3	3.8-5.3
	Child (2-12 yr)	3.6-5.2	3.6-5.2
	Adolescent: male	4.5-5.3	4.5-5.3
	Adolescent: female	4.1-5.1	4.1-5.1
Platelet count (thrombocyte count)		*×10³/mm³ (μL)*	*×10⁹/L*
	Infant/child/youth	150-450	150-450
	Critical values	<30 or >7100	<30 or >7100
Erythrocyte indexes Mean corpuscular volume (MCV)		*μm³*	*fL*
	Infant	70-86	70-86
	Child (6-12 yr)	77-96	77-96
	Adolescent: male (12-18 yr)	78-98	78-98
	Adolescent: female (12-18 yr)	78-102	78-102

		pg/Cell	fmol/Cell
Mean corpuscular hemoglobin (MCH)	Infant (2-6 mo)	25-35	0.39-0.54
	Infant/child (6-24 mo)	23-31	0.36-0.48
	Thereafter	25-34	0.39-0.54

		%Hb/Cell	mmol
Mean corpuscular hemoglobin concentration (MCHC)	Infant	30-36	4.65-5.58
	Thereafter	31-37	4.81-5.74

		%	Number Fraction
Reticulocyte count	Infant	0.3-3.1	0.003-0.031
	Thereafter	0.5-2.5	0.005-0.025

		mm/hr	mm/hr
Sedimentation rate (erythrocyte sedimentation rate—ESR)	Child	0-10	0-10
	Thereafter: male	1-15	1-15
	Thereafter: female	1-20	1-20

Continued

Table C-1 Hematology—cont'd

Test	Age/Sex	Reference Range	
		Conventional Values	International Units
White blood cell count (leukocyte count)		$\times 1000\ Cells/mm^3\ (\mu L)$	$\times 10^9\ Cells/L$
	Newborn	9.0-30.0	9.0-30.0
	Child (≤2 years)	6.2-17.0	6.2-17.0
	Child/adult	5.0-10.0	5.0-10.0
	Critical values	<2.5 or >30.0	
Differential white blood cell count		%	Number Fraction
Neutrophils (segmented and bands)	Infant	23	0.23
	Child	31-61	0.31-0.61
	Thereafter	54-75	0.54-0.75
Eosinophils		1-3	0.01-0.03
Basophils		0.5-1	0.005-0.01
Lymphocytes	Infant	61	0.61
	Child	28-48	0.28-0.48
	Thereafter	25-40	0.25-0.40

Monocytes	Infant	5	0.05
	Child	4-4.5	0.04-0.045
	Thereafter	2-8	0.02-0.08
		Time	*Time*
Bleeding time	Infant/child/adolescent	2-7 min	2-7 min
	Critical values	>12 min	>12 min
Clotting time	Infant/child/adolescent	5-8 min	5-8 min
Prothrombin time (PT): one stage, quick	Infant/child/adolescent	11-15 sec	11-15 sec
Partial thromboplastin time (PTT), nonactivated	Infant/child/adolescent	24-40 sec	24-40 sec
Activated partial thromboplastin time (APTT)	Infant (>6 mo)	<90 sec	<90 sec
	Thereafter	30-40 sec	30-40 sec
		mg/dl	*g/L*
Fibrinogen level (factor I, quantitative fibrinogen)	Infant/child/adolescent	200-400	2.0-4.0
	Critical values	<100	<1.0

Table C-2 Normal Cerebrospinal Fluid Values

Test	Age	Reference Range	
		Conventional Values	International Units
Appearance		Clear, colorless	
Pressure	Child	10-100 mm H_2O	10-100 mm H_2O
	Adult	90-180 mm H_2O	90-180 mm H_2O
Volume	Child	60-100 ml	60-100 ml
	Adult	90-150 ml	90-150 ml
Specific gravity		1.006-1.008	1.006-1.008
Neoplastic cells		Negative	Negative
Culture and sensitivity		No organisms	No organisms
		mmol/L	*mmol/L*
Chloride	Infant/child/adolescent	118-132	118-132
Sodium		138-154	138-154
		mg/dL	*mmol/L*
Glucose	Infant/child/adolescent	40-80 (fasting)	2.2-4.4 (fasting)

		g/dL	g/L
Protein, total		1.5-4.5	15-45
White blood cell count, total	Newborn	0-30 cells	
	1-5 years	0-20 cells	
	6-18 years	0-10 cells	
	Adult	0-5 cells	

	%	Number Fraction
Differential leukocyte count		
Lymphocytes	40-80	0.4-0.8
Monocytes	15-45	0.15-0.45
Neutrophils	0-6	0-0.6
Eosinophils	0-5	0-0.05
	μL	×10⁶/L
Erythrocytes	0-10	0-10

Table C-3 Blood, Serum, and Plasma Values

Test	Specimen	Age/Sex/Condition	Reference Range	
			Conventional Values	International Units
Acetone	Serum, plasma		*mg/dL*	*mmol/L*
Semiquantitative			Negative	Negative
Quantitative			0.3-2.0	0.05-0.34
Alkaline phosphatase (King-Armstrong method)	Serum		*U/dL*	*U/L*
		Infant (1 mo)	10-30	71-213
		Toddler (3 yr)	10-20	71-142
		Child (10 yr)	15-30	107-213
		Adult	4.5-13	32-92
Amylase (Somogyi method)	Serum	Infant/child/adult	*U/dL* 50-180	*U/L* 92-330
	Urine (24 hr)	Infant/child/adult	26-950 U/24 hr	
Bilirubin			*mg/dL*	*μmol/L*
Total	Serum	Infant/child/adolescent	<1.5	<25.6
Direct (conjugated)	Serum	Infant/child/adolescent	0.0-0.3	0-5.1

			_mg/dL_	_mmol/L_
Calcium				
Ionized	Serum, plasma whole blood	Infant/child/adolescent	4.48-4.92	1.12-2.70
Total	Serum	Child	8.8-10.8	2.2-2.70
		Thereafter	8.4-10.2	2.1-2.55
			mcg/dL	_µmol/L_
β-Carotene	Serum	Infant	20-70	0.37-1.30
		Child	40-130	0.74-2.42
		Thereafter	60-200	1.12-3.72
			µEq/L	_µmol/L_
Chloride	Serum, plasma	Infant/child/adolescent	97-107	97-107
	Critical values		<80 or >115	<80 or >115
	Urine	Infant	2-10	2-10
		Child	15-40	15-40
		Adolescent	36-176	36-176
	Sweat	Normal	5-35	5- 35
		Marginal	45-70	45-70
		Cystic fibrosis	60-200	60-200

Continued

Table C-3 Blood, Serum, and Plasma Values—cont'd

Test	Specimen	Age/Sex/Condition	Reference Range	
			Conventional Values	International Units
Cholesterol, total	Serum*		*mg/dL*	*mmol/L*
		Infant (≤4 yr)	112-203	2.9-5.25
		Child	121-205	3.13-5.30
		Adolescent	113-200	2.93-5.18
Copper	Serum		*mg/dL*	*mmol/L*
		Infant/child	30-190	4.7-29.83
		Adolescent	70-155	10.99-24.34
Cortisol	Serum, plasma		*mcg/dL*	*nmol/L*
		0800 hrs	5-23	138-635
		1600 hrs	3-16	83-441
Creatine kinase (CK, CPK)	Serum†		*U/L*	*U/L*
		Infant/child/adolescent: male	0-70	0-70
		Infant/child/adolescent: female	0-50	0-50

			mg/dL	*μmol/L*
Creatinine	Serum, plasma	Infant	≤0.5	≤44
		Child	≤0.6-0.9	≤53-80
		Adolescent	≤1.1-1.2	≤97-106
			mg/dL	*mmol/L*
Fatty acids, free	Serum, plasma	Children/obese adults	<31	<1.10
			g/day	*g/day*
Fecal fat	Feces	Breastfed infant	<1	<1
		Child (0-6 yr)	<2	<2
		Thereafter	<4	<4
			ng/ml	*mcg/L*
Ferritin	Serum	Infant	50-200	50-200
		Child	7-140	7-140
			ng/ml	*nmol/L*
Folate	Serum	Infant/child/adolescent	1.8-9	4.1-20.4
			mg/dL	*mmol/L*
Galactose	Serum	Infant/child/adolescent	<5	<0.28

Continued

Table C-3 Blood, Serum, and Plasma Values—cont'd

Test	Specimen	Age/Sex/Condition	Reference Range		
			Conventional Values		International Units
			mg/dL		*mmol/L*
Glucose	Serum	Child	60-100		3.3-5.5
		Adolescent	70-105		3.9-5.8
		Critical values	<40 or >700		<2.2 or >38.6
	Urine (qualitative)		Negative		Negative
Glucose tolerance test (GTT)	Dosage				
	2.5 g/kg	Infant (0-18 mo)			
	2.0 g/kg	Child (18 mo-3 yr)			
	1.75 g/kg	Child (3-12 yr)			
	1.25 g/kg (max. 100 g)	Adolescent (>12 yr)			
	Time (min)		*mg/dL*		*mmol/L*
	Fasting	Normal; diabetic	70-105; >115		3.9-5.8; >6.4
	60	Normal; diabetic	120-160; >200		6.7-8.8; ≥11
	90	Normal; diabetic	100-140; >200		5.6-7.8; ≥11
	120	Normal; diabetic	65-120; >140		3.6-6.7; ≥7.8

			mg/day	μmol/day
17-Hydroxycorticosteroid (17-OHCS)	Urine (24 hr)	Infant	0.5-1.0	1.4-2.8
		Child	1.0-5.6	2.8-15.5
		Adolescent: male	3.0-10.0	8.2-27.6
		Adolescent: female	2.0-8.0	5.5-22
			mg/dL	g/L
Immunoglobulin A (IgA)	Serum	Infant (1-6 mo)	7-46	0.07-0.46
		Infant/child (6 mo-2 yr)	19-74	0.19-0.74
		Child (3-5 yr)	66-120	0.66-1.20
		Child (6-11 yr)	71-191	0.71-1.91
		Adolescent (12-16 yr)	85-211	0.85-2.11
			mg/dL	μmol/L
Immunoglobulin D (IgD)	Serum	Child/adolescent	0-8	5-30
			IU/mL	mcg/L
Immunoglobulin E (IgE)	Serum	Newborn (6 wk)	0.1-2.8	0.24-9.6
		Infant (6 mo)	0.9-28	0.24-134.4
		Infant (1 yr)	1.1-10.2	0.24-199.2
		Child (4 yr)	2.4-34.8	0.96-345.6
		Child (10 yr)	0.3-215	4.56-1010.4
		Adolescent (14 yr)	1.9-159	3.84-1094.0

Continued

Table C-3   Blood, Serum, and Plasma Values—cont'd

Test	Specimen	Age/Sex/Condition	Reference Range	
			Conventional Values	International Units
Immunoglobulin G (IgG)	Serum		*mg/dL*	*g/L*
		Infant (1-6 mo)	250-900	2.5-9
		Infant/child (6 mo-2 yr)	220-1070	2.2-10.7
		Child (2-6 yr)	420-1200	4.2-12.0
		Child (>6 yr)	650-1600	6.5-16.0
Iron	Serum		*mcg/dL*	*μmol/L*
		Infant	40-100	7.16-17.90
		Child	50-120	8.95-21.48
		Adolescent: male	50-160	8.95-28.64
		Adolescent: female	40-150	7.16-26.85
		Intoxicated child	280-2550	50.12-456.5
		Fatally poisoned child	>1800	>322.2
Iron-binding capacity	Serum		*mcg/dL*	*μmol/L*
		Infant	100-400	17.90-71.60
		Thereafter	250-400	44.75-71.60

Test	Specimen		Conventional units	SI units
Lead	Whole blood	Child	*mcg/dL* <10	*μmol/L* <0.5
		Adult	<20	<1.0
		Levels associated with lead poisoning	>80	>3.86
Lipase (Tietz method)	Serum	Child/adolescent	*mcg/dL* 0.1-1.0	*μmol/L* 28-280
Magnesium	Serum	Infant/child/adolescent	*mEq/L* 1.3-2.1	*mmol/L* 0.65-1.05
Osmolality	Serum		*mOsm/kg H_2O* 275-295	
Phenylalanine	Serum	Infant/child/adolescent	*mg/dL* 0.8-1.8	*mmol/L* 0.05-0.11
Phenylketonuria	Serum	Infant	*mg/dL* Negative or <3	
Phosphorus, inorganic	Serum	Infant/child	*mg/dL* 4.5-6.5	*mmol/L* 1.45-2.1
		Adolescent	3.0-4.5	0.97-1.45

Continued

Table C-3 Blood, Serum, and Plasma Values—cont'd

Test	Specimen	Age/Sex/Condition	Conventional Values	International Units
Potassium	Serum		*mEq/L*	*mmol/L*
		Infant	4.1-5.3	4.1-5.3
		Child	3.4-4.7	3.4-4.7
		Adolescent	3.5-5.3	3.5-5.3
Protein, total	Serum		*g/dL*	*g/L*
		Child	6.2-8.0	62.0-80.0
		Adolescent	6.0-8.0	60.0-80.0
Salicylates	Serum, plasma		*mg/dL*	*mmol/L*
		Therapeutic	15-30	1.1-2.2
		Toxic	>30	>2.2
Sodium	Serum		*mEq/L*	*mmol/L*
		Infant	139-146	139-146
		Child	138-145	138-145
		Adolescent	135-148	135-148

			Conventional Units	SI Units
Thiamine (vitamin B$_1$)	Whole blood		mcg/dL 0-2.0	nmol/L 0.75-4
Thyroid-stimulating hormone (TSH)	Serum, plasma	Infant/child/adolescent	μIU/ml 2-11	mIU/L 2-11
Transferrin	Serum	Infant/child/adolescent	mg/dL 200-400	g/L 2.0-4.0
Triglycerides (TG; neutral fat)	Serum	Infant Adolescent Male Female	mg/dL 5-40 30-150 40-160 35-135	g/L 0.05-0.40 0.30-1.50 0.40-1.60 0.35-1.35
Tyrosine	Serum	Infant/child/adolescent	mg/dL 0.8-1.3	mmol/L 0.044-0.07
Urea nitrogen	Serum, plasma	Infant/child Adolescent	mg/dL 5-18 7-18	mmol urea/L 1.8-6.4 2.5-6.4

Continued

Table C-3 Blood, Serum, and Plasma Values—cont'd

Test	Specimen	Age/Sex/Condition	Reference Range	
			Conventional Values	International Units
Uric acid	Serum		*mg/dL*	*μmol/L*
		Child	2.0-5.5	119-327
		Adolescent: male	3.5-7.2	208-438
		Adolescent: female	3.0-8.2	178-488
Vitamin A	Serum		*μm/dL*	*μmol/L*
		Child	30-80	1.22-2.62
		Adolescent	30-65	1.05-2.27
Vitamin B_{12}	Serum	Infant/child/adolescent	*pg/ml*	*pmol/L*
			140-900	103-454
Vitamin C	Serum	Infant/child/adolescent	*mg/dL*	*μmol/L*
			0.6-2.0	34-113
Vitamin E	Serum	Infant/child	*mcg/mL*	*μmol/L*
			5-20	17.6-46.4

*Values are approximately 10% higher for African Americans.
†Values are higher after exercise and for African Americans.

Table C-4 Blood Gas Determinations

Determination	Age	Reference Range	
		Conventional Values	International Units
pH	Infant/child (2 mo-2 yr)	7.34-7.46	
	Child (>2 yr)	7.35-7.45	
	Critical values	<7.2 or ≥7.6	
O₂ saturation	Child/adolescent	96-100%	
	Critical values	<60%	
HCO₃, venous*		_mEq/L_	_mmol/L_
	Infant/child/adolescent	22-26	22-26
	Critical values	>40	>40
Base excess		_mmol/L_	_mmol/L_
	Infant	(−7)-(−1)	(−7)-(−1)
	Child	(−4)-(+2)	(−4)-(+2)
	Thereafter	(−3)-(+3)	(−3)-(+3)

*Arterial values are approximately 2 mmol/L lower.

Table C-5   Urinalysis

Test	Age	Reference Range		
		Conventional Values	International Units
Color		Pale yellow to amber	
Appearance		Clear to slightly hazy	
pH		4.5-8.0	
Specific gravity		1.002-1.025	
Bacteria	Infant/child	<1000 CFU/ml (clean catch)	
Bilirubin		Negative	Negative
Glucose, qualitative		Negative	Negative
Microscopic analysis		*Per high-power field*	
		0-4	
Leukocytes		Rare	
Erythrocytes		Rare	
Casts			
Occult blood		Negative	Negative
Osmolality		*mOsm/kg H_2O*	
Random	Infant/child/adolescent	50-1400	
24-Hour	Infant/child/adolescent	300-900	

Immunization Schedules for Infants and Children

Recommended Childhood and Adolescent Immunization Schedule UNITED STATES • 2005

Vaccine ▼ / Age ▶	Birth	1 month	2 months	4 months	6 months	12 months	15 months	18 months	24 months	4–6 years	11–12 years	13–18 years
Hepatitis B[1]	HepB #1	HepB #2			HepB #3						HepB Series	
Diphtheria, Tetanus, Pertussis[2]			DTaP	DTaP	DTaP		DTaP			DTaP	Td	Td
Haemophilus influenzae type b[3]			Hib	Hib	Hib	Hib						
Inactivated Poliovirus			IPV	IPV	IPV					IPV		
Measles, Mumps, Rubella[4]						MMR #1				MMR #2	MMR #2	
Varicella[5]						Varicella					Varicella	
Pneumococcal Conjugate[6]			PCV	PCV	PCV	PCV			PCV	PPV	PPV	
Influenza[7]					Influenza (Yearly)					Influenza (Yearly)		
Hepatitis A[8]										Hepatitis A Series		

Vaccines below this line are for selected populations

Range of recommended ages
Preadolescent assessment
Only if mother HBsAg(–)
Catch-up immunization

This schedule indicates the recommended ages for routine administration of currently licensed childhood vaccines, as of December 1, 2004, for children through age 18 years. Any dose not administered at the recommended age should be administered at any subsequent visit when indicated and feasible. ▓ Indicates age groups that warrant special effort to administer those vaccines not previously administered. Additional vaccines may be licensed and recommended during the year. Licensed combination vaccines may be used whenever any components of the combination are indicated and other components of the vaccine are not contraindicated. Providers should consult the manufacturers' package inserts for detailed recommendations. Clinically significant adverse events that follow immunization should be reported to the Vaccine Adverse Event Reporting System (VAERS). Guidance about how to obtain and complete a VAERS form is available at www.vaers.org or by telephone, **800-822-7967.**

The Childhood and Adolescent Immunization Schedule is approved by:
Advisory Committee on Immunization Practices www.cdc.gov/nip/acip
American Academy of Pediatrics www.aap.org
American Academy of Family Physicians www.aafp.org

FROM
DEPARTMENT OF HEALTH AND HUMAN SERVICES,
CENTERS FOR DISEASE CONTROL AND PREVENTION, 2005.

Footnotes
Recommended Childhood and Adolescent Immunization Schedule
UNITED STATES • 2005

1. **Hepatitis B (HepB) vaccine.** All infants should receive the first dose of HepB vaccine soon after birth and before hospital discharge; the first dose may also be administered by age 2 months if the mother is HBsAg negative. Only monovalent HepB may be used for the birth dose. Monovalent or combination vaccine containing HepB may be used to complete the series. Four doses of vaccine may be administered when a birth dose is given. The second dose should be administered at least 4 weeks after the first dose, except for combination vaccines which cannot be administered before age 6 weeks. The third dose should be given at least 16 weeks after the first dose and at least 8 weeks after the second dose. The last dose in the vaccination series (third or fourth dose) should not be administered before age 24 weeks.

   Infants born to HBsAg-positive mothers should receive HepB and 0.5 mL of hepatitis B immune globulin (HBIG) at separate sites within 12 hours of birth. The second dose is recommended at age 1–2 months. The final dose in the immunization series should not be administered before age 24 weeks. These infants should be tested for HBsAg and antibody to HBsAg (anti-HBs) at age 9–15 months.

   Infants born to mothers whose HBsAg status is unknown should receive the first dose of the HepB series within 12 hours of birth. Maternal blood should be drawn as soon as possible to determine the mother's HBsAg status; if the HBsAg test is positive, the infant should receive HBIG as soon as possible (no later than age 1 week). The second dose is recommended at age 1–2 months. The last dose in the immunization series should not be administered before age 24 weeks.

2. **Diphtheria and tetanus toxoids and acellular pertussis (DTaP) vaccine.** The fourth dose of DTaP may be administered as early as age 12 months, provided 6 months have elapsed since the third dose and the child is unlikely to return at age 15 to 18 months. The final dose in the series should be given at age ≥4 years. **Tetanus and diphtheria toxoids (Td)** is recommended at age 11–12 years if at least 5 years have elapsed since the last dose of tetanus and diphtheria toxoid-containing vaccine. Subsequent routine Td boosters are recommended every 10 years.

3. **Haemophilus influenzae type b (Hib) conjugate vaccine.** Three Hib conjugate vaccines are licensed for infant use. If PRP-OMP (PedvaxHIB® or ComVax® [Merck]) is administered at ages 2 and 4 months, a dose at age 6 months is not required. DTaP/Hib combination products should not be used for primary immunization in infants at ages 2, 4 or 6 months but can be used as boosters after any Hib vaccine. The final dose in the series should be administered at age ≥12 months.

4. **Measles, mumps, and rubella vaccine (MMR).** The second dose of MMR is recommended routinely at age 4–6 years but may be administered during any visit, provided at least 4 weeks have elapsed since the first dose and both doses are administered beginning at or after age 12 months. Those who have not previously received the second dose should complete the schedule by age 11–12 years.

5. **Varicella vaccine.** Varicella vaccine is recommended at any visit at or after age 12 months for susceptible children (i.e., those who lack a reliable history of chickenpox). Susceptible persons aged ≥13 years should receive 2 doses administered at least 4 weeks apart.

6. **Pneumococcal vaccine.** The heptavalent **pneumococcal conjugate vaccine (PCV)** is recommended for all children aged 2–23 months and for certain children aged 24–59 months. The final dose in the series should be given at age ≥12 months. **Pneumococcal polysaccharide vaccine (PPV)** is recommended in addition to PCV for certain high-risk groups. See *MMWR* 2000;49(RR-9):1-35.

7. **Influenza vaccine.** Influenza vaccine is recommended annually for children aged ≥6 months with certain risk factors (including, but not limited to, asthma, cardiac disease, sickle cell disease, human immunodeficiency virus [HIV], and diabetes), healthcare workers, and other persons (including household members) in close contact with persons in groups at high risk (see *MMWR* 2004;53[RR-6]:1-40). In addition, healthy children aged 6–23 months and close contacts of healthy children aged 0–23 months are recommended to receive influenza vaccine because children in this age group are at substantially increased risk for influenza-related hospitalizations. For healthy persons aged 5–49 years, the intranasally administered, live, attenuated influenza vaccine (LAIV) is an acceptable alternative to the intramuscular trivalent inactivated influenza vaccine (TIV). See *MMWR* 2004;53(RR-6):1-40. Children receiving TIV should be administered a dosage appropriate for their age (0.25 mL, if aged 6–35 months or 0.5 mL, if aged ≥3 years). Children aged ≤8 years who are receiving influenza vaccine for the first time should receive 2 doses (separated by at least 4 weeks for TIV and at least 6 weeks for LAIV).

8. **Hepatitis A vaccine.** Hepatitis A vaccine is recommended for children and adolescents in selected states and regions and for certain high-risk groups; consult your local public health authority. Children and adolescents in these states, regions, and high-risk groups who have not been immunized against hepatitis A can begin the hepatitis A immunization series during any visit. The 2 doses in the series should be administered at least 6 months apart. See *MMWR* 1999;48(RR-12):1-37.

*Immunization schedules are frequently updated. For up-to-date information on immunization schedules, you may visit www.cdc.gov/nip.

Recommended Immunization Schedule
for Children and Adolescents Who Start Late or Who Are More Than 1 Month Behind
UNITED STATES • 2005

The tables below give catch-up schedules and minimum intervals between doses for children who have delayed immunizations.
There is no need to restart a vaccine series regardless of the time that has elapsed between doses. Use the chart appropriate for the child's age.

CATCH-UP SCHEDULE FOR CHILDREN AGED 4 MONTHS THROUGH 6 YEARS

Vaccine	Minimum Age for Dose 1	Minimum Interval Between Doses				
		Dose 1 to Dose 2	Dose 2 to Dose 3	Dose 3 to Dose 4	Dose 4 to Dose 5	
Diphtheria, Tetanus, Pertussis	6 wks	4 weeks	4 weeks	6 months	6 months[1]	
Inactivated Poliovirus	6 wks	4 weeks	4 weeks	4 weeks[2]		
Hepatitis B[3]	Birth	4 weeks	8 weeks (and 16 weeks after first dose)			
Measles, Mumps, Rubella	12 mo	4 weeks[4]				
Varicella	12 mo					
Haemophilus influenzae type b[5]	6 wks	4 weeks if first dose given at age <12 months / 8 weeks (as final dose) if first dose given at age 12-14 months / No further doses needed if first dose given at age ≥15 months	4 weeks[6] if current age <12 months / 8 weeks (as final dose)[6] if current age ≥12 months and second dose given at age <15 months / No further doses needed if previous dose given at age ≥15 mo	8 weeks (as final dose) This dose only necessary for children aged 12 months–5 years who received 3 doses before age 12 months		
Pneumococcal Conjugate[7]	6 wks	4 weeks if first dose given at age <12 months and current age <24 months / 8 weeks (as final dose) if first dose given at age ≥12 months or current age 24–59 months / No further doses needed for healthy children if first dose given at age ≥24 months	4 weeks if current age <12 months / 8 weeks (as final dose) if current age ≥12 months / No further doses needed for healthy children if previous dose given at age ≥24 months	8 weeks (as final dose) This dose only necessary for children aged 12 months–5 years who received 3 doses before age 12 months		

*Immunization schedules are frequently updated. For up-to-date information on immunization schedules, you may also visit www.cdc.gov/nip. From Dept. of Health and Human Services, Centers for Disease Control and Prevention, 2005.

CATCH-UP SCHEDULE FOR CHILDREN AGED 7 YEARS THROUGH 18 YEARS

Vaccine	Minimum Interval Between Doses		
	Dose 1 to Dose 2	Dose 2 to Dose 3	Dose 3 to Booster Dose
Tetanus, Diphtheria[1]	4 weeks	6 months	**6 months**[8] if first dose given at age <12 months and current age <11 years **5 years**[8] if first dose given at age ≥12 months and third dose given at age <7 years and current age ≥11 years **10 years**[8] if third dose given at age ≥7 years
Inactivated Poliovirus[2]	4 weeks	4 weeks	IPV[2,3]
Hepatitis B	4 weeks	8 weeks (and 16 weeks after first dose)	
Measles, Mumps, Rubella[4]	4 weeks		
Varicella[10]	4 weeks		

Footnotes

Children and Adolescents Catch-up Schedules   UNITED STATES • 2005

1. **DTaP.** The fifth dose is not necessary if the fourth dose was administered after the fourth birthday.

2. **IPV.** For children who received an all-IPV or all-oral poliovirus (OPV) series, a fourth dose is not necessary if third dose was administered at age ≥4 years. If both OPV and IPV were administered as part of a series, a total of 4 doses should be given, regardless of the child's current age.

3. **HepB.** All children and adolescents who have not been immunized against hepatitis B should begin the HepB immunization series during any visit. Providers should make special efforts to immunize children who were born in, or whose parents were born in, areas of the world where hepatitis B virus infection is moderately or highly endemic.

4. **MMR.** The second dose of MMR is recommended routinely at age 4–6 years but may be administered earlier if desired.

5. **Hib.** Vaccine is not generally recommended for children aged ≥5 years.

6. **Hib.** If current age <12 months and the first 2 doses were PRP-OMP (PedvaxHIB® or ComVax® [Merck]), the third (and final) dose should be administered at age 12–15 months and at least 8 weeks after the second dose.

7. **PCV.** Vaccine is not generally recommended for children aged ≥5 years.

8. **Td.** For children aged 7–10 years, the interval between the third and booster dose is determined by the age when the first dose was administered. For adolescents aged 11–18 years, the interval is determined by the age when the third dose was given.

9. **IPV.** Vaccine is not generally recommended for persons aged ≥18 years.

10. **Varicella.** Administer the 2-dose series to all susceptible adolescents aged ≥13 years.

For additional information about vaccines, including precautions and contraindications for immunization and vaccine shortages, please visit the National Immunization Program Web site at www.cdc.gov/nip or call 800-CDC-INFO / 800-232-4636 (English or Spanish)

From Dept. of Health and Human Services, Centers for Disease Control and Prevention, 2005.

Sample Documentation of a Child Health History

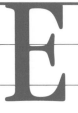

Name: *Sarah R.*   Age: *31 months*   Sex: *female*   Address: *214 Fifth Avenue*

Telephone: *567-9931* (parents' home)

Date of Admission: *December 1*

Telephone: *572-9771* (father's workplace)

Medical Diagnosis: *bilateral otitis media (BOM)*

Allergies: *None known*

Source of History: *mother (Meghan) and father (Jeff)*

Chief Complaints

"Pale for about 3 days… not eating… runny nose for a week… cranky." Doctor says Sarah might have an "earache." Child crying on admission and saying, "Owie, owie."

Present Illness

Child has been sick for about 1 week. "Ran temperature for 2 days" and "had cough and runny nose… Just didn't come around… Didn't eat." Mother says she is really tired because she has been up with Sarah for about 3 nights. Worried about effect of BOM on Sarah's hearing; had niece who had a "ruptured eardrum" and had "speech problems." Dad feels mother might be "babying" Sarah because she spends so much time with Sarah.

Past Health History

Birth History

Patient delivered by normal, uncomplicated, vaginal delivery. Mom and Sarah in hospital for 2 days following delivery. No obvious congenital abnormalities detected at birth.

Feeding History

Child "slow to gain" as an infant. Weight at birth 3.4 kg. Weight at 1 year 7.8 kg. "Picky eater" and "had to have formula changed a lot" because of "gas and crying." Cereal introduced at 4 months, fruits at 6 months, vegetables at 7 months, and full diet with homogenized milk by 9 months, with no adverse effects. Now eats nearly everything except peas. Eats "a lot." Takes a chewable multivitamin daily. Weaned from bottle at 18 months.

Dietary Recall

In the past 24 hours, child has had "about" 4 oz of milk, 8 oz of juice, bowl of soup, two crackers, an ice cream cone, and "two spoonfuls" of rice.

Elimination History

"Constipated a lot when on formula… poops were hard and smelly." "Since going on homogenized milk has been better… still has hard stools if she drinks too much milk." Mom "limits" milk intake to about 16 oz a day and encourages child to drink juice. Child prefers juice to fruit or vegetables.

Childhood Illnesses

Chickenpox at 1 year. Surgery for pyloric stenosis at 10 days.

Immunizations (No untoward reactions)

1 mo: HepB
2 mo: DTaP, IPV, HepB, Hib, PCV
4 mo: DTaP, IPV, Hib, PCV
6 mo: DTaP, PCV
12 mo: IPV, HepB, Hib, MMR, PCV
15 mo: DTaP

Current Medications

Tylenol 80 mg (liquid) at 2 PM (2 hours ago) for fever.

Growth And Development History

General Development

No delays noted on Denver II.

Physical Growth

Weight pattern noted under Feeding History. Current weight 14.8 kg; height 51 cm. All "baby teeth" in by 21 months. Completely toilet trained. Goes to bathroom on own; will ask to go "number one" or "number two."

Gross Motor Development

Rolled over from back to front and front to back by 5 months. Walked at 11 months. Able to jump with both feet and to stand on one foot momentarily.

Fine Motor Development

Holds crayon with fingers; able to copy circle; enjoys coloring.

Sleep

Child established uninterrupted nighttime sleep pattern at 6 months, but reverted to frequent night awakenings at 8 months. Mom says no changes in family or environment at this time. Since 8 months sleeps about 10 hours a night with frequent awakenings, which have no pattern. Child sometimes confused and crying when she awakens but at other times is calm. Mother responds to awakenings by taking child to bathroom and giving her a drink. If child does not immediately settle to crib after this, mom takes her into the family bed. Child does not have afternoon naps; goes down for night between 9 and 10 PM and gets up for day around 7:30 AM; generally is held and read to before bedtime; takes pink baby blanket to bed.

Language Development

First word at 9 months. First phrases after 24 months. Vocalization on admission limited primarily to "owie" and crying; however, mom states that child is usually very talkative and easy to understand. Has trouble with "l's" and "y's"; for example, says "lellow" for yellow. Uses sentences of four or five words. "Gets upset if you don't understand her and sulks."

Social Development

Recognizes familiar people, objects, and places. Initially shy with adults. Aggressive with other children; "bites and hits when she wants something." Parents use "time out" if child is aggressive or misbehaving. Dad feels spanking would be more effective; mom disagrees. Able to feed and dress self almost completely. "Very independent." "Occasional temper tantrums: screams and throws herself to ground . . . usually when meals are late." Has developed fear of "monsters."

Cognitive Development

Alert; follows instructions to "sit up here" or "lie down."

Personal/Social History

Family has well-defined parameters. Parents see themselves as "separate" from their families and able to set own patterns of discipline. Meghan sees her mother's depression as sometimes troublesome and says her mother demands Meghan's time but has little time for her granddaughter. Jeff and Meghan express conflict over discipline of Sarah. Both state that they have difficulty solving problems such as discipline because Jeff "gets mad and walks out" and then Meghan withdraws for "awhile," which makes Jeff mad. Family communication is "open" around matters involving household tasks and responsibilities but there is more difficulty with expressing emotion. Discipline of Sarah largely involves "time out." Father feels Sarah rules her mother sometimes, a perception not shared by Meghan. Couple states they have a wide network of friends, including Sarah's babysitter, to whom Sarah is "very attached." Meghan is a sales rep for a medical supply company; some college education. Jeff is an engineer and has a university degree. See genogram and ecomap (Figure E-1) for further information regarding internal and external family structures.

Systems Review

1. General

Pale, tired-looking child; alert; clings to mother when first
   approached; moves without difficulty.
Temperature: 38.2° C (axillary)
Pulse: 130/min (apical); regular
Respiration: 30/min
Blood pressure: 98/64 (right arm)
Weight: 14.8 kg (clothed)
Height: 51 cm (no shoes)

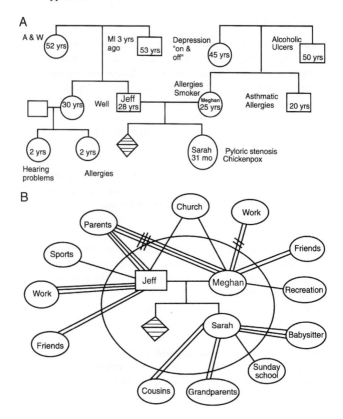

Figure E-1 **A,** Genogram. **B,** Ecomap

2. Integument

Skin: Pale, warm; slightly dry in arm creases; elastic; no edema.
  Lesion approximately 2.5 cm in diameter, red, dry, and raised
  on left medial forearm "due to fall from tricycle 2 weeks ago."
  Indented area "old chickenpox scar" (approximately 2 mm)
  near left eyebrow.

Mucous membranes: Reddened, moist.

Nailbeds: Pink, texture firm, no clubbing; tooth imprints on left
  index finger "due to sucking."

Hair/scalp: Hair clean, soft, abundant on scalp. Scalp clean,
  no lesions.

3. Head and Neck

Head: Normocephalic.

Neck: Full ROM, strong symmetrically; trachea at midline; thyroid not palpable. Firm, warm, diffuse nodes palpated in preauricular, submandibular, occipital, and cervical regions.

4. Ears

Auricle: No lesions; canals clean and free of cerumen.

Otoscopic examination: Drums bilaterally intact, red, and bulging; landmarks not present.

Hearing: Child asked for directions to be repeated on nearly every occasion. Rinne and Weber's tests: Unable to gain child's cooperation sufficiently to gain accurate assessments.

5. Eyes

Vision: Able to name four of seven cards on two tries at 4.6 m.

Extraocular movement: No deviation with cover test; light reflex equal. Unable to gain cooperation in fields of vision testing.

Conjunctivae: Clear.

Sclerae: Clear, white.

Iris: Blue, round.

Pupils: PERRLA.

Ophthalmoscopic examination: Disk round, creamy white; macular areas normal; normal veins and arteries.

Lacrimal system: No swelling or excess tearing.

Corneal reflex: Present.

6. Face, Nose, and Oral Cavity

Face, nose, and facial movements: Symmetric; child solemn but smiles with encouragement; marked shadows under both eyes; external nares excoriated, with green thick nasal discharge present; no pain on palpation of cheeks and areas above eyebrows; septum slightly deviated to left.

Oral cavity: Lips dry, pale, and slightly cracked; oral membranes moist, pink, no lesions.

Gums: No edema or swelling.

Teeth: Clean, all present. Both upper, central incisors protrude slightly.

Throat: Tonsils red and almost to uvula: adenoids visible; voice hoarse.

7. Thorax and Lungs

Thorax slightly oval, symmetric at rest. No indrawings. Respirations diaphragmatic. Tactile fremitus equal bilaterally. Vesicular sounds heard through lung fields. No adventitious sounds.

8. Cardiovascular System

Heart: PMI in fourth intercostal space; no abnormal pulsations palpated; $S_1 > S_2$ in mitral, tricuspid areas and at Erb's point. Systolic murmur heard in third intercostal space.

Vascular system: Radial and peripheral pulses equal, regular, and strong.

9. Abdomen

Healed scar in epigastric region (pyloric stenosis); abdomen protuberant, symmetric; no bulging; bowel sounds 4 to 5/min in each quadrant; firm mass palpated in lower left quadrant (last bowel movement 4 days ago); no hernias.

10. Genitourinary/Reproductive System

Breasts: Nipples symmetric, areola pink; no discharge.

Genitalia: Labia approximate and intact; vagina pink, no discharge.

11. Musculoskeletal System

Muscular development and mass normal for age; movements symmetric; gait normal; feet slightly flattened; all digits present; joints nontender, not swollen; full ROM; Kernig's sign negative.

12. Nervous System

Mental status: Child follows directions appropriately when direction repeated.

Cranial nerve function: Not done.

Motor function: Muscle strength equal and symmetric.

Related Nursing Diagnoses

Constipation: related to insufficient fluid intake, insufficient fiber intake.

Altered parenting: related to physical illness, unrealistic expectations for partner, lack of knowledge about parenting skills.

Fear: related to physical conditions, potential separation from support system.

Knowledge deficit: related to parenting practices, establishment of sleep patterns in toddlers.

Altered nutrition, less than body requirements: related to inability to ingest nutrients.

Pain: related to injury agent (biologic).

Sleep pattern disturbance: related to parent-infant interaction, fever, anxiety.

Bibliography

AACAP: Practice parameters for the assessment and treatment of children and adolescents with depressive disorders, *J Am Acad Child Adolesc Psychiatry* 37:63S-83S, 1998.

ACEP Clinical Policies Committee Subcommittee on Pediatric Fever: Clinical children policy for children younger than three years presenting to the emergency department with fever, *Ann Emerg Med* 42:530-546, 2003.

Adler J: Patient assessment: abnormalities of the heartbeat, *Am J Nurs* 77:647-673, 1977.

Ahmann E, Lawrence J: Exploring language about families, *Pediatr Nurs* 25:221-224, 1999.

All N, Siktberg L: Osteoporosis prevention in female adolescents: calcium intake and exercise participation, *Pediatr Nurs* 27:132, 135-138, 2001.

Ambrose MS, Quinless FW: Fundamental procedures. In Barnes ME: *Nursing Procedures,* ed 4, Philadelphia, 2004, Lippincott Williams & Wilkins.

American Academy of Pediatrics: *Caring for children with ADHD: a toolkit for clinicians,* Elk Grove Village, Ill, 2002, Author.

American Academy of Pediatrics: *Excessive sleepiness in adolescents may indicate more than just lack of sleep,* June 2005. Retrieved from http://www.aap.org/advocacy/releases/june05sleep.htm.

American Academy of Pediatrics: Policy statement: Eye examination in infants, children, and young adults by pediatricians, *Pediatrics* 111:902-907, 2003.

American Academy of Pediatrics: Year 2000 position statement: Principles and guidelines for early detection and prevention programs, 116:798-917, October 2000.

Amoateng-Adjepong Y et al: Accuracy of an infrared tympanic thermometer, *Chest* 115:1002-1005, 1999.

Androkites AL et al: Comparison of axillary and infrared tympanic membrane thermometry in a pediatric oncology outpatient setting, *J Pediatr Oncol Nurs* 15:216-222, 1998.

Arvidson CR: The adolescent gynecologic exam, *Pediatr Nurs* 25:71-74, 1999.

Baker N: Evaluation and management of infants with fever, *Pediatr Clin North Am* 46:1061-1072, 1999.

Ball J, Bindler R: *Pediatric nursing: caring for children,* ed 3, Upper Saddle River, NJ, 2003, Prentice Hall.

Beckenberg R, Sapala S: Pediatric management problems, *J Pediatr Nurs* 28:66-68, 2002.

Beckmann MR, Procter-Zentner J: *Nursing assessment and promotion: strategies across the lifespan,* Norwalk, Conn, 1993, Appleton & Lange.

Beecroft PC, Redick S: Possible complications of intramuscular injections on the pediatric unit, *Pediatr Nurs* 15:333-336, 1989.

Bellman M, Kennedy N: *Pediatrics and child health,* London, 2000, Churchill Livingstone.

Berk LE: *Infants, children, and adolescents,* ed 5, Boston, 2005, Pearson Education, Inc.

Bickley LS: *Bates' guide to physical examination and history taking,* ed 4, Philadelphia, 2004, Lippincott Williams & Wilkins.

Birbaum C et al: Assessing substance abuse in HIV-positive adolescents, *HIV Clin* 16(4):1, 4-5.

Blum RW, Nelson-Mmari K: The health of young people in a global context, *J Adolesc Health* 35:402-418, 2004.

Boszormenyi-Nagy I, Spark G: *Invisible loyalties,* New York, 1984, Brunner/Mazel.

Brennan A: Caring for children during procedures: a review of the literature, *Pediatr Nurs* 20:451-457, 1994.

Bresnahan K et al: Prenatal cocaine use: impact on infants and mothers, *Pediatr Nurs* 17:123-129, 1991.

Broome ME: Preparation of children for painful procedures, *Pediatr Nurs* 16:490-496, 1990.

Burten C, Metzger B: Childhood obesity and risk of cardiovascular disease: a review of the science, *Pediatr Nurs* 26:13-17, 2000.

Calamero CJ: Infant nutrition in the first year of life: tradition or science? *Pediatr Nurs* 26:211-215, 2000.

Centers for Disease Control and Prevention: *Avian influenza infections in humans,* November 2005. Retrieved from http://www.cdc.gov/flu/avian/gen-info/avian-flu-humans.htm.

Centers for Disease Control and Prevention: *Symptoms of West Nile virus,* August 2004. Retrieved from http://www.cdc.gov/ncidod/dvbid/westnile/qa/symptoms.htm.

Chernecky C, Berger BJ: *Laboratory tests and diagnostic procedures,* ed 3, Philadelphia, 2001, WB Saunders.

Clark MC: In what ways, if any, are child abusers different from other parents? *Health Visit* 62:268-270, 1989.

Clark MJ: *Community health nursing,* ed 4, Upper Saddle River, NJ, 2003, Prentice Hall.

Clubb R: Chronic sorrow: adaptation patterns of parents with chronically ill children, *Pediatr Nurs* 17:461-465, 1991.

Cohen SM: Lead poisoning: a summary of treatment and prevention, *Pediatr Nurs* 27:125-127, 2001.

Colby-Graham M, Chordes C: The childhood leukemias, *J Pediatr Nurs* 18:87-95, 2003.

Compton SN et al: Review of the evidence base for treatment of childhood psychopathology: internalizing disorders, *J Consult Clin Psychol* 70:1240-1266, 2002.

Cormier WH, Cormier LS: *Interviewing strategies for helpers: fundamental skills and behavioral interventions,* Pacific Grove, Calif, 1991, Brooks/Cole.

Cunha BA: The clinical significance of fever patterns, *Infect Dis Clin North Am* 10:33-44, 1996.

Danielson CB, Hamel-Bissel B, Winstead-Fry P: *Families, health, and illness: perspectives on coping and intervention,* St Louis, 1993, Mosby.

D'Apolito K: Substance abuse: infant and childhood outcomes, *Pediatr Nurs* 13:307-315, 1998.

De la Cuesta C: Relationships in health visiting: enabling and mediating, *Int J Nurs Stud* 31:451-459, 1994.

Denno DM et al: Etiology of diarrhea in pediatric outpatient settings, *Pediatr Infect Dis J* 24:142-148, 2005.

DeStefano Lewis K, Weiss SJ: Psychometric testing of an infant risk assessment for prenatal drug exposure, *J Pediatr Nurs* 18:371-378, 2003.

Doegnes M, Moorhouse M: *Nurse's pocket guide: nursing diagnoses with interventions,* ed 7, Philadelphia, 1998, FA Davis.

Downs MP, Silver NK: The ABCD's to HEAR: early identification in nursery, office, and clinic of the infant who is deaf, *Clin Pediatr* 11:563-565, 1972.

Drohan S: Managing early childhood obesity in the primary care setting: a behavior modification approach, *Pediatr Nurs* 28:599-607, 2002.

Dunst C et al: *Enabling and empowering families,* Cambridge, Mass, 1988, Brookline Books.

Engle MA: Heart sounds and murmurs in the diagnosis of heart disease, *Pediatr Ann* 10:18-31, 1987.

Faux SA et al: Intensive interviewing with children and adolescents, *West J Nurs Res* 10:180-194, 1988.

Frankenberg WK et al: The Denver II: a major revision and restandardization of the Denver Developmental Screening tool, *Pediatrics* 89:91-97, 1992.

Franzen MD, Berg RA: *Screening for brain impairment,* ed 2, New York, 1998, Springer.

Fischer J, Corcoran K: *Measures for clinical practice,* ed 2, New York, 1994, The Free Press.

Frohlich ED et al: Recommendations for human blood pressure determination by sphygmomanometers: report of special task force appointed by the steering committee, American Heart Association, *Circulation* 77:501A, 1988.

Froom J et al: A cross national study of acute otitis media: risk factors, severity and treatment at initial visit, *J Am Board Fam Pract* 14:406-417, 2001.

Fung K: *Tympanometry,* April 2005. Retrieved from http://www.nlm.nih.gov/medlineplus/ency/article/003390.htm.

Giedd JN et al: Brain development during childhood and adolescence, *Nat Neurosci* 2:861-863, 1999.

Gorsche R, Tilley P: The rash of West Nile virus infection, *CMAJ* 172:1440, 2005.

Goyan Kittler P, Sucher KP: *Cultural foods: traditions and trends,* Scarborough, Ont, 2000, Wadsworth.

Gryskiewicz JM, Huseby TC: The pediatric abdominal assessment: a multiple challenge, *Postgrad Med* 67:126-128, 1980.

Hall J, Driscoll P: The ABC of community emergency care: nausea, vomiting, and fever, *Emerg Med J* 22:200-204, 2004.

Hamrin V, Pachler MC: Depression in children and adolescents: the latest evidence-based psychopharmacological treatments, *J Psychosoc Nurs Ment Health Serv* 42(4):10-16, 2004.

Hartley B, Fuller CC: Juvenile arthritis: a nursing perspective, *J Pediatr Nurs* 12:100-106, 1997.

Haydel MJ, Shembaker AD: Prediction of intracranial injury in children aged five years and older with loss of consciousness after minor head injury due to nontrivial mechanisms, *Ann Emerg Med* 42:507-514, 2003.

Hays AD et al: The use of infrared thermometry for the detection of fever, *Br J Gen Pract* 54:448-450, 2004.

Hazell S, Rogers D: *Mosquito-borne flaviviruses and human disease,* May 2005. Retrieved from http://www.mlo-online.com/articles/0505/0505coverstory.pdf.

Heiney SP: Helping children through painful procedures, *Am J Nurs* 91(11):20-24, 1991.

Heresi GP et al: Giardiasis, *Semin Pediatr Infect Dis* 11:189-195, 2000.

Hockenberry MJ: *Wong's nursing care of infants and children,* ed 7, St Louis, 2003, Mosby.

Hoeckelman RA et al: *Primary pediatric care,* ed 4, St Louis, 2001, Mosby.

Hoffman C et al: Evaluation of three brands of tympanic thermometers, *Can J Nurs Res* 31:117-131, 1999.

Houck GM, King MC: Child maltreatment: family characteristics and developmental consequences, *Issues Ment Health Nurs* 10:193-208, 1989.

Houlder LC: The accuracy and reliability of tympanic thermometry compared to rectal and axillary sites in young children, *Pediatr Nurs* 26:311-314, 2000.

Jackson MM, McLeod RP: Tuberculosis in infants, children, and adolescents: an update with case studies, *Pediatr Nurs* 23:411-415, 1998.

Jackson S: Pediatric temperature measurement and child/parent/nurse preference using three temperature instruments, *J Pediatr Nurs* 18: 314-320, 2003.

Johnson TS et al: Reliability of three measurement techniques in term infants, *Pediatr Nurs* 25:13-17, 1999.

Johnstone HA, Marcinak JF: Sibling abuse: another component of domestic violence, *J Pediatr Nurs* 12:51-53, 1997.

Jones CT: Childhood autoimmune neurologic diseases of the central nervous system, *Neurol Clin* 21:745-764, 2003.

Jongsma AE et al: *The child and adolescent treatment planner*, New York, 1996, John Wiley & Sons, Inc.

Jordan R: *Autistic spectrum disorders*, London, 1999, David Fulton Publishers.

Josephs JE: Pertussis in the adolescent and adult: a primary care concern, *Clin Excell Nurse Pract* 4:361-365, 2000.

Kahn-D'Angelo L: Serious head injury during the first year of life, *Phys Occup Ther Pediatr* 9(4):49-59, 1989.

Kaslow FW: *Voices in family psychiatry,* Newbury Park, Calif, 1990, Sage.

Kelley SJ et al: Birth outcomes, health problems and neglect with prenatal exposure to cocaine, *Pediatr Nurs* 17:130-136, 1991.

Kim MJ et al: *Pocket guide to nursing diagnoses,* ed 7, St Louis, 1997, Mosby.

Knauth DG: Marital change during the transition to parenthood, *Pediatr Nurs* 27:169-172, 184, 2001.

Kools S et al: Psychosocial functioning of hospitalized adolescents and their families, *J Pediatr Nurs* 19:95-103, 2004.

Krantz C: Childhood fevers: developing an evidence-based anticipatory tool for parents, *Pediatr Nurs* 27:567-571, 2001.

Krowchuck H: Child abuser stereotypes: consensus among clinicians, *Appl Nurs Res* 2:35-39, 1989.

Kucik CJ et al: Common intestinal parasites, *Am Fam Physician* 69: 1161-1168, 2004.

Lagges AM, Dunn DW: Depression in children and adolescents, *Neurol Clin* 21:953-960, 2003.

LaMontagne L: Bolstering personal control in child patients through coping interventions, *Pediatr Nurs* 19:235-237, 1993.

Lanham DM et al: Accuracy of tympanic temperature readings in children under 6 years of age, *Pediatr Nurs* 25:39-42, 1999.

LeClerc S: Recommendations for grading of concussion in athletes, *Sports Med* 31:629-636, 2001.

Lefrancois GR: *Of children,* Belmont, Calif, 1977, Wadsworth.

Leung A, Sigalet DL: Acute abdominal pain in children, *Am Fam Physician* 67:2321-2326, 2003.

Leung C, Chui K: Clinical picture, diagnosis, and treatment of acute respiratory syndrome in children, *Paediatr Respir Rev* 5:275-288, 2004.

Leung C et al: Severe acute respiratory syndrome among children, *Pediatrics* 113:535-635, 2004.

Lewin L: Establishing a therapeutic relationship with an abused child, *Pediatr Nurs* 16:263-264, 1990.

Linnard-Palmer L, Kools S: Parents' refusal of medical treatment based on religious and/or cultural beliefs: the law, principles, and clinical implications, *J Pediatr Nurs* 19:351-356, 2004.

Loranger N: Play intervention strategies for the Hispanic toddler with separation anxiety, *Pediatr Nurs* 18:571-574, 1992.

Louters LL: Don't overlook childhood depression, *JAAPA* 17(9):18-24, 2004.

Loveys A: Measuring temperatures, *Pediatr Infect Dis J* 17:920-921, 1998.

Manian FA, Griesenauer S: Lack of agreement between tympanic and oral measurement in adult hospitalized patients, *Am J Infect Control* 26:428-430, 1998.

Marino BL, Lipshitz M: Temperament in infants and toddlers with cardiac disease, *Pediatr Nurs* 17:445-448, 1991.

McCance KL, Huether SE: *Pathophysiology: the biologic basis for disease in adults and children*, ed 3, St Louis, 1998, Mosby.

McFarlane J, Soeken K: Weight gain of infants, age birth to 12 months, born to abused women, *Pediatr Nurs* 25:19-22, 1999.

McGee ZA, Gorby GL: The diagnostic value of fever patterns, *Hosp Pract* 22:103-110, 1987.

Meeropol E: Parental needs assessment: a design for nurse specialist practice, *Pediatr Nurs* 17:456-458, 1991.

Meissner HC: Reducing impact of viral respiratory infection in children, *Pediatr Clin North Am* 52:695-710, 2005.

Montville NH, White MA: Diagnosis and pharmacological management of acute otitis media, *Pediatr Nurs* 23:423-425, 1998.

Moon TD et al: Balance and gait abnormalities of a child with West Nile virus infection, *Pediatr Infect Dis J* 24:568-570, 2005.

Mosby's medical, nursing and allied health dictionary, ed 6, St Louis, 2002, Mosby.

Murphy MJ: Immune reconstitution disease (IRD) increasing; recognition, management important, *HIV Clin* 16(4):1-3, 2004.

Murry S et al: Screening families with young children for child maltreatment potential, *Pediatr Nurs* 26:47-51, 2000.

Muscari ME, Milks CJ: Assessing acute abdominal pain in females, *Pediatr Nurs* 21:215-220, 1995.

Nittina SM: *Lippincott manual of nursing practice*, ed 7, Philadelphia, 2000, Lippincott Williams & Wilkins.

North American Nursing Diagnosis Association: *NANDA nursing diagnoses: definitions and classification, 1999-2000,* Philadelphia, 1999, Author.

O'Brien E: Detection and removal of head lice with an electronic comb: zapping the louse! *J Pediatr Nurs* 13:265-266, 1998.

Onusko E: Tympanometry, *Am Fam Physician* 70(9):1713-1720, 2004.

O'Ryan M et al: A millennium update on pediatric diarrhea: illness in the developing world, *Semin Pediatr Infect Dis* 16:265-236, 2005.

Pagana K, Pagana TJ: *Diagnostic testing and laboratory test reference,* ed 5, St Louis, 2001, Mosby.

Pantell RH: Management and outcomes of fever in early infancy, *JAMA* 291:1203-1212, 2004.

Patrick PD et al: DSM-IV: diagnosis of children with traumatic brain injury, *NeuroRehabilitation* 17:123-129, 2002.

Perry AG et al: *Pocket guide to basic skills and procedures*, ed 5, St Louis, 2003, Mosby.

Pillitteri A: *Child health nursing: care of the child and family,* Philadelphia, 1999, JB Lippincott.

Pillsbury D: *Manual of dermatology,* Philadelphia, 1971, WB Saunders.

Potter PA: *Pocket guide to health assessment,* ed 4, St Louis, 1998, Mosby.

Potter PA, Perry AG: *Fundamentals of nursing,* ed 6, St Louis, 2004, Elsevier Health Sciences.

Quick G, Sicilio M: When should you suspect child abuse? A photographic guide: part 1: cutaneous lesions, *Consultant* 29(7):31-39, 1989.

Quick G, Sicilio M: When should you suspect child abuse? A photographic guide: part 3: neurologic manifestations, *Consultant* 29(7):70-76, 1989.

Ramirez M: *Psychotherapy and counseling with minorities: a cognitive approach to individual and cultural differences,* Toronto, 1991, Pergamon Press.

Rice R: *Manual of home health nursing procedures,* ed 2, St Louis, 1999, Mosby.

Robertson J: Pediatric pain assessment: validation of a multidimensional tool, *Pediatr Nurs* 19:209-213, 1993.

Schreck KA et al: A comparison of eating disorders between children with and without autism, *J Autism Dev Disord* 34:433-438, 2004.

Schultz A et al: Preverbal, early verbal pediatric pain scale (PEPPS): development and early psychometric testing, *J Pediatr Nurs* 14:19-26, 1999.

Sganga A et al: A comparison of four methods of normal newborn temperature measurement, *MCN Am J Matern Child Nurs* 25:76-79, 2000.

Sharer VW, Ryan-Wenger NA: School-aged children self-reported stress symptoms, *J Pediatr Nurs* 28:21-27, 2002.

Sheff B: Norwalk virus, *Nursing 2003* 33(9):70, 2003.

Sherwen LN et al: *Maternity nursing: care of the childbearing family,* Stamford, Conn, 1999, Appleton & Lange.

Shier D et al: *Hole's essentials of human anatomy and physiology,* ed 7, Toronto, 2002, McGraw-Hill Higher Education.

Silverman BG et al: The use of infrared ear thermometers in pediatric and family practice offices, *Public Health Rep* 113:268-272, 1998.

Sivberg B: Parent's detection of early signs in their children having an autistic spectrum disorder, *J Pediatr Nurs* 18:433-439, 2003.

Smith J: Are electronic thermometry techniques suitable alternatives to traditional mercury thermometers in the pediatric setting? *J Adv Nurs* 28:1030-1039, 1998.

Spector RE: *Cultural diversity in health and illness,* Upper Saddle River, NJ, 2000, Prentice Hall.

Stanhope M, Knollmueller RN: *Handbook of public and community nursing,* ed 2, St Louis, 2000, Elsevier Health Sciences.

Stanhope M, Lancaster J: *Community and public health nursing: process and practice for promoting health,* ed 6, St Louis, 2003, Mosby.

Stevens S: Attention deficit/hyperactivity disorder: working the system for treatment and diagnosis, *J Pediatr Nurs* 20:47-51, 2005.

Stewart MJ: *Community nursing: promoting Canadians' health,* ed 2, Toronto, 2000, Saunders.

Stuart G, Laraia M: *Stuart and Sundeen's principles and practice of psychiatric nursing,* ed 6, St Louis, 1998, Mosby.

Stulginsky M: Nurses' home health experience: part II: the unique demands of home visits, *Nurs Health Care* 14:476-485, 1993.

Sutter K et al: Reliability of head circumference measurements in preterm infants, *Pediatr Nurs* 23:485-486, 1997.

Terkelson K: Toward a theory of family life cycle. In Carter EA, McGoldrick M, editors: *The family life cycle: a framework for family therapy,* New York, 1980, Gardner.

Tessler MD et al: Pain behaviors: postsurgical responses of children and adolescents, *J Pediatr Nurs* 13:41-46, 1998.

Thapar N, Sanderson IR: Diarrhea in children: an interface between developing and developed countries, *Lancet* 363:641-653, 2004.

Turner D: Acute otitis media in infants less than two months of age: microbiology, clinical presentation, and therapeutic approaches, *Pediatr Infect Dis J* 21:669-674, 2002.

Van Baalen B et al: Traumatic brain injury: classification of initial severity and determination of functional outcome, *Disabil Rehabil* 25:9-18, 2003.

Vessey J: Developmental approaches to examining young children, *Pediatr Nurs* 21:53-57, 1995.

Vincent PH et al: Use of active surveillance to validate International Classification of Diseases Code: estimates of rotavirus hospitalizations in children, *Pediatrics* 115:78-83, 2005.

Wadsworth BJ: *Piaget's theory of cognitive and affective development,* ed 4, New York, 1989, Longman.

Washburn P: Identification, assessment, and referral of adolescent drug abusers, *Pediatr Nurs* 17:137-140, 1991.

Waxler-Morrison N, Anderson J, Richardson E: *Cross-cultural caring: a handbook for professionals in Western Canada,* Vancouver, 1990, UBC Press.

Weber J, Kelley J: *Health assessment in nursing,* Philadelphia, 1998, JB Lippincott.

Weiss ME et al: A comparison of temperature measurements using three ear thermometers, *Appl Nurs Res* 11:158-166, 1998.

Williams SR: *Nutrition and diet therapy,* ed 8, St Louis, 1998, Mosby.

Wilson CJ, Mason M: Preparation for routine physical examination, *Child Health Care* 19:178-182, 1990.

Wong DL, Perry SE, Hockenberry MJ: *Maternal child nursing care,* ed 2, St Louis, 2001, Mosby.

Wong DL et al: *Whaley & Wong's nursing care of infants and children,* ed 6, St Louis, 1999, Mosby.

Wright L, Leahey M: *Nurses and families: a guide to family assessment and intervention,* Philadelphia, 2000, FA Davis.

Yim R et al: Spectrum of clinical manifestations of West Nile virus infection in children, *Pediatrics* 114:1673-1675, 2004.

Zator Estes ME: *Health assessment & physical examination,* ed 2, New York, 2002, Thomson Delmar Learning.

Index

A

Abdomen, 238-273
  anatomy of, 238-240, 267f
  assessment of, 264-271
    dehydration in, 263t
    diarrhea in, 254t-262t
    equipment for, 240
    pain in, 247t-252t
    preparation for, 240-241, 264
    rationale for, 238
    sequence for, 63, 238
    stool in, 253t
    vomiting in, 241t, 242t-246t
  nursing diagnoses for, 273
  review of, 454
Abdominal breathing, 201, 204-205
Abdominal reflex, 323t
Abducens nerve, 319t
Abuse. *See* Child abuse; Drug abuse.
Accessory nerve, 320t
Achilles reflex, 323t
Acne vulgaris, 140t
Acoustic nerve, 320t
Activity, vital signs and, 97t, 105t,
    108t, 113t
Adenoids, 189, 198
Adolescent pediatric pain tool, 331t
Adolescents
  breast examination in, 283,
    286-288
  communicating with, 7
  eating habits of, 80, 84t-85t
  families with, 46-47
  genitalia examination in, 282-283

Adolescents—cont'd
  growth and development of, 74t,
    362-364t
  growth charts for, 407f-420f
  hearing assessment for, 161-164
  height for, 78
  pain responses by, 330t
  physical assessment of, 71-72
  vital signs in, 96t, 104t, 107t,
    112t
  weight for, 75-76
Adventitious breath sounds, 207,
    218t-219t
Age
  blood pressure and, 112t
  body temperature and, 96t
  physical growth and, 74t
  pulse rates and, 104t
  respirations and, 107t, 108t, 201
  visual acuity and, 170t
Aging families, 47
Alcohol poisoning, 243t
Alcohol use or abuse
  assessment of, 383
  behavior associated with, 380,
    381, 385t
Allen cards, 182
Allergies
  cough with, 210t-211t
  history of, 39
  lesions related to, 135t-136t
Alliances/coalitions, family, 56
Allis' sign, 305t
Alopecia, 143
Alternating pulse, 106t
Alveoli, 200-201
Amnesia, posttraumatic, 312
Amphetamines, 387t

Note: Page numbers followed by f indicate
figures; t, tables; b, boxes.

Anal area, 239, 264, 272
Anal reflex, 272, 323t
Anorexia nervosa, 86t-87t
   behavior in, 380-381
   eating habits in, 85t
   weight in, 75-76
Aortic area, 227, 230f
Aortic regurgitation and stenosis, 229, 233t
Aortic valve, 221
Apical pulse, 105, 106, 225-226
Apnea, 109t
Appearance, 378
Appendicitis
   pain in, 251t, 268, 270, 271
   vomiting in, 243t
Areola, 286
Arrhythmia, 106t, 227-228
Asian Indian culture, 10t-11t
Assessment. *See* Physical assessment;*specific type.*
Asthma, 213t
Ataxic breathing, 109t
Athlete's foot, 139t
Atopic dermatitis, 135t
Attention deficit hyperactivity disorder, 378-379
Audiometry, 164
Auricle, 156-157, 159
Auscultation, 65, 67
   of abdomen, 266
   of blood pressure, 114, 116-118
   of breath sounds, 206-207
   of heart sounds, 226-230
Autism, 379
Axillary hair, 287
Axillary temperature, 100t, 103

B

Babinski's sign, 325t
Bacterial endocarditis, 98t
Bacterial meningitis, 242t-243t
Bacterial pneumonia, 98t, 214t
Bacterial skin infections, 137t
Ballottement test of knee, 302

Barbiturates, 385t
Barlow's test, 305t
Bartholin's glands, 279, 289
Behavior, 343
   assessment of, 378-384
   in drug and alcohol abuse, 385t-389t
Biceps reflex, 321f, 322t
Bigeminal pulse, 106t
Bimanual pelvic examination, 290
Biot's respiration, 109t
Birth history, 36-37, 449
Birthmarks, 141t
Black culture, 12t-13t
Blackbird Preschool Vision Screening System, 182
Bladder, 240, 267, 270
Bleeding
   abnormal uterine, 290
   rectal, 272
Blink reflex, 170, 180, 325t
Blood gas values, 441t
Blood pressure, 111-119
   age and, 112t
   dehydration and, 263t
   influences on, 113t
   measurement of, 114-115
      auscultation for, 116-118
      cuff sizes for, 114, 115t
      equipment and preparation for, 113
      flush method for, 119
      palpation for, 118-119
      rationale for, 111
      sites for, 115f
   nursing diagnoses for, 119
   regulation of, 111, 113
Blood transfusion, fever and, 98t
Blood values, 430t-440t
Body mass index
   formula for, 76
   growth charts for, 412f, 420f
Body odors, 64t
Body righting reflex, 327t

Body temperature. *See* Temperature.
Bones, 296
Boundaries, family, 45, 49-50, 370t
Bowel sounds, 266
Bowleg, 301
Boys, growth charts for, 414f-421f
Brachioradialis reflex, 322t
Bradycardia, 106t
Bradypnea, 109t
Brain, 309-310
Brain injuries, traumatic, 312-313.
    See also Concussion.
Brain tumor, 245t, 334t
Brainstem, 310
Breasts
    assessment of, 204, 283,
        286-288
    development of, 282, 284f
Breath sounds
    adventitious, 218t-219t
    auscultation of, 206-207
    normal, 217t
Breathing. *See also* Respirations.
    abdominal or thoracic, 201,
        204-205
    nasal, 185-186, 201
Bronchi, 200
Bronchial and bronchovesicular
        breath sounds, 217t
Bronchitis, 211t
Brudzinski's sign, 299
Bruising, 127, 130, 133t
Buccal mucosa, 194-195
Bulimia nervosa, 85t, 86t-87t
Bulla, 131t

C

Cambodian culture, 14t-15t
Campylobacter jejuni, 256t
Candidiasis, 138t
Cannabis, 388t
Canthal distance, inner,
    171, 172f
Capillaries, lymphatic, 274
Cardiac output, 111, 113

Cardiovascular system, 221-237
    anatomy of, 221-222
    assessment of
        equipment for, 222
        heart in, 223t, 224-230, 231t,
            233t-234t
        preparation for, 222, 224
        rationale for, 221
        vascular system in, 232,
            235f-236f
    nursing diagnoses for, 236-237
    nutritional status and, 91t
    review of, 454
Caries, dental, 197
Celiac disease, 262t
Cellulitis, 137t
Central cyanosis, 110, 126
Cerebellum, 310, 318
Cerebrospinal fluid values,
    428t-429t
Cerebrum, 310
Cerumen, 153, 157-158
Cervical lymphadenopathy, 150
Cervix, 279
Chest circumference, 144, 203.
    See also Thorax.
Chest retractions, 204, 216f
Cheyne-Stokes respiration, 109t
Chickenpox, 137t
Chief complaint, 34-35, 448
Child abuse, 369-375
    assessment of, 369-371
    development of, 369
    family characteristics in, 370t
    indicators of, 372b-374b
    nursing diagnoses for, 374-375
    risk factors for, 371b
Child rearing practices, 10t-31t
Childhood illnesses, history of,
    37-38, 38, 449
Chinese culture, 15t-17t
Cholecystitis, 252t
Cholera, 256t
Circular communication, 54
Clitoris, 278, 279f, 289

Clubbing
assessment of, 141, 203, 225
stages of, 216f
Clubfoot, 301
Cluster headaches, 335t
Cocaine, 386t
Cognitive development,
346t-364t, 451
Color vision, 179-180
Communication, 3-4
with adolescents, 7
cultural diversity in, 8-9
with families, 47-48
impairments of, 365, 366t-367t
in-family, 53-54, 61, 370t
with infants, 4-5
during interview, 32-34
with parents, 7-8
with preschoolers, 6
with school-age children, 6-7
with toddlers, 5-6
Concrete operations stage,
360t-362t
Concussion, 310
grading system for, 316t
headache in, 338t
mental status in, 312-313,
314, 380
symptoms of, 311b
Conduction hearing loss, 159, 162
Congenital heart defects, 229,
233t-234t
Congestive heart failure,
209t-210t, 224, 225
Conjunctivae, 169f, 170, 175-176
Consciousness, level of, 312, 315f
Constipation, 241, 249t
Contact dermatitis, 136t
Control in family, 55-56, 370t
Cornea, 168, 169f
Corneal light reflex test, 177,
178, 325t
Corrigan's pulse, 106t
Cough, 202, 208t-215t
Cover test, 177, 178

Crackles, 207, 218t
Cradle cap, 140t
Cranial nerves, 310, 318, 319t-320t
Craniotabes, 148
Crawling reflex, 325t
Cremasteric reflex, 323t
Crepitation, thoracic, 206, 219t
Crohn's disease, 250t, 260t
Croup, 212t
Crust, skin, 132t
Cuffs, blood pressure, 114, 115t
Culture
communication and, 8-9
family, 50-51, 61
family and health practices and,
10t-31t
Cyanosis, 110
heart disease and, 224
lip color in, 194
nailbeds in, 203
skin color in, 126
Cystic fibrosis, 211t, 261t
Cystitis, 247t

D

Dance reflex, 325t
Deep tendon reflexes, 318, 321f,
322t-323t
Dehydration, 103, 263t
Dentition, 91t, 187-189, 197
Denver Developmental Screening
Test II, 311, 344-345,
400f-404f
Depression, 376-377
manifestations of, 314, 380,
382, 390t
suicide risk in, 381, 383-384
Dermatitis, 135t-136t, 140t
Dermis, 123, 124f
Development, family, 46-47, 52
Developmental assessment,
343-368, 399-404
age-related, 345, 346t-364t
Denver II screening for, 311,
344-345, 400f-404f

Developmental assessment—cont'd
nursing diagnoses for, 368
preparation for, 343-344
rationale for, 343
speech and language in, 365,
366t-367t
Developmental dysplasia of hip
assessment of, 301, 305t-306t
gait in, 297, 307f
Developmental history, 39-41,
450-451
Diabetic ketoacidosis, 251t
Diarrhea
etiologies of, 254t-262t
stool in, 241, 253t
Diastolic murmur, 230f
Dietary history, 37, 449.
See also Nutritional
assessment.
Direct percussion, 65
Discharge
auricular, 159
nasal, 192-193
ocular, 174
vaginal, 290
Diurnal variation
in blood pressure, 113t
in temperature, 97t
Documentation, health history,
448-455
Dorsalis pedis pulse, 232, 236f
Down syndrome, 148, 172,
176, 299
Drooling, 186-187, 196
Drug abuse. *See also* Medications.
behavior associated with, 314,
379, 380, 381, 383,
385t-389t
pupil size and, 312
suicide risk and, 384
Dull percussion sound, 66t, 206,
266-267
Duodenal ulcer, 252t
Dysfunctional uterine bleeding, 290
Dyspnea, 109t

E
Ears, 153-167
anatomy of, 153-154
assessment of
equipment for, 154
external, 156-159
hearing acuity in, 159-164
otoscopic, 164-167
preparation for, 154-155
rationale for, 153
nursing diagnoses for, 167
review of, 453
Eating disorders, 86t-87t
behavior in, 380-381
eating habits in, 84t-85t
weight in, 75-76
Eating practices
age and, 82t-85t
assessment of, 78-80, 380-381
Ecchymosis, 127, 130, 133t
Ecomap, 50f, 452f
Ecstasy, 387t
Ectopic pregnancy, 248t
Ectropion, 173
Eczema, 135t
Edema, 129-130, 224
Elimination pattern
assessment of, 241, 382
history for, 241, 382
Emesis, types of, 241t
Emotional abuse, 369, 372b
Emotional communication in
family, 53
Endocarditis, bacterial, 98t
Endometriosis, 248t
Entamoeba histolytica, 258t
Entropion, 173
Environment
body temperature and, 97t
family, 51-52
home, 59-61
preparation of, 68
Epicanthal folds, 172
Epidermis, 123, 124f
Epididymis, 280, 281

Epidural hemorrhage, 336t-337t
Epispadias, 292
Erb's point, 227, 230f
Erosion, skin, 132t
Erythema chronicum migrans, 139t
Erythema infectiosum, 137t
Escherichia coli, diarrheagenic, 255t
Esophagitis, 251t
Eustachian tube, 154
Examination. *See* Physical
    assessment.
Exercise, vital signs and, 97t, 105t,
    108t, 113t
Expressive functioning of family,
    53, 370t
Extended family, 52
External ear, 153, 154, 156-159
Extraocular movement, 177-179
Extremities
    lower, 300-303, 305t-306t, 307f
    upper, 299-300, 304f
Extrusion reflex, 186, 325t
Eyebrows, 174
Eyelids, 169f, 170, 173-174
Eyes, 168-184
    anatomy of, 168-170, 172f
    assessment of
        color vision in, 179-180
        equipment for, 170-171
        external, 171-177
        extraocular movement in,
            177-179
        ophthalmoscopic, 183-184
        preparation for, 171
        rationale for, 168
        visual acuity in, 180-183
    headache related to, 335t
    nursing diagnoses for, 184
    nutritional status and, 90t
    review of, 453

F

Face, 185-186
    assessment of, 185, 190-193
    nursing diagnoses for, 199
    review of, 453

Facial nerve, 319t
Families
    abusive and violent, 369,
        370t, 371b
    communicating with, 47-48
    cultural variations in, 8-9,
        10t-31t
    developmental stages for, 46-47
    extended, 52
    interviewing, 32-34
    step-, 47
Family assessment, 44-57
    components of, 48-56
    concepts for, 44-45
    in-home, 58-62
    nursing diagnoses for, 56-57
    rationale for, 44
Family history, 41-42, 43f,
    451, 452f
Fecal incontinence, 382
Feeding practices, infant
    assessment of, 78, 79, 82t
    history of, 37, 449
Femoral hernia, 271
Femoral pulse, 232, 235f
Fetal alcohol syndrome, 191, 314,
    378, 379
Fever, 98t-99t
    assessment of, 95, 96-97
    vital signs and, 105t, 108t
Field of vision, 177, 179
Fifth disease, 137t
Filipino culture, 18t-19t
Fissures
    anal, 272
    skin, 132t
Flat percussion sound, 66t
Flush method of blood pressure
    measurement, 114, 119
Fontanels, 144-145
    assessment of, 148-149
    location of, 145f
Foreskin, 280, 291
Formal operational stage,
    362t-364t
Fovea centralis, 168, 184

Fremitus, tactile, 205-206
Fungal infections
  of nail, 142
  of skin, 138t-139t

G

Gag reflex, 198, 320t
Gait
  assessment of, 297-298
  Trendelenburg, 306t, 307f
Galant's reflex, 326t
Galeazzi's sign, 305t
Gamma hydroxybutyrate, 385t
Gastroenteritis, 250t
Gastroesophageal reflux, 244t
Gastrointestinal system.
      See also Abdomen.
  anatomy of, 238-239
  nutritional status and, 91t
Genitalia. *See also* Reproductive
      system.
  female, 278-279
    assessment of, 288-290
    development of, 281f,
      282, 285f
  male, 280-281
    assessment of, 290-293
    development of, 281-282, 294f
Genitourinary system, 238, 239-
      240. *See also* Abdomen;
      Reproductive system.
Genograms
  examples of, 43f, 452f
  purpose of, 41, 48
Genua varum and valgum, 301
German measles, 136t
Giardia lamblia, 258t
Gingivae
  assessment of, 194, 195-196
  in newborn, 187
  nutritional status and, 91t
Girls, growth charts for, 406f-413f
Glasgow Coma Scale, 312, 315f
Glial cells, 310
Glossopharyngeal nerve, 320t
Grooming, 314

Growth
  assessment of, 345, 346t-364t
  history of, 39, 450-451
  nutritional status and, 88t
  weight/height gain in, 74t
Growth charts, 405-421f
Gums. *See* Gingivae.
Gynecomastia, 204

H

Hair, 124f
  assessment of, 142-143
  axillary, 287
  nutritional status and, 89t
  pubic, 281-282, 285f, 288,
      292, 294f
Halitosis, 64t, 195, 196
Hallucinogens, 387t
Handedness, 317
Head, 144-145
  assessment of, 144,
      147-149, 316
  nursing diagnoses for,
      151-152
  nutritional status and, 89t
  review of, 453
Head circumference, 144
  growth charts for, 413f, 421f
  measurement of, 146-147
Head injury. *See* Concussion.
Headache, 334t-338t
  assessment of, 324
  migraine, 244t-245t
Health history, 32-43
  communication guidelines
      for, 3-9
  documentation of, 448-455
  information for, 34-42, 43f
  interview guidelines for,
      32-34
  setting for, 9
Health practices, cultural
      variations in, 10t-31t
Hearing acuity, 159-164.
      See also Ears.
Hearing loss, 159-160, 162

Heart
  anatomy of, 221-222
  assessment of, 221, 223t,
      224-230, 231t, 233t-234t
Heart defects, congenital, 229,
    233t-234t
Heart disease
  murmurs in, 229
  signs of, 224-225
Heart failure, congestive, 209t-210t,
    224, 225
Heart sounds, 221-222
  auscultation of, 226-230
  types of, 223t
Height
  average gain in, 74t
  growth charts for, 409f, 411f,
      417f, 419f
  measurement of, 77-78
  nutritional status and, 88t
Hemangioma, 141t
Hematology values, 423t-427t
Hematoma, subdural, 336t
Hemorrhage, epidural, 336t-337t
Henoch-Schönlein purpura, 140t
Hepatitis, 251t
Hernias
  femoral or inguinal, 271
  umbilical, 266
Herpes simplex, 134f, 138f
Herpes zoster, 138f
Hip, developmental dysplasia of
  assessment of, 301, 305t-306t
  gait in, 297, 307f
Hirschsprung's disease, 259t
Hispanic culture, 20t-21t
History. *See* Health history.
Hoarseness, 202
Hodgkin's disease, 98t
Home visits, 58-62
  environmental assessment in,
      59-61
  guidelines for, 58
  initial, 59
  nursing diagnoses for, 61-62

HOTV test, 182
Hydrocephalus, 316
Hygiene
  home, 60
  personal, 314, 378
Hyperpnea, 109t, 205
Hyperresonance, 66t, 206
Hypertelorism, 171
Hypoglossal nerve, 320t
Hypopnea, 205
Hypospadias, 292
Hypotelorism, 171

I
Illnesses, history of, 37-38, 449
Immunizations
  history of, 38, 449
  schedules for, 443-447
Impetigo contagiosa, 137t
Indirect percussion, 65
Infants or neonates
  bladder of, 240
  breathing in, 107, 108,
      185-186, 201
  communicating with, 4-5
  digestive tract of, 239
  face and mouth of, 185-187
  families with, 46
  feeding practices of, 78, 79, 82t
  gait of, 297
  growth and development of, 74t,
      346t-354t
  growth charts for, 406f-421f
  head and neck of, 144-145
  head assessment for, 147-149
  head circumference of, 144,
      146-147
  hearing in, 154, 160-161
  heart of, 222
  history for, 36-37, 449
  length for, 77-78
  lungs and thorax of, 201
  oral examination in, 190
  otoscopic examination in, 155
  pain responses by, 330t

Infants or neonates—cont'd
  pain scale for, 324, 332b-333b
  physical assessment of, 69-71
  reflexes in, 161, 170, 180, 186, 324, 325t-329t
  speech and language development in, 366t
  visual acuity in, 170, 180, 183
  vital signs in, 96t, 104t, 107t, 112t
  weight for, 73, 75
Infections
  diarrhea in, 254t-257t
  fever in, 98t-99t
  nail, 142
  skin lesions in, 137t-139t
  vomiting in, 242t-243t
Inguinal hernia, 271
Inhalant abuse, 388t
Injuries. *See also* Concussion.
  abuse-related, 372b-373b
  history of, 37-38
  musculoskeletal, 297
Inner ear, 154
Insomnia, 381
Inspection, guidelines for, 63
Instrumental functioning of family, 52-53, 370t
Integument, 123-143.
      See also Hair; Nails; Skin.
  anatomy of, 123-124
  assessment of
    hair in, 142-143
    nails in, 141-142
    preparation for, 124-125
    rationale for, 123
    skin in, 125-141t
  nursing diagnoses for, 143
  review of, 452
Interactions, family, 61
Interview, guidelines for, 32-34.
      See also Health history.
Intestines, 239, 269
Intussusception, 243t-244t
Iranian culture, 22t-23t

Iris, 168, 169f, 176-177
Ishihara's test, 179

J
Japanese culture, 23t-25t
Jaundice, 125, 126, 265
Joints
  assessment of, 299-303, 305t-306t
  range of motion in, 317

K
Kernig's sign, 301
Ketoacidosis, diabetic, 251t
Kidneys, 239-240, 269
Knee, 302-303
Knee jerk reflex, 322t
Knock-knee, 301
Koplik's spots, 195
Korean culture, 26t-27t
Kussmaul's respiration, 109t
Kyphosis, 298

L
Labia majora and minora, 278, 279f, 288-289
Laboratory values, 422-442t
Labyrinth righting reflex, 327t
Lactose intolerance, 250t, 260t-261t
Language, 365. *See also* Speech and language development.
Laotian culture, 14t-15t
Laryngitis, acute spasmodic, 212t
Laryngotracheobronchitis, 212t
Larynx, 200
Length, infant
  growth charts for, 408f, 416f
  measurement of, 77-78
Lens of eye, 168, 169f
Lesions, skin. *See* Skin lesions.
Level of consciousness, 312, 315f
Lice, 139t, 142, 143, 293
Lichenification, 133t
Limping, 297

Lips
assessment of, 194
nutritional status and, 90t
Liver
assessment of, 266-267, 269, 270
functions of, 238
Lower extremities, 300-303,
305t-306t, 307f
Lungs
anatomy of, 200-201
assessment of, 202-207, 216f
breath sounds in, 217t-219t
cough in, 208t-215t
equipment for, 201
preparation for, 202
rationale for, 200
nursing diagnoses for, 220
review of, 454
Lyme disease, 134f, 139t
Lymphadenopathy, 150, 275
Lymphatic system, 274-277
anatomy of, 274-275, 276f
assessment of
equipment and preparation
for, 275
lymph nodes in, 275-276
rationale for, 274
spleen in, 277
nursing diagnoses for, 277

M

Macewen's sign, 149
Macula, 168, 169f, 184
Macule, 130t
Major depressive disorder,
376-377, 390t
Malnutrition, signs of, 80, 88t-92t
Marijuana, 388t
Marriage, 46
Mastoid, 159
McGill concussion grading
system, 316t
McMurray's test, 302
Measles, 134f, 136t
Meckel's diverticulum, 259t

Medical history, 36-39, 449
Medications
current, history of, 39, 449
vital signs and, 97t, 105t,
108t, 113t
Memory, 313
Meningeal irritation, 299, 301,
314, 317
Meningitis
bacterial, 242t-243t
headache in, 337t
Menstruation, 282, 283
Mental health assessment, 376-391
appearance in, 378
behavior in, 378-384
depression in, 390t
drug and alcohol abuse in,
385t-389t
nursing diagnoses for, 390-391
preparation for, 377-378
rationale for, 376-377
Mental status, 311-314,
315f, 316t
Methamphetamines, 387t
Microcephaly, 316
Middle-age families, 47
Middle ear, 153-154
Migraine, 244t-245t, 338t
Mitral area, 227, 230f
Mitral regurgitation, 229, 234t
Mitral stenosis, 229, 233t
Mitral valve, 221
Mixed hearing loss, 159
Molluscum contagiosum, 136t
Mongolian spot, 141t
Mononucleosis, infectious, 99t
Mons pubis, 278, 288
Mood, 314, 379-380
Moro's reflex, 326t
Motor behavior, 313-314
Motor development,
346t-364t, 450
Motor function, 316-318
Mottling, 224
Mouth. *See* Oral cavity.

Mucous membranes
  buccal, 194-195
  dehydration and, 263t
  nasal, 191-192
Mumps, 136t
Murmurs, heart
  assessment of, 221, 229
  cardiac defects with, 233t-234t
  innocent, 231t
  timing of, 230f
Muscle, 296-297
Muscle strength, 300, 302, 317
Musculoskeletal system, 296-308
  anatomy of, 296-297
  assessment of, 297-303, 304f
    hip dysplasia in, 305t-306t, 307f
    preparation for, 297
    rationale for, 296
  nursing diagnoses for, 307-308
  nutritional status and, 92t
  review of, 454
Myelinization, 310

N

Nails
  assessment of, 141-142
  clubbing of, 141, 203, 216f, 225
Narcotics, 386t
Nares. See also Nose.
  assessment of, 192-193
  flaring of, 203
Nasal discharge, 192-193
Nasal mucosa, 191-192
Native American culture, 28t-29t
Neck
  assessment of, 144, 149-151
  of infant and toddler, 145
  nursing diagnoses for, 151-152
  nutritional status and, 89t
  review of, 453
Neck righting reflex, 327t
Neglect, 369
  assessment of, 369-371
  indicators of, 372b-373b
  risk factors for, 371b

Neonates. See Infants or neonates.
Nervous system, 309-339
  anatomy of, 309-310
  assessment of
    cranial nerves in, 318,
      319t-320t
    deep tendon reflexes in, 318,
      321f, 322t-323t
    equipment and preparation
      for, 310
    infant reflexes in, 324,
      325t-329t
    mental status in, 311-314,
      315f, 316t
    motor function in, 316-318
    pain in, 324, 330t-338t
    rationale for, 309
    sensory function in, 318
  nursing diagnoses for, 339
  nutritional status and, 92t
  review of, 454-455
Neurons, 310
Nevi, 141t, 174
Newborns. See Infants or neonates.
Nicotine, 389t
Nipple, 286-287
Nodule, 131t
Norwalk virus, 254t-255t
Nose, 185-186
  assessment of, 185, 190-193
  nursing diagnoses for, 199
  nutritional status and, 90t
  review of, 453
Numeric pain scale, 331t
Nursing diagnoses
  for abdomen, 273
  for cardiovascular system,
    236-237
  for child abuse, 374-375
  for development, 368
  for ears, 167
  for eyes, 184
  for face, nose, and oral cavity, 199
  for family assessment, 56-57
  for head and neck, 151-152

Nursing diagnoses—cont'd
  for home visits, 61-62
  for integument, 143
  for lymphatic system, 277
  for mental health, 390-391
  for musculoskeletal system,
      307-308
  for nervous system, 339
  for nutritional assessment,
      80-81
  for reproductive system, 295
  for thorax and lungs, 220
  for vital signs, 110, 119
Nutritional assessment, 73-92
  eating practices in, 78-80
  height in, 74t, 77-78
  history for, 37, 449
  in-home, 60
  nursing diagnoses for, 80-81
  physical signs in, 80, 88t-92t
  weight in, 73-77
Nystagmus, 170, 177, 179

O
Obesity, 75, 76
Oculomotor nerve, 319t
Odors
  body, 64t
  breath, 195, 196
  skin, 125
Olfactory nerve, 319t
Ophthalmoscopic examination,
    183-184
Optic disk, 168, 169f, 183-184
Optic nerve, 168, 169f, 319t
Oral cavity, 186-189
  assessment of, 185, 190,
      194-199
  nursing diagnoses for, 199
  nutritional status and, 90t-91t
  review of, 453
Oral temperature, 101t, 103
Orientation, 313
Ortolani's test, 305t
Otitis media, 242t

Otoscopic examination, 164-167
  nasal, 192
  position for, 155f
Oxygen saturation, 203

P
Pain
  abdominal
    assessment of, 240, 241, 264,
        268-269, 270, 271
    etiologies of, 247t-252t
  assessment of, 324, 331t,
      332b-333b
  developmental responses to, 330t
  headache, 244t-245t, 324,
      334t-338t
  musculoskeletal, 297, 300,
      302, 303
  vital signs and, 105t, 108t
Palate, 189f, 194-195
Pallor, 127, 194
Palmar creases, 299, 304f
Palmar grasp, 328t
Palpation, 63-65
  of abdomen, 264, 268-271
  of blood pressure, 114, 118-119
  of breast, 287-288
  in heart assessment, 225-226
  of knee, 302-303
  of lymph nodes, 275-276
  of mastoid, 159
  of pulses, 232, 235f-236f
  for Skene's and Bartholin's
      glands, 289
  of skin, 128-130
  of skull, 148-149
  of spleen, 269, 270, 277
  of testes, 292-293
  of thorax, 205-206
  of trachea and thyroid, 150-151
Palpebral slant, 172, 173f
Pancreatitis, 252t
Papule, 129, 130t
Parachute reflex, 327t
Paradoxical pulse, 106t

Parasites
  diarrhea related to, 257t-258t
  lesions related to, 134f, 139t
Parents, communicating with, 7-9.
  See also Families.
Parietal bone, 149
Parotid swelling, 150
Patella, 302
Patellar reflex, 322t
Patent ductus arteriosus, 234t
Pediculosis corporis, 139t, 142,
  143, 293
Pelvic examination, 283, 290
Pelvic inflammatory disease, 248t
Penis, 280
  assessment of, 290-291, 292
  development of, 281, 294f
Peptic ulcer disease, 245t
Percussion, 65
  of abdomen, 266-267
  finger position for, 67f
  of heart, 226
  of parietal bone, 149
  sounds heard in, 66t
  of thorax, 206
Perineum, 278, 279f
Periodic breathing, 109t
Peripheral cyanosis, 110, 126
Peripheral vascular resistance,
  111, 113
Peristalsis, 239, 265
Pertussis, 208t-209t
Petechiae, 130, 133t, 195
pH of skin, 124
Pharyngitis, streptococcal, 249t
Physical abuse, 370, 372b-373b
Physical assessment, 63-67
  age-related, 70-72
  auscultation in, 65, 67
  communication guidelines for, 3-9
  completion of, 395
  cultural factors for, 10t-31t
  environment for, 68
  equipment for, 68-69
  guidelines for, 69-70

Physical assessment—cont'd
  inspection in, 63, 64t
  palpation in, 63-65
  percussion in, 65, 66t, 67f
  setting for, 9
Physical development, normal, 74t,
  346t-364t
Pigmentation, skin, 125-127
Pinna, 156-157, 159
Placing reflex, 328t
Plasma values, 430t-440t
Pleural friction rub, 206, 219t, 230
Pneumonia
  abdominal pain in, 250t
  bacterial, 98t, 214t
  viral, 208t
Point of maximal impulse, 106,
  225-226
Polydactyly, 299
Popliteal pulse, 232, 235f
Port-wine stain, 141t
Postconcussion syndrome, 310,
  311b, 314, 380
Posterior tibial pulse, 232
Posttraumatic amnesia, 312
Posttraumatic stress disorder,
  379-380
Posture, 313-314
Precordial friction rub, 226, 230
Pregnancy
  ectopic, 248t
  history of, 36-37
Preoperational stage, 355t-360t
Prepuce, 280, 291
Preschool-age children
  communicating with, 6
  eating habits of, 80, 83t-84t
  families with, 46
  growth and development of, 74t,
    358t-360t
  growth charts for, 407f-420f
  hearing assessment for, 161
  height for, 78
  pain responses by, 330t
  physical assessment of, 71

Preschool-age children—cont'd
  speech and language
      development in, 367t
  visual acuity in, 170t
  vital signs in, 96t, 104t,
      107t, 112t
  weight for, 75
Present illness, history of,
    35-36, 448
Preverbal, Early Verbal Pediatric
    Pain Scale, 324, 332b-333b
Problem solving in family, 54-55
Pruritus, 130
Psoas muscle test, 271
Psoriasis, 140t
Psychogenic pain, 249t
Psychosocial history, 40-41, 451
Ptosis, 173
Pubic hair
  female, 282, 285f, 288
  male, 281-282, 292, 294f
Puerto Rican culture, 29t
Pulmonary vascular resistance, 222
Pulmonic area, 227, 230f
Pulmonic stenosis, 233t
Pulmonic valve, 221
Pulse
  age and, 104t
  apical, 105, 106, 225-226
  dehydration and, 263t
  deviations in, 106t
  grading of, 107t
  influences on, 105t, 228
  measurement of, 104-106
  nursing diagnoses for, 110
  peripheral, 232, 235f-236f
Pulse oximetry, 203
Pulsus alternans, 106t
Pupils, 168, 169f
  assessment of, 176-177
  distance between, 172f
  drugs affecting, 312
Purpura, 133t, 140t
Pustule, 131t
Pyloric stenosis, 246t, 265, 270

R
Radial pulse, 105, 106, 232
Rales, 207, 218t
Random-dot-E stereoscopic test,
    177, 178-179
Range of motion, 300, 317
Rank order in family, 48-49
Rash. *See* Skin lesions.
Rectal prolapse, 272
Rectal temperature, 97,
    100t-101t, 103
Red reflex, 183, 184
Reflexes
  anal, 272
  corneal light, 177, 178
  deep tendon, 318, 321f, 322t-323t
  gag, 198, 320t
  infant, 161, 170, 180, 186, 324,
      325t-329t
  red, 183, 184
  superficial, 318, 323t
Refractive errors, 180-181, 335t
Religion, family, 51, 61
Reproductive system, 278-295
  assessment of, 278, 282-283
  female, 278-279
    assessment of, 283, 286-290
    development of, 281f, 282,
        284f-285f
  male, 280-282
    assessment of, 290-293
    development of, 281-282, 294f
  nursing diagnoses for, 295
  review of, 454
Resonance, 66t, 206
Respirations. *See also* Lungs;
    Thorax.
  age and, 107t, 185-186, 201,
      204-205
  altered patterns of, 109t
  assessment of, 202-207
  heart disease and, 225
  influences on, 108t
  measurement of, 106-110
  nursing diagnoses for, 110

Respiratory disorders, 200
  breath sounds in, 217t-219t
  cough in, 208t-215t
  fever in, 98t
  signs of, 202-207, 216f
Respiratory syncytial virus, 213t
Retina, 168, 169f
Retractions, chest, 204, 216f
Rheumatic fever, 98t
Rheumatic heart disease, 229
Rhonchi, 207, 218t
Rinne's test, 162
Rohypnol, 385t
Roles, family, 55, 370t
Romberg's test, 318
Rooting reflex, 186, 328t
Roseola, 98t, 134f
Rotavirus, 254t
Rubella, 136t
Rubeola, 134f, 136t

S
Safety, home and personal, 59-60
Salmon patch, 141t, 174
Salmonella, 256t-257t
Scabies, 134f, 139t
Scale, skin, 128-129, 132t
Scarlet fever, 99t, 137t
School-age children
  communicating with, 6-7
  eating habits of, 80, 84t
  families with, 46
  growth and development of, 74t, 360t-362t
  growth charts for, 407f-420f
  hearing assessment for, 161-164
  height for, 78
  pain responses by, 330t
  physical assessment of, 71
  speech and language development in, 367t
  vital signs in, 96t, 104t, 107t, 112t
  weight for, 75-76
Sclerae, 168, 169f, 175-176
Scoliosis, 298, 303f

Scrotum, 280
  assessment of, 292
  development of, 281, 294f
Seborrheic dermatitis, 140t
Sensorimotor stage, 346t-355t
Sensorineural hearing loss, 159, 162
Sensory function, 318
Serum values, 430t-440t
Severe acute respiratory syndrome, 98t, 215t
Sexual abuse, 369, 370, 373b-374b
Sexual development
  female, 282, 284f-285f
  male, 281-282, 294f
Shigella, 255t
Shingles, 138f
Sigmoid colon, 269
Simian crease, 299, 304f
Sinus arrhythmia, 106t, 227-228
Sinuses, 185, 186f, 193
Sinusitis, 335t
Skeleton, 296
Skene's glands, 279, 289
Skin, 123-124
  abdominal, 265, 268
  assessment of, 123, 125-130
  birthmarks on, 141t
  dehydration and, 263t
  nursing diagnoses for, 143
  nutritional status and, 88t-89t
  temperature of, 102t
Skin color, 125-127
Skin lesions, 130t-133t
  anal, 272
  arrangement of, 134f
  assessment of, 124-125, 130
  disorders with, 135t-140t
Skinfold thickness, 76-77
Skull, 144-145, 148-149
Sleep pattern, 381, 450
Smell, sense of, 186, 193
Snellen letter chart, 180-182
Snoring respirations, 202
Social class of family, 51

Social development, 346t-364t, 451
Social history, 40-41, 451
"Soft signs" of brain
     dysfunction, 313
Speculum examination
  nasal, 192
  vaginal, 290
Speech and language development
  assessment of, 365
  history of, 450
  impairments in, 366t-367t
  normal, 346t-364t
Sperm, 280-281
Spina bifida occulta, 298, 316
Spine
  assessment of, 298-299, 316
  lateral curvature of, 298, 303f
Spleen
  anatomy of, 275
  palpation of, 269, 270, 277
Staphylococcus, diarrhea related
    to, 257t
Startle reflex, 161, 329t
Stepfamilies, 47
Stepping reflex, 325t
Steroid abuse, 389t
Stethoscope, 65, 67
Stomach, 239
Stool, 241, 253t
Strabismus, 170, 178, 335t
Strawberry nevus, 141t
Strength, muscle, 300, 302, 317
Streptococcal pharyngitis, 249t
Striae, 133t, 265, 286
Stridor, 202, 219t
Strongyloidiasis, 257t
Subcutaneous tissue, 123, 124f
Subdural hematoma, 336t
Substance abuse. *See* Drug abuse.
Subsystems, family, 44-45, 49
Sucking reflex, 329t
Suicide, 376-377
  risk assessment for, 383-384
  warning signs for, 380,
    381, 384b

Sunset sign, 173
Superficial reflexes,
    318, 323t
Support networks, family, 61
Surgery, history of, 37-38
Sutures, cranial, 144,
    145f, 148
Sydney line, 299, 304f
Syndactyly, 299
Systems
  family, 44-45, 49-50
  review of, 42, 451-455
Systolic murmur, 229, 230f

T

Tachycardia, 106t
Tachypnea, 109t
Tactile fremitus, 205-206
Tanner stages
  female, 284f-285f
  male, 294f
Taste, sense of, 187
Teenagers. *See* Adolescents.
Teeth
  eruption of, 187, 188f, 189
  inspection of, 197
  nutritional status and, 91t
Temperature
  age and, 96t
  factors influencing, 97t
  measurement of, 95-103
    guidelines for, 97, 103
    preparation for, 96-97
    rationale for, 95
    sites for, 100t-102t
  nursing diagnoses for, 110
  regulation of, 95-96
  skin, 128
Tension headache, 334t
Testes, 280-281
  development of, 282, 294f
  palpation of, 292-293
Tetralogy of Fallot, 234t
Thoracic breathing,
    201, 204

Thorax
  anatomy of, 201
  assessment of, 202-207, 216f
    breath sounds in, 217t-219t
    cough in, 208t-215t
    equipment for, 201
    preparation for, 202
    rationale for, 200
  nursing diagnoses for, 220
  review of, 454
Thready pulse, 106t
Thrills, cardiac, 226
Thrush, 195
Thyroid gland, 145, 150-151
Tinea, 138t-139t
Toddler diarrhea, 260t
Toddlers
  communicating with, 5-6
  eating habits of, 80, 82t-84t
  gait in, 297
  growth and development of, 74t,
    354t-358t
  growth charts for, 419-421f
  height for, 77-78
  pain responses by, 330t
  pain scale for, 324, 332b-333b
  physical assessment of, 69-70, 71
  speech and language
    development in, 366t-367t
  visual acuity in, 170t
  vital signs in, 96t, 104t, 107t, 112t
  weight for, 75
Tongue, 186, 189f
  assessment of, 194, 196
  nutritional status and, 90t
Tonic neck reflex, 329t
Tonsils, 189, 197-198
Trachea, 150, 200, 201
Tracheitis, 212t
Transportation, family, 60
Trendelenburg gait, 306t, 307f
Triceps reflex, 321f, 322t
Trichuriasis, 258t
Tricuspid area, 227, 230f
Tricuspid valve, 221

Trigeminal nerve, 319t
Trochlear nerve, 319t
Tuberculosis, miliary, 98t
Tumbling E chart, 182
Tumor
  brain, 245t, 334t
  skin, 131t
Tuning fork tests, 162
Turgor, skin, 129
Tympanic membrane, 153, 154
  examination of, 165-167
  landmarks in, 166f
Tympanic temperature, 102t
Tympanometry, 163
Tympany, 66t, 206, 267

U
Ulcer
  duodenal, 252t
  peptic, 245t
  skin, 132t
Ulcerative colitis, 248t, 259t
Umbilical hernia, 266
Umbilicus, 265-266
Upper extremities, 299-300, 304f
Urethra and urinary meatus
  female, 278, 279f, 289-290
  male, 280, 292
Urinalysis, 442t
Urinary obstruction, 247t
Urinary tract infection, 99t
Urolithiasis, 247t
Urticaria, 135t
Uterus, 279
Uvula, 189f, 198

V
Vagina, 279, 289-290
Vaginal discharge, 290
Vagus nerve, 320t
Valves, cardiac, 221-222
  auscultation of, 227, 230f
  defects in, 233t-234t
Varicella zoster, 137t
Vas deferens, 280, 281

Vascular system, 221, 232, 235f-236f. *See also* Cardiovascular system.
Venereal disease, 289, 291
Ventricular septal defect, 234t
Verbal communication in family, 53-54
Vesicle, 131t
Vesicular breath sounds, 217t
Vestibule, 278
Vietnamese culture, 30t-31t
Viral infections
  of skin, 138t
  upper respiratory, 98t
Viral pneumonia, 208t
Vision. *See also* Eyes.
  binocular, 177-179
  color, 179-180
  field of, 177, 179
  headache related to, 335t
Visual acuity
  age and, 170t
  assessment of, 168, 179, 180-183
  in infants, 170
Vital signs. *See* Blood pressure; Pulse; Respirations; Temperature.

Voice quality, 199
Vomiting, 242t-246t
  assessment of, 240, 241
  emesis types in, 241t
Vulva, 278

W

Water-hammer pulse, 106t
Wax, ear, 153, 157-158
Weber's test, 162
Weight
  average gain in, 74t
  dehydration and, 263t
  growth charts for, 406f-407f, 410f-411f, 414f-415f, 418f-419f
  measurement of, 73, 75-77
  nutritional status and, 88t
West Nile virus, 138f
Wheal, 131t
Wheezes, 202, 207, 218t-219t
Whooping cough, 208t-209t
Wong-Baker FACES Pain Rating Scale, 331t

Y

Yersinia enterocolitica, 257t